ANNUAL REVIEW OF GERONTOLOGY AND GERIATRICS

Volume 21, 2001

ANNUAL REVIEW of
Gerontology and Geriatrics

Volume 21, 2001

Focus on Modern Topics in the Biology of Aging

Vincent J. Cristofalo, PhD
Richard Adelman, PhD
Volume Editors

K. Warner Schaie, PhD
Series Editor

SPRINGER PUBLISHING COMPANY

Springer Publishing Company, Inc.
536 Broadway
New York, NY 10012-3955

Acquisitions Editor: Helvi Gold
Production Editor: Pamela Lankas
Cover design by Susan Hauley

02 03 04 05 06 / 5 4 3 2 1

ISBN 0-8261-1448-2
ISSN 0-198-8794

Printed in the United States by Maple Vail.

Dedication

This volume of the *Annual Review of Gerontology and Geriatrics* is dedicated to the memory of M. Powell Lawton (1923–2001), who served as series editor for volumes 10 to 21 (1990 to 2001). Lawton, who was recognized as one of the pioneers and major contributors to behavioral gerontology, died of a brain tumor on January 29, 2001. At the time of his death he was senior research scientist and director emeritus of the Polisher Research Institute at the Philadelphia Geriatric Center. Dr. Lawton made seminal contributions to the psychology of aging and gerontology in general with his influential work on the interface between the aging individual and his/her changing environment. He was one of the first to recognize the importance of designing supportive living environments for older persons and those with Alzheimer's disease. His work on activities of daily living and instrumental activities of daily living provided objective standards for determining levels of care required for dependent older persons. One of his last major contributions (to be published posthumously) was a seminal chapter on end-of-life issues, which will appear in the 5th edition of the *Handbook of the Psychology of Aging*. Dr. Lawton served as president of the Gerontological Society of America and he received that society's prestigious Kleemeier Award for distinguished research contributions.

Many tributes have appeared indicating Lawton's numerous scientific contributions and his qualities as a caring friend and mentor to many current gerontologists. What should be specifically mentioned here is his important role in the dissemination of gerontological knowledge throughout our interdisciplinary community. During his tenure as associate editor of *Psychology and Aging* he did yeoman's work to broaden the definition of that field beyond the experimental psychology of aging. And as an editor for this series of Annual Reviews he astutely selected a broad range of current topics in gerontology and geriatrics, always successfully selecting the best informed colleagues to serve as editors of volumes on specific topics. His judgment and wisdom will be sorely missed. We have lost one of the giants of our field.

K. WARNER SCHAIE
Series Editor

Publisher's Tribute

Powell Lawton was an author and dear friend of Springer Publishing Company for nearly 20 years. We published some of his early research on elder housing and environment, and were fortunate that in 1989 he agreed to become chief editor of the *Annual Review of Gerontology and Geriatrics.*

It was a joy to work with Powell: He was cooperative and helpful, dependable, and so wise. He shared with us insights from his profound knowledge of gerontological research. We miss him and deeply mourn Powell Lawton, scholar, author, friend.

URSULA SPRINGER

Contents

Preface

This volume is the twenty-first in a series, begun in 1980, entitled the *Annual Review of Gerontology and Geriatrics*. True to the series title, the various volumes span the breadth of the field from very fundamental to applied studies.

The last volume in this series that addressed the biology of aging appeared in 1990 and was entitled *Special Focus on the Biology of Aging* (V. J. Cristofalo, Ed.). In the Preface to that volume, the editor wrote, "The biological mechanisms by which aging occurs remain one of the great unsolved problems of biology." Here, 11 years later, the nature of the biological mechanisms of aging still eludes us. This is not to infer the absence of advances. In fact, major advances have occurred, especially conceptually, as we begin to understand that the important theoretical issues about aging concern not so much the aging phenotype per se, but rather the basis for why species live as long as they do.

In 1990's volume there was emphasis on tissue-specific alterations with age, whereas the present volume is devoted much more to the why and how of aging. In general, gerontologists recognize three general paradigms of aging research: demographic studies, evolutionary studies, and studies of biological mechanisms. In this volume, we have tried to combine these three approaches by selecting authors whose expertise and clarity of expression can communicate the subtleties and value of their approaches. Furthermore, three of the chapters (K. G. Manton; G. E. McClearn; and S. J. Olshansky & B. A. Carnes) provide a view of contemporary paradigms of research on the biology of aging from the perspective of the social and behavioral sciences.

In chapter 1 Manton justifies the collection of standardized, human longitudinal data in the context of currently available theoretically motivated models of aging, such as cause-specific morbidity statistics. He also documents the critical need for new analytical tools, such as nonstandard statistical inference and engineering models of complex systems, which are able to account for multiple existing data sources and information gaps and to inspire knowledge-based synthesis of data sources within and between national boundaries.

In chapter 2 Austad discusses how the comparative analysis of natural patterns across and within species reveals underlying biological mechanisms. He specifically focuses on the longevity relationships of body size and gender differences for animals that age in nature. He also encourages the exploration of cellular correlates of organismic aging rates.

In chapter 3 Kirkwood presents the evolutionary basis of aging and longevity in the context of a guide to pursuit of its underlying mechanisms. He refutes the commonly held notion that aging is driven by an evolved genetic program, instead casting it as an indirect consequence of natural selection. Furthermore, he segregates and analyzes two distinct categories of nonadaptive theory: that aging occurs either as the power of natural selection declines across the life span or as the byproduct of selection for some other trait.

In chapter 4 Masoro begins to address the questions of how aging works. He puts the well-known physiological deterioration that occurs into the context of genetics and environment, and simultaneously integrates the confounding impacts of cohort effects and diseases. He also advocates replacement of the notion of "successful aging" with the more accurate view that marked individual differences in age of physiological decline reflect individual differences in the rate of deterioration.

In chapter 5 Allen, Balin, and Cristofalo discuss the contributions of human cells in culture as a model of human aging. They review environmental and genetic factors that probably contribute to the loss of proliferative capacity in later-passage cultures. Especially intriguing is the refutation by this laboratory of previous claims by others of a relationship between donor age and life span, thereby necessitating a change in interpretation of data from a senescence model.

In chapter 6 Zakeri and Lockshin review evidence that apoptosis, the decision of any cell to die, remains intact during aging. In contrast, however, the threshold for activation of the physical machinery of cell death changes. Therapeutic potential of intervention in this system awaits enhanced understanding of its structure and regulation.

In chapter 7 Gershon and Gershon critically analyze the use of models for understanding human aging. With characteristic skepticism and candor, they offer numerous examples of misleading results and conclusions that probably are attributable to artificial conditions employed in the maintenance of experimental models. They conclude with specific recommendations for more sophisticated experimental design, for example, nutrition, ambient temperature, diurnal fluctuations, and lighting.

In chapter 8 Jazwinski reviews genetic studies in *Drosophila, C. elegans* and yeast, and summarizes the contribution of these models to our understanding of the fundamental molecular genetics of aging. Of special interest is the correspondence between genetic regulation of physiological mechanisms, for example, caloric restriction, which underlie aging in a broad variety of organisms. He then tackles the potential relevance of these recent genetic studies to human aging.

In chapter 9 Joseph et al. discuss nutritional modification of the pathway of neurodegenerative diseases. Numerous types of changes in neuronal function during aging, such as signaling, apparently result in behavioral deficits and may be the consequence of increased brain vulnerability to oxidative stress and inflammation. The authors emphasize possible underlying mechanisms, as well as possible dietary intervention in these processes by fruits, vegetables, or other natural products.

In chapter 10 McClearn reviews a broad array of research designs and analytical techniques that support a strong hereditary influence on behavioral aging. He then projects future directions of research that embody complex biological systems. The eventual capability to identify quantitative trait loci, to manipulate individual genes, to assemble specific genotypes, and to monitor gene expression across life-span development promises to reveal the dynamics of interactions between genetics and environment.

Lastly, in chapter 11, Olshansky and Carnes tackle the questions of why humans die when they do and whether the life tables contain biology. They show that inherent to each species is a fundamental link between timing of sexual maturation, length of reproductive window, and onset and rate of increase in the death rate from biological causes of death. They then project that more sophisticated understanding of biological mechanisms of aging may reveal how demographic shifts in a population's age structure alter expression of aging in a rapidly growing and more diverse older population.

We have compiled these chapters so as to put aging research in a new perspective. We hope that both students and professionals in the biomedical, social, and behavioral sciences will gain a better perspective of the inroads into our understanding of aging.

We wish to thank the authors for their outstanding contributions. We also wish to express our appreciation for the excellent editorial assistance of Janet Berens of the Lankenau Institute for Medical Research.

The work of putting together this volume was supported in part by USPHS AG00378, the Lankenau Hospital Foundation, and Research Incentive Funds of the University of Michigan Institute of Gerontology.

VINCENT J. CRISTOFALO, PHD
RICHARD C. ADELMAN, PHD

Contributors

Richard C. Adelman, PhD
Institute of Gerontology and Department of Biological Chemistry
University of Michigan
Ann Arbor, MI

R. G. Allen, PhD
Lankenau Institute for Medical Research
The Sally Balin Medical Center for Dermatology, Cosmetic Surgery and Longevity Medicine
Media, PA

Steven N. Austad, PhD
Department of Biological Sciences University of Idaho
Moscow, ID

Arthur K. Balin, MD, PhD, FACP
Lankenau Institute for Medical Research
The Sally Balin Medical Center for Dermatology, Cosmetic Surgery and Longevity Medicine
Media, PA

Donna Bielinski, PhD
USDA Human Nutrition Research Center on Aging
Tufts University
Boston, MA

Bruce A. Carnes, PhD
NORC/Center on Aging
University of Chicago
Chicago, IL

Vincent J. Cristofalo, PhD
Lankenau Institute for Medical Research
Wynnewood, PA
Thomas Jefferson University
Philadelphia, PA

Natalia Denisova, PhD
USDA Human Nutrition Research Center on Aging
Tufts University
Boston, MA

Derek Fisher, BS
USDA Human Nutrition Research Center on Aging
Tufts University
Boston, MA

David Gershon, PhD
Faculty of Biology
Technion/Israel Institute of Technology
Haifa, Israel

Harriet Gershon, PhD
Department of Immunology
Rappaport Faculty of Medicine
Technion/Israel Institute of Technology
Haifa, Israel

S. Michal Jazwinski, PhD
Department of Biochemistry and Molecular Biology
Louisiana State University Health Sciences Center
New Orleans, LA

James A. Joseph, PhD
USDA Human Nutrition Research
Center on Aging
Tufts University
Boston, MA

Thomas B. L. Kirkwood, PhD
Department of Gerontology
University of Newcastle upon Tyne
Newcastle, UK

Richard A. Lockshin, PhD
Department of Biological Sciences
St. John's University
New York, NY

Kenneth G. Manton, PhD
Center for Demographic Studies
Duke University
Durham, NC

Edward J. Masoro, PhD
Department of Physiology
University of Texas
Health Science Center
San Antonio, TX

Gerald E. McClearn, PhD
Center for Developmental
and Health Genetics
Pennsylvania State University
University Park, PA

S. Jay Olshansky, PhD
School of Public Health
University of Illinois at Chicago
Center on Aging
University of Chicago
Chicago, IL

Barbara Shukitt-Hale, PhD
USDA Human Nutrition
Research Center on Aging
Tufts University
Boston, MA

Kuresh Youdim, PhD
USDA Human Nutrition Research
Center on Aging
Tufts University
Boston, MA

Zahra Zakeri, PhD
Department of Biology
Queens College and Graduate
Center of City University
of New York
Flushing, NY

Forthcoming

ANNUAL REVIEW OF GERONTOLOGY AND GERIATRICS

Volume 22: Economic Outcomes in Later Life: Public Policy, Health, and Cumulative Advantage

Editor-in-Chief: K. Warner Schaie

Volume Editors: Stephen Crystal and Dennis Shea

Contents

CHAPTER 1

Demography of Populations and Global Aging: Societal Implications of the Old–Old

KENNETH G. MANTON
CENTER FOR DEMOGRAPHIC STUDIES
DUKE UNIVERSITY

A major limitation in the cross-national study of aging and chronic disease is the lack of standardized longitudinal data on morbidity, disability, and mortality and changes in aging biomarkers in most developing, and many developed, countries. In attempting to address the problem by increased investment in data collection, one is immediately faced with the question of what data to collect. That is, to invest efficiently in collecting population data it is necessary to have theoretically motivated models of aging processes (Manton, 1999). This can help determine both the type of data to collect as well as help in the design of the process of data collection, for example, identify the necessary length of follow-up, frequency of assessments, and the age ranges to cover. It will also aid in determining which population groups (e.g., gender, race, genotype, cohort) should be differentially sampled in one's observational design. We will argue here that sufficient biomedical and epidemiological research on physiological aging processes has now been conducted in the U.S. and other developed countries so that such theoretical models of aging can be developed.

Parallel to the issue of the needing appropriate theoretical models to guide the construction of data collection systems, models that might be constructed from a compendium of existing biomedical research results and extant population data (e.g., cause-specific morbidity statistics), there is the problem of developing analytic tools that will most efficiently use the multiple existing data sources, deal with significant gaps in information, and allow the knowledge based synthesis of data sources to improve the credibility of, within, and between other country's analyses and results.

This implies that nonstandard methods of statistical inference like Bayes and Empirical Bayes models could be necessary to combine effectively various types of empirical evidence and expert judgment. Additionally, lessons could be learned from the modeling in engineering studies of complex systems, where no single data collection is adequate to describe total system dynamics. Other areas of application where data sources and theoretical knowledge are combined to analyze complex biological systems are the use of stochastic compartment models to evaluate drug metabolism (Jacquez, 1972; Manton & Stallard, 1988).

Those approaches involve positing a general mathematical framework for the complex, dynamic system and using that multi-equation (possibly nonlinear) model to synthesize parameters that are estimated from a wide range of data sets, and then performing plausible simulations of system performance and structural evolution. Finally, it is useful to include true (not simply statistical or sampling) uncertainty in the models by using "fuzzy set" concepts (e.g., Manton, Woodbury, & Tolley, 1994) and various types of physical diffusion processes (Risken, 1996). This has been recently called for by Finch and Kirkwood (2000) who believe the ability to explain, at best, 25% to 50% of the variance of longevity from genetic factors is due to true stochasticity in the expression of proteins from genes due to intracellular molecular dynamics (e.g., translation effects from ^{t}RNA, ^{m}RNA, ribsome functioning, and the operation of such factors as heat shock proteins [Georgopulos & Welch, 1993]).

RECENT POPULATION EVIDENCE ON TEMPORAL CHANGES IN CHRONIC DISABILITY

Perhaps the best evidence of recent changes in chronic disability in the older adult population in a developed country is the U.S. data from the National Long Term Care Survey (NLTCS). Evidence of a decline in chronic disability in the older U.S. population was first cited from the 1982–1989 NLTCS (Corder, & Stallard, 1993). That evidence was the subject of a special National Academy of Science analysis and report (Freedman & Soldo, 1994), which concluded that though there was evidence of a decline in chronic disability prevalence, any conclusions about policy or public health responses to make to the observed decline should await its confirmation in the 1994 NLTCS.

The decline was observed not only to be continuing in the 1994 NLTCS, but also the relative rate of decline in chronic disability increased from 1.0% in 1982–1989 to 1.5% in 1989–1994 (Corder, & Stallard, 1997). Analyses of the rate of decline (1.5% per annum) showed that its continuation could alleviate much of the concern about the future fiscal solvency of Medicare and Social Security (Singer & Manton, 1998)—especially if economic trends and federal actions are favorable. This was further supported by analyses showing large differentials in Medicare expenditures across disability levels in the 1982–1994 NLTCS (Manton & Singer, 2000).

Since the 1982–1994 NLTCS data was reported, another NLTCS has been conducted (1999). It showed a further acceleration in the rate of decline in chronic disability to 2.6% per annum from 1994 to 1999. The relative rates of decline for 1982–1989, 1989–1994, and 1994–1999 are recorded in Table 1.1.

We see that declines are manifest at most levels of functional impairment. For example the prevalence of persons with IADL impairments declined from 5.7% in 1982 to 3.2% in 1999. Institutional residents (who averaged 4.8 ADLs impaired) declined from 6.8% in 1982 to 4.2% in 1999.

In Table 1.2 we analyze these declines by age. We see that declines accelerate most rapidly at ages 85+. The nondisabled population aged 85+ increased by 9.9% from 36.2 to 46.1% from 1982 to 1999. Not only is the improvement at ages 85+ highly significant, but it is also more than twice as large for the oldest old group than for the 65–74 age group.

Analyses of factors associated with the acceleration of decline in chronic disability suggests the potential importance of (a) increased levels of education in the oldest-old (age 85 years or more), (b) declines in the prevalence of severe dementia (Manton & Gu, 2001; Manton, Stallard, & Corder, 1998), (c) improved management of sensory impairments such as cataracts and glaucoma (Manton & Corder, 2000), and (d) improved pain management (Manton & Gu, 2001).

The ultimate validation of such disability declines in the U.S. is whether the findings can be replicated in other large longitudinal surveys. Replication was forthcoming in the 1984–1993 Survey of Income and Program Participation (Freedman & Martin, 1998), which found that four measures of disability declined from 0.9% to 2.3% per annum, that is, in some cases declines were more rapid than in the NLTCS. Additional confirmation of declines in chronic disability in the older American population come from studies of the 1993–1996 Current Medicare Beneficiary Surveys (Waidmann & Liu, 1998) and from studies of the National Health Interview Survey (NHIS) (Crimmins, Saito & Reynolds, 1997). Recently, confirmation of a decline was also found by comparing the 1984 and 1994/1995 supplement to the NHIS (Freedman & Martin, 2000).

Alternate sources of confirmation are several studies by Fogel (1993) and Costa (1998) of Union Army Civil War veterans. This data was generated during medical examinations of Civil War veterans aged 65+ who were applying for a federal pension in 1910. These veterans represented the birth cohorts of 1825 to 1844. The prevalence of chronic morbidity in this population was compared to chronic morbidity reported by W.W. II

TABLE 1.1 Population Distribution (Age standardized to 1999) of Disabilities from 1982 to 1999

Year	1982	1989	1994	1999
Nondisabled (%)	73.8	75.6	77.5	80.3
IADL only	5.7	4.8	4.4	3.2
1-2ADLs	6.9	6.7	6.1	6.0
3-4 ADLs	3.0	3.7	3.4	3.5
5-6 ADLs	3.7	3.0	3.0	2.9
Institutional	6.8	6.1	5.7	4.2
Total (%) disabled standardized by 1999 age population distribution	26.2	24.4	22.5	19.7
Relative decline rates (%) (per year)		(82–89) 1.0	(89–94) 1.6	(94–99) 2.6

veterans in the 1985–1988 NHIS. Those analyses showed that chronic morbidity prevalence declined 0.62% per annum (6% per decade) over the 75-year period. Costa (1998) analyzed select measures of disability reported in the 1910 medical exams; compared to assessments of disability in the 1990–1994 National Health and Nutrition Examination Survey the prevalence of disability declined at a rate similar to that for chronic morbidity (National Center for Health Statistics, 2000). These long-term declines were hypothesized to be due to improvements in maternal and early-life nutrition, which affected late-life chronic disease risks (Fogel, 1994). Fogel and Costa (1997) later postulated a more comprehensive model of "technophysiological" evolution to suggest that many sources of change in the individual's physical and social environment contributed to the long-term improvements in health and functioning.

With these observations about disability decline in the U.S., it is interesting to examine cross-national studies to determine if other countries shared in the decline of disability in the older adult population. The results were mixed with few clear trends found in Australia (e.g., Mathers, 1994) and Canada (Wilkins & Adams, 1983; Wilkins, Chen, & Ny, 1994). There was clear evidence of declines in disability in several longitudinal studies done in France (Robine, 1994) and for select age groups in some health surveys in Britain (Bebbington, 1988). On the occasion of the G-8 economic conference in Denver, Colorado, Waidmann and Manton (1998) conducted a broader analysis of declines for the U.S. Assistant Secretary for Policy and Evaluation and found evidence suggestive of significant

TABLE 1.2 Changes in Age-Specific Estimates of Chronic Disability Risk 1982 to 1999

Disability and age-status	1982 %	1999 %	Difference %	*t*-test for change 1982 to 1999
1. Nondisabled				
65-74	86.0	90.4	4.4	5.9
75–84	69.4	76.8	7.4	16.1
85+	36.2	46.1	9.9	19.4
2. IADL only				
65–74	4.3	2.4	–1.9	–10.6
75–84	7.1	3.7	–3.6	–15.7
85+	8.0	5.4	–2.6	–10.4
3. 1–2 ADLs				
65–74	4.1	3.2	–0.9	–4.7
75–84	8.4	8.0	–0.4	–1.4
85+	14.3	12.4	–1.9	–5.4
4. 3–4 ADLs				
65–74	1.8	1.8	0.0	0.0
75–84	3.5	4.1	0.6	3.0
85+	6.8	8.9	2.1	7.5
5. 5–6 ADLs				
65–74	2.1	1.3	–0.8	–6.2
75–84	4.2	3.3	–0.9	–4.7
85+	8.9	8.5	–0.4	–1.4
6. Institutional				
65–74	1.8	0.9	–0.9	–8.2
75–84	7.4	4.1	–3.3	–13.8
85+	25.9	18.8	–7.1	–16.9

declines in chronic disability in several less developed countries like Taiwan. Data collected by the World Health Organization (WHO) evidenced a mixed pattern with large variations across countries due to survey differences (WHO, 2000).

A more comprehensive effort to assess changes in chronic disability has been sponsored by REVES, an international consortium whose purpose is develop methodologies to calculate and conduct population studies to assess changes in disability weighted life expectancy, or "active life expectancy" globally (Robine, Blanchet, & Dowd, 1992; Robine & Ritchie, 1991; Robine and Michel, 1990). REVES has been in existence now for 10 years and has succeeded in sensitizing governments and WHO to the need for examining functional decline with age as a primary measure of changes in the human potential resident in aging populations (Manton, 2000; Manton & Land, 2000).

Another widely available though not universal, data resource is national vital statistics on cause specific mortality (National Center for Health Statistics, 2000). Though maintained for many national populations, such records relate only indirectly relate to specific dimensions of age-related biological and health processes. For example, cancer mortality data and cross-national data on site specific cancer incidences from tumor registries gathered by International Agencies for Research on Cancer (1997), have been combined in biologically motivated models to examine the age dependence of specific major types of cancer (e.g., breast and lung; Manton & Stallard, 1988). The models generally utilize the multihit/stage model of carcinogenesis in their construction (Armitage & Doll, 1961; Whittemore et al., 1977). Cause-specific mortality data for a number of countries have likewise been combined with dynamic-risk-factor models estimated from major epidemiological studies like the Framingham Heart Study's (Dawber, Meador, & Moore, 1951), to better assess premortal changes in risk-factor profiles by age and gender (Dowd & Manton, 1990). Perhaps the most comprehensive effort to combine vital statistics and other data sets in mathematical models is the Global Burden of Disease (GBD) Study conducted by WHO (Murray & Lopez, 1996), which attempted to assess the burden of all major disease entities in developed and developing countries. Unfortunately, the results of that study have proven quite controversial among WHO member states because the perception of the major health problems in each country often differed from the GBD estimates.

LONGITUDINAL POPULATION DATA ON BIOLOGICAL STATE VARIABLES UNDERLYING AGING

There are relatively few studies with the necessary length of follow-up of a large population with sufficiently detailed physiological measures to support dynamic modeling of degenerative disease and senescent processes. Perhaps the best illustration of such a study is the classic Framingham Heart Study, started in 1949–1950 and continuing through at least 50 years of follow-up of the original cohort of 5,209 persons. A battery of basic physiological measurements were assessed in the cohort every 2 years along with disease-specific morbidity and mortality endpoints and select clinical assessments (e.g., EKG). The basic measurements included diastolic and systolic blood pressure; hematocrit; serum cholesterol; vital capacity;

body weight and height, blood sugar, smoking, pulse rate, and measures of cardiovascular function such as left ventricular hypertrophy. In 1949–1950 the initial age range of the cohort was 29 to 62 years of age so surviving participants may now be more than 100 years of age (the oldest person observed so far was 103 years of age). The risk-factor measures, though not encompassing all desired biomarkers, include a wide range of physiological measures which are correlated with a broader range of underlying factors (e.g., blood pressure and kidney function). As we will describe in the next section, this type of longitudinal study is well suited for establishing parameters of a detailed model of physiological aging changes for the analysis of population aging.

Measurements in the later waves of the Framingham cohort have recently been expanded to include additional physiological measures (HDL, LDL, triglycerides, ApoE), as well as measures of functional status and genotype by drawing blood samples. In addition, the value of the study has been greatly enhanced by the collection of similar data on a large ($N = 5{,}142$) sample of offspring of the original Framingham cohort. The offspring cohort in Framingham now more than 26 years of biennial follow-ups. Blood data and detailed information on offspring make this a very valuable data set for studying age changes in the phenotypic manifestation of genotypes.

One limitation of the Framingham Heart Study is that it is of a relative genetically select population in homogeneous socioeconomic conditions (i.e., it was drawn from a White middle-class suburban community near Boston). Hence, in order to examine the variation of aging processes across genetically distinct populations and in a variety of cultures and socioeconomic conditions, it is necessary either to compare the Framingham study to other similar longitudinal studies or to identify longitudinal studies that were collected in multiple distinct community populations. Both types of analytic strategies are now possible due to recent federal (NIH) efforts to increase access to such longitudinal population studies.

For example, long-term follow-up studies containing many of the same types of risk-factor assessments that were made in Framingham have been done in Honolulu (the Honolulu Heart Study) (Curb, Read, Yano, Kauto, & Albers, 1986) and in Charleston, South Carolina (the Charleston Heart Study) (Keil et al., 1993). Though these studies have many similar measurements, each has major design differences. The advantage of comparing the Framingham and Honolulu heart studies is that the Honolulu population is a reasonably homogenous Japanese male population. This allows the identification of select genetic differences between males in Framingham and males in Honolulu. A disadvantage is that only males were studied in Honolulu. In the Charleston study, one major advantage is that there is a large representation in the study population of both male and female African Americans who were selected to represent variation in socioeconomic status. One disadvantage, as in the Honolulu study, is that the assessed risk factors are not as complete as in the later stages of Framingham and the periods of reassessment are 5 (or 10) rather than 2, years. In addition, neither blood data or functional status assessments have yet been made in the Charleston and Honolulu studies.

Two other studies that could be assessed are the ARIC study (Arteriosclerosis Risk In Communities) and CHS (Cardiovascular Health Study). There are detailed longitudinal assessments of risk factors in both studies, but the length of follow-up is shorter than in Framingham, Honolulu, and Charleston. An advantage of the CHS is that the entire study population was older than age 65. In both studies, multiple communities were evaluated (for example, 4 in ARIC and 4 in CHS), both blacks and whites were represented, and the study population was large (approximately 5,888 in CHS and 15,792 in ARIC). Given the common observational plan in each community, study aspects of age-dependent-state variable modeling are greatly simplified.

There are also some national surveys of risk-factor assessments that extend over a significant period of time. In the U.S. the best-known epidemiological survey is the National Health and Nutrition Examination Surveys, which were started in 1960–1962. The most recent survey was conducted for 1990–1994 and is distinguished by virtue of having used blood samples for genotyping. A second national survey that is truly longitudinal in design is the 1982–1999 National Long-Term Care Survey, in which all persons had to be aged 65 or over. Few physiological risk factors were assessed in the 1982–1994 NLTCS, but detailed measures of functional states were made for the 17-year period. In the 1999 NLTCS, blood data was drawn both for survey respondents and for their older adult siblings. The NLTCS design will be replicated in Sweden and is now being considered for replication by certain Organization for Economic Cooperation and Development member states after discussion of the NLTCS results in the G7 and G8 economic meetings.

Two other major longitudinal U.S. studies are the Multiple Risk Factor Intervention Trial (MRFIT) (1996, 1997) and the National Cancer Institute's Surveillance of Epidemiology and End Results (SEER) studies. The MRFIT study was very large (360,000 persons screened; 25,000 in the intervention phase) but with a relatively short follow-up with few follow-up assessments. The SEER data for 1973 to 1998 (Ries et al., 2001), is detailed and of national scope, but it only examined cancer endpoints and did not assess physiological changes prior to death.

Some longitudinal population studies have been done in Europe and Japan that made physiological assessments. For example, there is the well-known seven-country study (Keys, 1980) in which three countries

(Finland, the Netherlands, and Italy) have continued risk-factor assessments for up to 30 years and for which functional assessments were made in the later waves. In the Finnish study cross-sectional risk-factor surveys were conducted in the North Karelia province. One continuing longitudinal study of some recent interest is the Rotterdam study (Hofman et al., 1997).

A more common observational plan are risk-factor surveys conducted in a large number of countries with relatively short-term follow-up that usually focuses on cardiovascular disease. Major sets of such surveys coordinated by WHO were done in 32 collaborating centers in 21 countries in the MONICA Project (monitoring of cardiovascular disease); (Tunstall-Pedoe, 1988; Tunstall-Pedoe et al., 1994; Tunstall-Pedoe et al., 2000). The lack of a lengthy follow-up period, a focus on heart disease and stroke endpoints, and little exposure at ages 75+ reduce the value of those surveys for modeling aging processes cross-nationally.

SPECIFICATION OF A THEORETICAL DYNAMIC MODEL OF HUMAN DISEASE AND AGING

A theoretically motivated model of aging and mortality that we have applied to longitudinal data on physiological risk factors is based on a stochastic process model of both physiological state changes and the age-dependence of mortality (Woodbury & Manton, 1977; Manton, Stallard & Singer, 1992; Manton & Yashin, 2000). In this model the risk of an adverse health event is modeled as a quadratic function of state variables, where $x(t)$ is a vector of J state variable measured at age t,

$$\mu(t,x(t)) = (x(t))^T Qx(t))$$

where μ is the mortality rate expressed as a function of age t and age-specific risk factors $x(t)$ and Q is a matrix of hazard coefficients relating the level of each of J risk factors to the risk of death or to an age-dependent morbidity event. When there are D specific events competing with one another (for example, death due to cancer and CVD), the quadratic function can be estimated for each of the events and the D independent Quadratic forms summed, that is

$$\mu = \sum_{d=1}^{D} \mu_d (t,x(t)) = \sum_{d=1}^{D} (x(t)^T Q_D x(t)).$$

To describe the dynamics of each of the J variables among survivors to age t, it is necessary to also estimate a set of linear dynamic equations,

$$x(t) = C_0 + \beta x(t-1) + e(t-1),$$

which, if the dynamics matrix β (i.e., the regression coefficients describing the dependence of each of J factors at time t on their prior values at $t-1$) is dependent on the age of each person the equation can be generalized to

$$x(t) = C_0 + \beta\,(Age_i\,(t))\;(x(t-1)) + e(t-1)$$

or

$$x(t) = C_0 + [\beta \cdot Age_i\,(t)]\;(x(t-1) + e(t-1)),$$

where β is made an explicit function of age. The evolution of the set of J state variables in a population is described by the evolution of two equations, the hazard and mortality, as they interact.

A more interesting model of age-related health events can be generated by describing the effects of unobserved variables because the J measurements will almost never be the true state variables. This is done by examining such standard hazard processes used to describe the age-related risk of death as the Gompertz or Weibull functions (Strehler, 1977). The Gompertz function can be written simply as the exponential function,

$$\mu(t) = \alpha e^{\theta t}$$

where α represents the hazard rate at age = 0 and θ represents the percentage increase in mortality for each year of age. In this Gompertz function no state variables, $x(t)$, are observed. This is of interest in that both Strehler (Strehler & Mildvan, 1960) and Sacher (Sacher & Trucco, 1962) developed their theoretical models of mortality as a function of physiological variables (Strehler, 1977). Unfortunately, they did not have sufficient longitudinal data to directly estimate the parameters of the dynamic equations, β, so they examined estimates of temporal changes in physiological functions made for example, by Shock, Greulich, & Andres (1984) and then attempted to analyze mathematically how the temporal rate of decline in physiological function would be related to changes in α and θ estimated in multiple human populations (Strehler & Mildvan, 1960) using thermodynamic and other arguments (Rosenberg, Kemeny, Smith, Skurnick, & Bandurski, 1973). We substitute instead a multivariate diffusion process in α in the Gompertz function, which we can directly estimate from longitudinal data (for instance, the Framingham 40-year follow-up),

$$\mu(t,x,\theta) = (x(t)^T Q_G x(t))e^{\theta^{\bullet} t}$$

where obviously α has been replaced by Q_G, i.e., the quadratic hazard function. The $\theta^{\bullet}$ estimated in this function will generally be lower than θ in the standard Gompertz function in that some of the age dependence of θ will be explained by the diffusion process in the variables x (Tolley & Manton, 1991; Manton et al., 1994). Thus, the physiological state dynamics are directly represented in this model by taking advantage of the longitudinal data on risk factor changes.

The important aspect of this model is that the population-level process represented by the generalized hazard function can be interpreted in terms of the cellular failure processes. That is, the parameters of the hazard model can be interpreted in terms of the cellular thermodynamics (e.g., protein denaturation by heat stress) of aging and mortality processes. The use of a thermodynamic metaphor is important because it leads to critical tests of mathematically (and theoretically) distinct aging processes. For example, an alternative to the diffusion process-dependent Gompertz is the generalized Weibull hazard process,

$$\mu(t,x,m) = \left(x(t)^T Q_W x(t)\right)t^{m-1}$$

where m represents the number of mutations, or intracellular events, necessary for a lethal disease process to be triggered by cell failure. The Weibull versus Gompertz form leads to quite distinct interpretations of the thermodynamics failure process at the level of the cell (Rosenberg et al., 1973). It also leads to very different conclusions about the age-related effects of the latent state variables described by either $e^{\theta t}$ or t^{m-1}. Both of those models differ from the simple quadratic form (i.e., with $e^{\theta t}$ or t^{m-1}) where the effects of unobserved variables (i.e., variables affecting mortality not in $x(t)$) cause a random dispersion of mortality points in the risk factor space (Woodbury & Manton, 1977). Instead of a distribution of *points* where death occurs, the generalized Gompertz and Weibull models lead to a random dispersion of *lines* or *geodesics* of elevated mortality risk where the lines are determined by the age functions $e^{\theta t}$ and t^{m-1} and the distribution of the time lines is determined by the state variable diffusion process.

There is a fundamental mathematical distinction to be made between the Weibull and Gompertz models of aging dynamics. If we believe there is a scale invariance across levels of biological organization, then there should be a fractal relation between the population of individuals, the population of cells, and the population of proteins subject to intracellular dynamics and diffusion. This fractal relation leads naturally to the Weibull formulation where m is not an integer power (Dewey, 1997). Consistency with a fractal relation across levels of biological organization allows us to take advantage of a series of powerful mathematical tools developed by

Mandelbrot (1982). This may allow us to reflect the impact of protein structure and function on cellular thermodynamics up to the macro-level manifestation of aging changes on individual mortality. The use of the fractal structure (utilizing, say, Julia sets) also has the advantage that we can further generalize the Weibull model to represent the effects of complex variables, that is,

$$\mu(x,t,m,i) = (x(t)^T\, Q(x(t))t^{(m_1 + m_2)}$$

where m_1, reflects the failure of certain components of the cell and im_2 represents the effects of cell repair mechanisms reversing those errors. This then allows us to describe regenerative treatments by m_2 which, effectively, reverse the age accumulation of damage on the cell. In the classical application of the Weibull model to carcinogenesis using a multihit or stage formulation (Armitage & Doll, 1961) the estimated value of m confounds the effects of m_1, and m_2 (Watson, 1977). To describe not the empirical function but the parameters of the actual compensating biological processes, estimates of both m_1 and m_2 must be made.

The use of complex variables in our model can also aid us in cross-study population evaluations. By generalizing the complex factors we can compare the biological invariants of degenerative and regenerative processes across populations. This generalization of complex variables is called quaternions at the simplest levels (Hamilton, 1844). A more complex set of such factors are called octonions (i.e., four pairs of complex numbers in a system). Richard Feynman, the Nobel prize–winning physicist, railed against the use of unnecessary mathematical concepts—in particular the Octonions—in the development of certain physical theories. However, the biophysical system we are attempting to describe, involving the functional implications of 3D protein topology, are intrinsically more complex than the physical systems to be dealt with. It is also informative, for example, that quaternions and octonions are routinely used in computer games for children. They are necessary for rotating complex topologies like graphic figures in three dimensions.

EXAMPLES

The examples we present are in the nature of "thought" experiments because the practical applications of the model proposed earlier require solving difficult problems in numerical analyses. We have successfully estimated a complex variable Gompertz model from the 40-year follow-up of the Framingham data (Manton & Dowd, 2000). However, full implementation of the model requires our dealing with nonsymmetric matrices with both positive and negative roots. We are working on practical algorithms for the implementation of such models in a 12-dimensional space (i.e., $J = 12$ the number of measured physiological state variables). We are also working on the more difficult problem of estimating the generalized Weibull process where the m_1 and m_2 estimates are confounded with the state dynamics.

In Figure 1.1 we graphically illustrate the conceptual structure of the mathematical functions to demonstrate the opposition of regenerative and degenerative forces.

In the figure we represent mortality as a function of risk factors *x(t)*. In the first figure we describe mortality at an early age *t* (say age 50). The second figure represents it at an advanced age $x + \Delta x$ (say age 85). In both figures (i.e., at both ages) the Gompertz parameter θ_1, for degeneration, and θ_2, for regeneration, are the same. The curvature of the two lines A and C differ because of the age difference. Lines A and C in both figures represent not probabilities, but probability amplitudes, which can be summed to describe the actual change in the probability of death as a function of *x* at a given age. That is, in contrast to probabilities that are defined as positive quantities, probability amplitudes can be negative or positive. This is a standard concept in physics. Generally one will expect $\theta_1 > \theta_2$. Thus, the effects of degeneration are expected to increase with age factors. However, to the extent that the *x(t)* describe the effects of θ_1 and θ_2 we have identified variables whose values, if they can be controlled appropriately, might decrease degeneration—or accelerate regeneration.

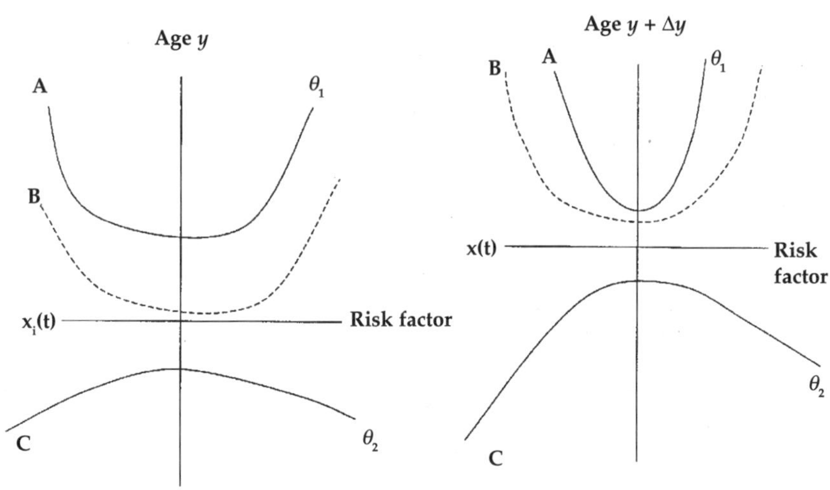

FIGURE 1.1 Degenerative and regenerative age-dependent processes.

SUMMARY

We reviewed longitudinal human population data sets that might be used to estimate models of human aging processes, as well as their cross-national variation. In addition we presented a set of theoretically motivated models of aging humans that may identify the biological invariants of those multivariate stochastic processes. Such general, theoretically motivated models of physiological aging can more efficiently target interventions in aging processes in a broader range of circumstances. Such models may help us understand, for example, declines in chronic disability such as observed in the U.S. and France and help determine how such declines might be promoted in other countries. They may help us also to better explain the variation of aging processes across population.

REFERENCES

Armitage, P., & Doll, R. (1961). Stochastic models for carcinogenesis. In: Biology and Problems of Health Berkeley, In *Proceedings of the Fourth Berkeley Symposium on Mathematical Statistics and Probability* (Vol. IV). University of California Press.

Bebbington, A. (1988). The expectation of life without disability in England and Wales. *Social Sciences Medicine, 27*, 321–326.

Costa, D. (1998). Understanding the twentieth century decline in chronic conditions among older men. University of Chicago Pres: *National Bureau of Economic Research*, 1–40.

Crimmins, E., Saito, Y., & Reynolds, S. (1997). Further evidence on recent trends in the prevalence and incidence of disability among older Americans from two sources: The LSOA and the NHIS. *Journals of Gerontology. Series B, Psychological Sciences and Social Sciences, 52*, S59–S71.

Curb, J., Reed D., Yano, K., Kauta, J., & Albers, J. (1986). Plasma lipids and lipoproteins in elderly Japanese-American men. *Journal of the American Geriatrics Society, 34*, 773–780.

Dawber, T., Meadors, G., & Moore, F. (1951). Epidemiological approaches to heart disease: The Framingham Study. *American Journal of Public Health*, 41, 279–286.

Dewey, T. G. (1997). In D. G. Truhlar (Ed.), *Fractals in molecular biophysics* (p. 268). New York: Oxford University Press.

Dowd, J. E., Manton, K. G. (1990). Forecasting chronic disease risks in developing countries. *International Journal of Epidemiology, 19*, 1018–1036.

Finch, C., & Kirkwood, T. (2000). *Chance, development, and aging*. New York: Oxford University Press.

Fogel, R. (1993). *The relevance of Malthus for the study of mortality today: Long-run influences on health, mortality, labor force participation, and population growth.* Presentation to the Population-Environment-Development seminar, The Royal Swedish Academy of Sciences, Stockholm, Sweden.

Fogel, R. (1994). Economic growth, population theory, and physiology: The bearing of long-term processes on the making of economic policy. *American Economic Review, 84,* 369–395.

Fogel, R., & Costa, D. L. (1997). A theory of technophysiological evolution, with some implications for forecasting population, health care costs, and pension costs. *Demography, 34,* 49–66.

Freedman, V., & Martin L. (1998). Understanding trends in functional limitations among older Americans. *American Journal of Public Health, 88,* 1457–1462.

Freedman, V., & Martin, L. (2000). Contribution of chronic conditions to aggregate changes in old-age functioning.

Freedman, V., & Soldo, B. (1994). *Trends in disability at older ages.* Washington, DC: Committee on National Statistics.

Georgopulos, C., & Welch, W. (1993). Role of the major heat shock proteins as molecular chaperones. *Annual Review of Cell Biology, 9,* 601–634.

Hamilton, W. (1844). On a new species of imaginary quantities connected with a theory of quaternions. *Proceedings of the Royal Irish Academy, 2,* 424–434.

National Center for Health Statistics. (2000). *Health, United States, 2000.* Hyattsville, MD, Public Health Service.

Hofman, A., Ott, A., Breteler, M., & Bots, M., Slooter, A. N., Van Harskamp, F., Van Dujin, C., Van Broekhoven, C., & Grobbee, D. (1997). Atherosclerosis apolipoprotein E and prevalence of dementia and Alzheimer's disease in the Rotterdam study. *Lancet, 349,* 151–154.

International Agency for Research on Cancer. (1997). Cancer incidence in five continents. In D. Parkin, S. Whelan, J. Ferlay, L. Raymond, and J. Young (Eds.), Vol. VII: *International Agency for Research on Cancer* Scientific Publications, 1240.

Jacquez, J. (1972). *Compartmental analysis in biology and medicine.* Amsterdam: Elsevier.

Keil, J., Sutherland, S., Knapp, R., Lackland, D., Gazes, P., & Tyroler, H. (1993). Mortality rates and risk factors for coronary disease in black as compared with white men and women. *New England Journal of Medicine, 329,* 73–78.

Keys, A. (1980). Wine, garlic, and CHD in seven countries. *Lancet, 1,* 145–146.

Mandelbrot, B. (1982). *The fractal geometry of nature.* New York: W. H. Freeman.

Manton, K. G. (1999). Dynamic paradigms for human mortality and aging. *Journal of Gerontology: Biological Sciences, 54A,* B247–B254.
Manton, K. G. (2000). Aging and health in old age. *International encyclopedia of the social and behavioral science.* Oxford, England: Elsvier Science.
Manton, K. G., & Corder, E. H. (in review). Changes in the prevalence of dementia 1982 to 1999. *New England Journal of Medicine.*
Manton, K. G., Corder, L. S., & Stallard, E. 1993). Changes in the use of personal assistance and special equipment 1982 to 1989: Results from the 1982 and 1989 NLTCS. *The Gerontologist, 33,* 168–176.
Manton, K. G., Corder, L., & Stallard, E. (1997). Chronic disability trends in the U.S. elderly populations 1982 to 1994. *Proceedings of the National Academy of Sciences, 94,* 2593–2598.
Manton, K. G., & Dowd, J. E. (2000, October). *A multidimensional stochastic generalization of the multi-stage model.* Presented at the Impact of Biotechnology on Cancer Diagnostic and Prognostic Indicators Symposium, Geneva, Switzerland.
Manton, K. G., & Gu, X., (2001, May 8). Changes in the prevalence of chronic disability in the U.S. Black and non-Black population aged 65+ from 1982 to 1999. *Proceedings of the National Academy of Sciences, USA.*
Manton, K. G., & Land, K. C. (2000). Active life expectancy estimates for U.S. elderly population: Multidimensional continuous mixture model of functional change applied to completed cohorts, 1982 to 1996. *Demography, 37(3),* 253–265.
Manton, K. G., & Singer, B. (in press). Variation in disability decline and Medicare expenditures. *Proceedings of the National Academy of Sciences.*
Manton, K. G., & Stallard, E. (1988). *Chronic disease risk modelling: Measurement and evaluation of the risks of chronic disease processes.* In the Griffin Series of the Biomathematics of Diseases. London: Charles Griffin.
Manton, K. G., Stallard, E., & Corder, L. S. (1998). The dynamics of dimensions of age-related disability 1982 to 1994 in the U.S. elderly population. *Journal of Gerontology: Biological Sciences , 53A*(1), B59–B70.
Manton, K. G., Stallard, E., & Singer, B. H. (1992). Projecting the future size and health status of the U.S. elderly population. *International Journal of Forecasting, 8,* 433–458.
Manton, K. G., Woodbury, M. A., & Tolley, H. D. (1994). *Statistical applications using fuzzy sets.* Wiley-Interscience Publication.
Manton, K. G., & Yashin, A. I. (2000). Mechanisms of aging and mortality: Searches for new paradigms. *Monographs on Population Aging, 7.*
Mathers, C. (1994). Health expectancies in Australia 1993: Preliminary results. In C. Mathers, J. McCallum, & J. Robine, (Eds.), *Advances in Health Expectancies* (pp. 198–212). Canberra, Australia: Australian Institute of Health and Welfare.

Murray, C., & Lopez, A. (1996). The global burden of disease: A comprehensive assessment of mortality and disability from diseases, injuries, and risk factors in 1990 and projected to 2020. *Global burden of disease and injury: Vol. 1.* Geneva, Switzerland: World Health Organization.

Multiple Risk Factor Intervention Trial. (1996). Mortality after 16 years for participants randomized to the Multiple Risk Factor Intervention Trial. *Circulation, 94,* 946–951.

Multiple Risk Factor Intervention Trial. (1997). Multiple risk factor intervention trial: Risk factor changes and mortality. *Journal of the American Medical Association, 277,* 582–594.

Ries, L., Eiser, M., Kosary, C., Hankey, B., Miller, B., Clegg, L., & Ewards, B. (2001) *SEER cancer statistics review, 1973–1998.* Bethesda, National Cancer Institute.

Risken, H. (1996). *The Fokker-Planck equation.* New York: Springer Publishing Co.

Robine, J. (1994). Disability-free life expectancy trends in France: 1981–1991, international comparison. In C. Mathers, J. McCallum, and J. Robine (Eds.), *Advances in Health Expectancies* (pp. 43–52). Canberra, Australia: Australian Institute of Health and Welfare.

Robine, J., Blanchet, M., & Dowd, J. (1992). *Health expectancy: First workshop of the international healthy life expectancy network.* (REVES). Paris: Office of Population Censuses and Surveys.

Robine, J., & Michel, J., (1990). *Recommendations for international guidelines for comparisons of healthy life expectancy.* Geneva, Switzerland: World Health Organization.

Robine, J., & Ritchie, K. (1991). Healthy life expectancy: Evaluation of global indicator of change in population health. *British Medical Journal, 302,* 457–460.

Rosenberg, B., Kemeny, G., Smith, L., Skurnick, I., Bandurski, M. (1973). The kinetics and thermodynamics of death in multicellular organisms. *Mechanisms of Aging and Development, 2,* 275–293.

Sacher, G., & Trucco, E. The stochastic theory of mortality. *Annals of the New York Academy of Sciences,* 96, 985.

Shock, N., Greulich, R., & Andres, R. (1984). *Normal human aging: The Baltimore longitudinal study on aging.* Washington, DC: National Institutes of Health.

Singer, B., & Manton, K. G. (1998). The effects of health changes on projections of health service needs for the elderly population of the United States. *Proceedings of the National Academy of Science, 95,* 15618–15622.

Strehler, B. (1977). *Time, cells and aging.* New York: Academic Press.

Strehler, B., & Mildvan, A. (1960). General theory of mortality and aging. *Science, 132,* 14–21.

Tolley, H. D., & Manton, K. G. (1991, April). A grade of membership method for partitioning heterogeneity in a collective. *Scientific Committee on Oceanic Research Notes,* 121–151.

Tunstall-Pedoe, H. (1988). The World Health Organization MONICA project (monitoring trends and determinants in cardiovascular disease): A major international collaboration. *Journal of Clinical Epidemiology, 41,* 105–113.

Tunstall-Pedoe, H., Kuulasmaa, K., Amouyel, P., Arveiler, D., Rajakangas, A., & Pajak, A. Myocardial infarction and coronary deaths in the world health organization MONICA Project. Registration procedures, event rates, and case-fatality in 38 populations from 21 countries in four continents. *Circulation, 90,* 583–612.

Tunstall-Pedoe, H., Vanuzzo, D., Hobbs, M., Mahonen, M., Cepaitis, Z., Kuulasmaa, K., & Keil, U. (2000). WHO MONICA Project. *Lancet, 2000,* 688–700.

Waidmann, T., & Liu, K. (2000). Disability trends among the elderly and implications for the future. *Journal of Gerontology: Social Sciences 55B*(5): S298–S307.

Waidmann, T., & Manton, K. G. (1998). *International evidence on disability trends among the elderly.* Final Report for the Department of Health and Human Services.

Watson, G. (1977). Age incidence curves for cancer. *Proceedings of the National Academy of Science, 74,* 1341–1342.

Whittemore, A. (1977). The age distribution of human cancer for carcinogenic exposures of varying intensity. *American Journal of Epidemiology, 106,* 418–432.

Wilkins, R., & Adams, O. (1983). Health expectancy in Canada, late 1970s: Demographic, regional, and social dimensions. *American Journal of Public Health, 73,* 1073–1080.

Wilkins, R., Chen, J., & Ny, E. (1994). Changes in health expectancy in Canada from 1986 to 1991. *Advances in Health Expectancies* (pp. 115–132). Canberra, Australia: Australian Institute of Health and Welfare.

Woodbury, M. A., & Manton, K. G. (1977). A random walk model of human mortality and aging. *Theoretical Population Biology, 11,* 37–48.

World Health Organization (2000). *Health systems: Improving performance,* pp. 1–18 (overview). Geneva, Switzerland. Author.

CHAPTER 2

The Comparative Biology of Aging

STEVEN N. AUSTAD
DEPARTMENT OF BIOLOGICAL SCIENCES
UNIVERSITY OF IDAHO

The study of natural patterns can suggest or reveal underlying biological mechanisms. For instance, the trend to inversely correlate body size and mass-specific metabolism in mammals led to the understanding that heat loss across body surfaces was a key physiological constraint on the rate of metabolism in homeotherms (birds and mammals) (Kleiber, 1961). Similarly, the conservation of amino acid sequences in proteins of similar function across an assortment of distantly related species indicates general structural constraints on efficient protein function (Hochachka & Somero, 1984).

Comparative biology may be defined as the search for instructive patterns across species or populations and their analysis. Comparative studies of aging have a long history, and the most general patterns—such as the positive relation between mammal body size and longevity—and the superior longevity of birds as compared with mammals—have been documented for centuries (e.g., Bacon, 1638). Modern comparative studies have focused more on particular predictions from specific theories. For instance, despite the putative ubiquity of aging among multicellular animals, Bell (1984) noted that, consistent with a prediction from evolutionary theory, senescence was not observed among two asexual invertebrate species, which reproduced by fission, in contrast with four asexual invertebrates, which reproduced by laying parthenogenetic eggs.

Comparative biology need not be confined to studies among species. Within species, comparisons may be similarly informative. The fact that a mountain lion's body length nearly doubles between equatorial and temperate zones (McNab, 1972) suggests the general selection pressures, climatic in this case, on the evolution of body size. Similarly, small domestic dog breeds typically live longer than large breeds (Li, Deeb, Pendergrass, & Wolf, 1996). Such a trend, particularly if it also found in other species, might reveal something about the effect of the action of growth hormone or some other mechanistic component of growth rate on aging and longevity.

Some of the main conclusions that can be drawn to date from a comparative perspective on aging will be outlined in the text that follows. I will also consider how a comparative approach can contribute to future aging research.

COMPARATIVE PATTERNS IN AGING AND LONGEVITY

Animals Aging in Nature

It has long been conjectured that animals do not age in nature (Comfort, 1979; Hayflick, 2000; Medawar, 1952). We now know that this is not correct. Promislow (1991), for instance, examined 56 published life tables of mammals in the wild and found statistically significant evidence for senescence (measured by an increase in mortality rate with age) in 44% (26) of the species and a trend in the same direction in another 34% (20) of the species. Similarly, Holmes and Austad (1995) examined 59 life tables of natural bird populations and noted that 25% of the populations exhibited statistically significant senescence, whereas 80% of the populations evidenced a trend toward increasing mortality with age. Thus, among published studies of birds and mammals, there is suggestive evidence of aging in nature in more than three fourths of the species studied and statistically persuasive evidence in more than one third of the species. Although animals in nature are unlikely to reach a state of advanced decrepitude as they often do in captivity, aging *does* occur in wild populations and is detectable with simple demographic analysis.

Evolutionary senescence theory (reviewed in Kirkwood, in this volume) assumes that aging evolves as a consequence of the waning force of natural selection with increasing age. The rate of this waning force is a function of the probability of dying due to extrinsic causes, as well as the particular reproductive schedule of the organism in question, and the trade offs between growth, development, reproduction, and somatic maintenance. The age-related erosion of natural selection's power is predicted to lead to aging by one or both of two genetic mechanisms: (1) the passive genomic accumulation of alleles, which are effectively neutral because they have no impact on early-life fitness but have a deleterious late-life effect; and (2) positive selection for alleles with beneficial effects early in life when the force of selection is powerful and detrimental effects later on when selection is weak. Evidence to date strongly supports the latter mechanism, also known as antagonistic pleiotropy, whereas evidence for the former is weak to nonexistent (Kirkwood & Austad, 2000). One implicit consequence of these findings, assuming that manageably few physiological processes present beneficial short-term consequences but detrimental long-term consequences, is that aging processes are less likely to be purely idiosyncratic within species or genetic lineages, and more likely to be "public," that is relatively general across species and populations (Martin, Austad, & Johnson, 1996).

Evolutionary Biology: The Body Size–Longevity Relationship

Evolutionary theory provides a conceptual foundation for understanding certain long-observed interspecies patterns in longevity. One prediction stemming from the theory which has been confirmed in the laboratory, field, and by comparative analysis is that populations subjected to historically lower (or higher) levels of environmentally imposed mortality will evolve slower (or faster) aging rates (Austad, 1993; Edney & Gill, 1968; Ricklefs, 1998; Stearns, Ackermann, Doebeli, & Kaiser, 2000). This prediction and its empirical confirmation lead to a new interpretation of the well-known positive relationship between body size and captive longevity (Figure 2.1).

A traditional interpretation of this relationship has to do with the putative constancy of lifetime energy use per unit body mass, the so-called lifetime energy potential (Cutler, 1978; Lindstedt & Calder, 1981; Stahl, 1962). Such constancy is suggested by the fact that the negative slope of the line relating body size to mass-specific basal metabolic rate is almost exactly the opposite of the positive slope of the body size–longevity line. However, such constancy is illusory when the data are examined in detail. First, there exists substantial scatter about the body mass–longevity regression line, which explains only 38% of the variation in longevity using the most recent data on 610 species. Second, far from constancy in lifetime energy potentials, a greater than 40-fold range of lifetime energy potentials is observed among mammals (Austad & Fischer, 1991). Moreover, some of the highest energy values come from field populations, indicating that the range might be considerably greater under uniformly captive conditions. Suggestively, outliers above and below the line are clustered in certain taxonomic groups. Bats, for instance, are much longer lived than expected from this relationship and marsupials are shorter-lived (Figure 2.1; Austad & Fischer, 1991).

Another explanation for this relationship assumes that body mass itself may be a surrogate for some other variable. One such variable that has been mentioned repeatedly in the literature is brain weight, or relative brain weight (brain weight as a proportion of body weight; Hofman, 1983; Mallouck, 1976; Sacher, 1959; Western, 1979). In contrast to the link between aging and metabolism in which the generation of damaging reactive oxygen species provides a plausible mechanistic link, there is no

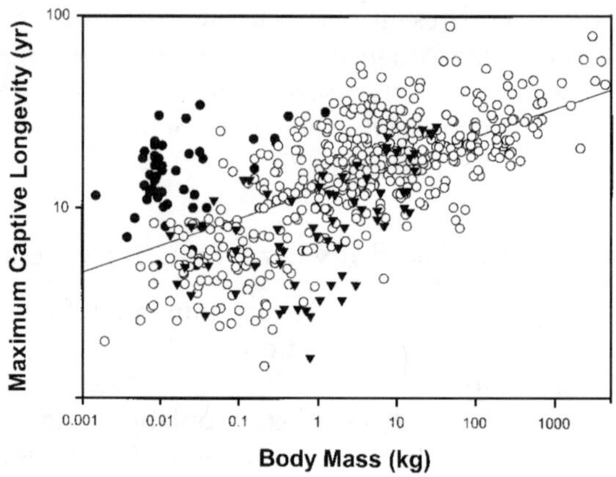

FIGURE 2.1 Maximum captive longevity and body mass of 606 mammal species. Note that bats (•) are exceptionally long-lived even though they are the only group from which longevity records are derived primarily from field studies rather than captive studies. Marsupials (▼) by contrast are a particularly short-lived group. ○ = all other mammals.

Note: From "Longevity of Captive Mammals," by L. Jones, 1982, *Zoologische Garten, 52,* pp. 113–128. Adapted with permission.
From *Walker's Mammals of the World* (6th ed.), by R. M. Novak, 1999. Baltimore: Johns Hopkins University. Adapted with permission.

clear functional hypothesis about why relative brain mass might be related to longevity. An argument could be made that the brain controls physiological maintenance and homeostasis, and therefore relatively larger brains would be able to better preserve homeostatic processes, which in turn might lead to longer life. There is in fact little suggestive evidence to support this idea, beyond the mere fact that relative brain weight correlates more closely with longevity than does body weight itself.

Correlation, as every introductory statistics text emphasizes, is not causation regardless of the correlative strength of the relationship. One explanation of the better correlation between brain size and longevity compared to body size is that brain size varies much less among individuals than does body size, and it is less affected by seasonal and environmental factors (Calder, 1984). It may therefore be a better indicator of body size than is body weight.

Fundamental scientific procedure dictates that sound analyses should include appropriate controls whenever possible. A reasonable control for the relative brain size–longevity hypothesis might include how well longevity correlates with the weight of other organs. A comparative analysis of the relative brain size–longevity hypothesis across nearly 600 species of mammals found that relative brain mass indeed significantly correlated with maximum captive longevity *among primates* (Austad & Fischer, 1992). However, a more recent analysis found only marginally significant statistical support for a relative brain size–longevity hypothesis (Judge & Carey, 2000). The study included updated longevity records and average longevity maxima of genera (as opposed to species) to help reduce bias due to species sample composition and poor characterization of some species. The two major outliers among primates—those of the genus *Homo* and *Cebus*—both exhibit exceptionally large brains, but the relationship is weak among the rest of the primates. Parenthetically, it should be noted that recent information on longevity in the genus *Cebus* (55 years in the 3 kg *C. capuchinus* [Nowak, 1999]) now makes it as exceptionally long-lived as humans for its body size. On the other hand, no relation between relative brain size and longevity was observed among nonprimates; in well-represented orders (bats, carnivores, insectivores, marsupials, rodents, and even-toed ungulates); nor was brain mass more closely correlated with longevity than was heart, liver, kidney, or spleen weight (Austad & Fischer, 1992). Furthermore, bats, which do not have exceptionally large brains, were by far the longest-lived taxonomic group of mammals for their body size. In fact, the brains of bats are somewhat smaller than the mammalian average for their body size (Austad & Fischer, 1991). Therefore, although some statistical evidence may still suggest that exceptionally large brains may be functionally related to long life in primates, there is no support for this idea among mammals generally.

Another explanation for this relationship from evolutionary senescence theory is that for many mammals, body size may correlate inversely with susceptibility to environmental hazards such as food shortages, temperature extremes, and predation. According to this hypothesis, larger animals have historically lived in a safer environment than smaller animals, leading to the evolution of retarded senescence in large animals compared with small animals. This explanation could also be expanded to explain exceptions to the general trend: Flying mammals (bats) experience reduced environmental hazards compared with nonfliers of similar body size due to their enhanced ability to escape predators and local environmental catastrophes (Austad & Fischer, 1991). In fact, similar logic may explain otherwise anomalous patterns such as sailing mammals (e.g., "flying" squirrels and gliding marsupials) outliving nongliders in captivity, arboreal rodents outlasting terrestrial rodents, and species protected by spines or hard carapaces living longer than their unprotected relatives.

The preceding analysis of mammalian trends in longevity ignores phylogeny, the evolutionary relationships among organisms, which for several reasons, should always be considered in comparative studies. First, inferences can be biased due to sampling artifacts. For instance, if the species used in comparative analysis of mammalian body size and longevity were heavily weighted toward bats, which are small but long-lived, and marsupials, which tend to be larger and much shorter-lived, one could erroneously conclude that larger mammals don't live as long as smaller species (Figure 2.1). Second, a key assumption of most parametric statistics is that individual data points are independent of one another. Because of phylogenetic inertia—the tendency for related species to resemble one another as a consequence of genetic similarity—data points in comparative analyses cannot legitimately be considered independent of one another, which invalidates traditional statistical tests (Harvey & Pagel, 1991). In recent years, a panoply of analytic techniques has been developed that incorporates phylogenetic information into correlational analyses (e.g., Felsenstein, 1985; Garland, Harvey, & Ives, 1992). These techniques should be used when a reasonable phylogeny can be constructed for the species in question. Fortunately, generalizations formulated from a broad analysis of taxonomically diverse species rarely have been overturned when phylogenetically appropriate techniques have been implemented (Ricklefs & Stark, 1996). Therefore, the very broad generalizations mentioned above are likely to remain valid even as more refined phylogenetic information about mammals becomes available (see Judge & Carey, 2000 for such an analysis). Note, however, that phylogenetically appropriate analyses may call into question more specific generalizations, such as the evolution of an arboreal life history in rodents leading to the evolution of retarded aging (Austad & Holmes, 1999).

Whereas the general trend to associate increasing body size with increasing longevity *between species* is well established and satisfactorily explained by susceptibility to environmental hazards, there is no similar satisfactory explanation for an emerging trend for *genetically* smaller individuals *within a species* to be longer-lived. Such a trend has been reported in fruit flies (Hillesheim & Stearns, 1992), *C. elegans* (van Voorhies & Ward, 1999), dogs (Deeb & Wolf, 1994), mice (reviewed in Miller, 2001), and, more anecdotally, in horses and humans (Samaras & Elrick, 1999, but see Davey et al., 2000). *Nutritionally* smaller individuals are longer-lived in laboratory rats and mice (Turturro et al., 1999).

A possible evolutionary explanation for this trend derives from the effect of small body size on reproductive capacity, as predicted by the mechanism of antagonistic pleiotropy. Small, long-lived mutants have a reduced reproductive rate in the fruit flies (Hillesheim & Stearns, 1992), *C. elegans* (Van Voorhies & Ward, 1999), dogs (Robinson, 1973), and mice (Miller, 2001) mentioned previously. Nutritionally smaller laboratory rodents also have compromised reproductive function (Holehan & Merry, 1986). Recently,

Sgró and Partridge (1999) showed that genetically selected long life in *Drosophila* could be completely explained by a reduction in reproductive rate.

Mechanistically, the basis of longevity enhancement by genetic dwarfism is best understood in laboratory mice. Mutations in two genes (*Pit1* and *Prop1*) involved in proper development of the anterior pituitary extend life by about 50% in Snell and Ames dwarves, respectively (Miller, 2001). These mutations lead to multiple hormone deficiencies, including growth hormone, thyroxine, and prolactin, and to infertility as well as dwarfism. Hypothyroidism in these mice suggests they may be hypometabolic relative to normal-sized littermates. As with the caloric restriction effect, however, the dwarfism effect seems unlikely to be due to reduced metabolic rate, because Ames dwarves consume more calories per gram of body mass than controls (Miller, 2001). The impact of infertility on longevity in these dwarf mutants can be experimentally assessed, because fertility can be restored with appropriate hormonal interventions. However, the effect of such treatments on longevity are not yet available.

The growth hormone–IGF-1 pathway seems a particularly promising candidate for understanding the mechanism underlying this effect. Disruption of the growth hormone receptor, with attendant reduction in body size and IGF-1 level, has recently been shown to extend life in mice (Coschigano, Clemmons, Bellush, & Kopchick, 2000), suggesting these hormones may be implicated in the life-extension effect. Interestingly, the effect of caloric restriction on growth hormone dynamics is still unclear, with some reports of increased levels (Sonntag et al., 1999), some of decreased levels (Koizumi et al., 1989). Yet studies uniformly find that caloric restriction decreases IGF-1 levels (Kari, Dunn, French, & Barrett, 1999; Sonntag et al., 1999). Combining this information with the life-extending impact of mutations in the insulin/IGF-1 pathway in *C. elegans* (Guarente & Kenyon, 2000) suggests that further investigation of IGF-1 dynamics may yield considerable insight into the dynamics of aging.

Sex Differences in Longevity

Sex differences in longevity, which can be substantial, is a woefully understudied aging phenomenon and potentially could lead to insights on basic mechanisms of aging. Most of the largest sex differences in longevity occur among invertebrates. For instance, female tarantulas can live decades as adults whereas males live only a matter of months, and eusocial insect queens can live many years yet males live a matter of weeks. Considerable sex differences may be found among mammals as well. In one population of short-finned pilot whales, for example, males live about 12 years and females live about 23 years, with the oldest female in the study 17 years older than the oldest male (Kasuya & Marsh, 1984). Female killer whales also live substantially longer than males in the wild (50-year life expectancy versus 29 years) (Olesiuk, Bigg, & Ellis, 1990), as do diverse other mammal species such as red deer, African lions, vervet monkeys (Clutton-Brock, 1988), and macaques (Dittus, 1975).

In humans, of course, it has long been noted that males do not survive as long as females, starting at conception and continuing throughout life, in both long-lived populations from industrialized regions as well as in short-lived populations in pretechnological societies (Neel, 1990; Smith, 1993). This difference is generally on the order of 5%–15% of life expectancy (United Nations, 1990). One or a few single causes of death do not account for the difference (Hazzard, 1994).

The ubiquity of superior female longevity in humans, together with the assertion that a similar phenomenon is nearly universal among animals (Comfort, 1979; Hamilton, 1948; Hazzard, 1994), has fostered several theories that attempt to explain longer female survival in general terms. One group of theories invokes the chromosomal difference between the sexes. I call these the "heterogametic sex hypotheses," because they predict that the heterogametic sex should age more rapidly.

Female mammals typically have two X chromosomes, whereas males—the XY heterogametic sex—have only one. The sex longevity difference could in principle be caused by life-shortening genes on the Y chromosome. However, the Y chromosome bears few genes, and most of these have to do with sex determination and fertility. In humans, for instance, only 32 genes have been identified on the Y chromosome compared with 424 on the X chromosome (National Center for Biotechnology Information, 2001).

The difference could also have to do with having two copies of the X chromosome, which could prevent phenotypic exposure of deleterious sex-linked recessive alleles. Even though one of the two X chromosomes is typically randomly inactivated during embryogenesis in female somatic cells, genetic mosaicism on the cellular level could allow functional compensation for defects in one X by the normal allele on the other. Males, being hemizygous for such alleles, would lack the same compensatory advantage (Smith & Warner, 1990). Such a mechanism is suggested by the fact that sex-linked phenotypes, such as hemophilia and red-green colorblindness, typically are not apparent in heterozygous females.

In addition to cellular mosaicism, there may also be positive selection during the course of a lifetime for proliferative descendants of cells with the better X chromosome activated. Such a view is supported by a recent observation that as women age, one X chromosome tends to become increasingly prevalent in peripheral blood cells. If the "better" X chromosome is the one that predominates over time, enhanced female longevity could possibly be due to this sort of cellular selection on the basis of which X is activated (Christensen et al., 2000).

One clear prediction of these sex chromosome theories is that among organisms such as birds and butterflies in which the female is the heterogametic sex, males would be predicted to live longer (Christensen et al., 2000). Among field populations, there is no such clear trend in birds. Although males indeed appear to live longer in song sparrows, great tits, indigo buntings, and red-billed gulls, females live as long or longer than males in blue tits, pied flycatchers, kingfishers, kittiwakes, fulmars, and sparrow hawks (Clutton-Brock, 1988; Newton, 1989). Similarly among captive birds, males live longer among pigeons, Japanese quail, Bengalese finches, and cockatiels, but not in chickens and a variety of parrots (Ottinger, Nisbet, & Finch, 1995; Purdue Veterinary Medical Database, 1994; Smith, 1993). Thus there is no clear pattern of superior male longevity in either captive or field populations.

Although longevity patterns in birds do not seem to fit the sex chromosome hypothesis, it is conceivable that birds and mammals differ in this respect. Male birds, for instance, do not exhibit gene dosage compensation via inactivation of one Z chromosome (Smith, 1993) as female mammals do, and the W chromosome in birds is larger than the analogous Y in mammals. Focusing on mammals alone, two groups would make intriguing case studies of relevance to the hypothesis of cellular selection for the better X-chromosome explanation of the sexual survival difference. One such group is the marsupials, which unlike other mammals do not inactivate one X chromosome randomly. In marsupials, it is always the paternal X which is inactivated (Graves, 1996), thus no X-chromosome selection would occur. Thus the prediction would be that female survival superiority would be lost in marsupials; males should live as long as females. Although data are not available for a large number of marsupial species, females in species with sudden, population-wide male death do clearly live longer than males in the wild (Halley, 1992; McDonald, Lee, Bradley, & Than, 1981). However, this male mortality reflects a physiological response to sexual competition that is somewhat unique to this group of animals. On the other hand, under well-controlled captive conditions, male Leadbeater's possums significantly outlive females (Myroniuk & Seebeck, 1992). So until more data become available, it is probably premature to reject or accept the X-chromosome selection hypothesis based on data from marsupials.

Another group of interest from this perspective would be lemmings of the genera *Dicrostonyx* and *Myopus*, in which two types of X chromosomes exist, one normal form and one mutated form (deemed X*). Phenotypically normal females can have the genotypes XX, XX*, or X*Y (Bulmer, 1988). The X-chromosome selection hypothesis would predict that the latter type of female would be shorter-lived than the other two, because only one X chromosome is available. Unfortunately no appropriate data are available for these taxa.

Sex chromosome explanations, whatever their mechanistic basis, suggest that superior female longevity should be a fairly general mammalian trait. It is always possible, of course, that humans are somehow atypical compared with other mammals, but a first approach to validating these sex chromosome hypotheses might be simply to ask, How general is superior longevity among female mammals? As previously mentioned, a number of field studies in a diverse assemblage of mammalian species find females to be longer-lived. For instance, at age 13 greater than 25% of a population of female red deer were alive compared to about 6% of males (Clutton-Brock, Albon, & Guinness, 1988). Similarly, the long-term study of Serengeti lions found that nearly 20% of females were still alive at 13 years of age compared with less than 5% of males (Packer et al., 1988). Similar patterns have been observed in a number of primate species (Dunbar, 1987), in addition to the very large differences observed in the whale species mentioned earlier in this section.

Females in nature do not always live longer, however. Long-term studies of elephant seals and kangaroo rats found no sexual difference in survival (LeBoeuf & Reiter, 1988: Waser & Jones, 1991), and male chimpanzees in the wild have been reported to have a substantially higher life expectancy (Teleki, Hunt, & Pfifferling, 1976); studies of other populations have found the reverse (Nishida, 1990).

Interpretations of sexual differences in longevity from the field are difficult, because any intrinsic sexual differences in resistance to aging could easily be masked by environmental or behavioral factors. For instance, males of most mammal species are the sex most likely to disperse from their natal area prior to breeding, an activity associated with exceptional danger (Waser, Austad, & Keane, 1986). Males also are more likely to be injured in fights than are females. So intrinsic differences between the sexes in the ability to survive are better inferred from captive studies where behavioral and environmental differences are minimized.

Carey, Liedo, Orozco, Tatar, & Vaupel (1995) present a useful conceptual dissection of the difficulties associated with interpreting data on sexual survival differences, relevant to interpreting captive versus field data. They break the differences into three components: (1) constitutional endowment for survival, which includes resistance to disease, stress, physiological challenge, and intrinsic deterioration; (2) reproductive biology, which focuses on the differential impact of reproduction on survival; and (3) behavioral predispositions. (1) and (2) are most relevant to understanding basic mechanisms of aging, whereas survival in the field may often be the result primarily of (3). Implicit in this formulation is that studies designed to investigate sexual survival differences should ideally control reproductive opportunities.

Captive studies present no uniform trend in sexual survival differences either. Many, but not all, inbred mice strains exhibit somewhat greater male survival (e.g., Goodrick, 1975; Turturro et al., 1999) as do some, but not all, rat strains (Committee on Animal Models for Research on Aging, 1981; Turturro et al., 1999). Data on dogs are conflicting, with reports finding greater female longevity (Hamilton, 1948; Waters, Shen, & Glickman, 2000); no difference (Albert, Benjamin, & Shukla, 1994); and greater male longevity (Bronson, 1982). A small study of gerbils suggests a slight female survival advantage, whereas males seem to live longer in guinea pigs, multimammate rats, and most hamsters (Committee on Animal Models for Research on Aging, 1981). Females outlive males in number of species of captive primates, but not all species (Allman, Kumar, & Hasenstaub, 1998). Although data are not in hand to make inferences about the relative frequency of male versus female longevity advantage, it is clear that females are not inevitably the longer-lived sex even under protected conditions. Moreover, even the magnitude of survival differences between the sexes does not clearly favor one sex only (Table 2.1). Thus little empirical support exists for hypotheses that suggest generally increased resistance to aging in the homogametic sex.

Other explanations for sexual differences in longevity have to do with evolutionary/ecological factors. For instance, Allman et al. (1998) have suggested that in slowly developing species with single births, the sex that bears the greater burden in offspring care will tend to survive longer. Relative investment in offspring care is difficult to quantify. How might the relative contributions of investment in lactation be assessed compared with carrying the infant? Nevertheless, Allman et al. find that females of most primate species live longer than males, except for siamangs, owl monkeys, and titi monkeys in which males have primary responsibility for carrying infants and also tend to live longer. This explanation apparently does not extend to nonprimate mammals. Although male guinea pigs and hamsters are longer lived than females, they contribute no discernible parental care (Nowak, 1999).

One final explanation, evolutionary in nature, seeks to address the sex-longevity differential as a consequence of historical disparities between the sexes in their pattern of susceptibility to environmental hazards and breeding opportunities (Rose, 1991; Williams, 1957). Most mammals are polygynous, so male competition for access to females can be fierce, with males being killed or injured in sexual competition more often than females. In addition, because normally only the most vigorous males will win access to females, reproduction will be skewed toward younger individuals more so in males than in females. In addition, male mammals more frequently disperse from their natal territory to breed, and if both sexes disperse, males typically disperse farther (Greenwood, 1980). Dispersal through unfamiliar territory is a period of exceptional danger in nature and is associated with exceptionally high mortality (Waser et al.,

TABLE 2.1 Relative Longevity in a Sample of Mammal Species

Species	*Ln* Female/male life expectancy	Reference
Short-finned pilot whale *(Globicephala macrorhynchus)*	0.651	Kasuya & Marsh (1984)
Killer whale *(Orcinus orca)*	0.545	Olesiuk et al. (1990)
Chimpanzee *(Pan troglodytes)*	0.349	Dyke et al. (1995)
Human *(Homo sapiens)*	0.095	Smith (1993)
Chinese hamster *(Cricetulus griseus)*	– 0.095	CAMRA (1981)
Guinea pig *(Cavia porcellus)*	– 0.418	CAMRA (1981)
Golden hamster *(Mesocricetus auratus)*	– 0.651	CAMRA (1981)

Note: Natural logarithm of the ratio is used in order that equal deviations from unity in opposite directions will be represented by equal positive deviations from zero. Data represent life expectancy or median longevity as available. CAMRA = Committee on Animal Models for Research on Aging. Note the range of differences is virtually identical in either direction.

1986). In sum, these factors suggest that for prototypical mammals, the force of natural selection should decline more rapidly for males than for females, hence females should evolve slower aging in prototypical species. On the other hand, certain aspects of the evolutionary ecology of a species, such as higher female dispersal rates or a monogamous or polyandrous mating system, could weaken or reverse this prediction.

The easiest way to evaluate this line of reasoning might be to examine so-called atypical species such as those with primarily female dispersal and relaxed male-male competition, or else species such as guinea pigs, hamsters, and titi monkeys in which greater male constitutional endowment for longevity seems most convincingly established.

Such an examination offers little support for this idea. When compared with mammals, birds are much more frequently monogamous and females more frequently are the dispersing sex, suggesting (like the heterogametic sex hypotheses) that males should age more slowly. As we have seen, this is frequently but by no means universally true. Titi and owl monkeys, in which captive males live longer, live in monogamous social groups and both sexes disperse (Nowak, 1999), so there would seem to be little obvious sex difference in the force of natural selection. Female chimpanzees are the primary dispersing sex, yet they live longer in captivity (Dyke, Gage, Alford, Swenson, & Williams-Blangero, 1995), although this case is difficult to interpret since males are more frequently killed in intergroup encounters (Nishida, 1990). Male guinea pigs live longer, but experience severe male–male conflicts over mating opportunities (Rood, 1972). Too little is known about the biology of hamsters in the wild to assess the relative force of natural selection on the sexes.

Sexual differences in aging and longevity can be substantial, and can favor either males or females. It is a phenomenon that deserves more rigorous study, but one for which there are no generally satisfying explanations.

Cellular Correlates of Organismic Aging Rate

If organismal aging could be studied in the short term on the cellular level, it would greatly accelerate and simplify research into fundamental aging mechanisms. Comparative analyses have been invoked to establish cellular correlates of aging rate for many years. For instance, longevity across species has been correlated with cellular proliferative potential (Röhme, 1981), radiation induced ADP-ribosyl transferase activity (Pero, Holmgren, & Persson, 1985), DNA excision repair rate (Hart & Setlow, 1974), superoxide dismutase activity (Tolmasoff, Ono, & Cutler, 1980), and resistance to oxidative and nonoxidative chemical challenges (Kapahi, Boulton, & Kirkwood, 2000).

Such correlations should be interpreted cautiously for the usual reasons associated with correlation versus causation. An additional cautionary note concerns the impact of body size on these correlations. As Promislow (1994) noted, larger body size is expected to lead to enhanced damage resistance of somatic cells even in the absence of any difference in longevity. In a simple model, he deduced the following: assuming that the malignant transformation of any single cells can lead to a fatal neoplasm, because a larger organism has more cells at risk one would expect elephant cells to have evolved greater resistance to transformation, even if elephants and mice both lived the same length of time. Similarly Miller (1997) pointed out that the additional proliferative potential required to build and maintain a large organism (as compared with a small one) from a single fertilized egg suggests that greater proliferative potential may be more relevant to body size than to aging.

Two ways to address this issue are (1) make some reasonable correction to the data to account for body size; or (2) employ species comparisons in which body size is controlled. The most biologically relevant method for accounting for body size affects is unclear. Promislow (1994) used partial correlation to remove the effects of body size on DNA repair rates in four studies, all of which had previously found statistically significant correlations between repair rate and maximum longevity. In the corrected analysis of body size, only two of the four studies still exhibited significant effects. Humans contributed as substantial outliers in all studies, and Promislow pointed out several lines of argument for why the use of humans is problematic in this sort of analysis. If humans are removed, only one study retains statistical significance. If phylogenetic corrections are also included in the analysis, even this one study becomes only marginally significant ($0.05 < p < 0.1$) (Promislow, 1994).

Removal of the effects of body size by partial correlation also reduces the strength of the published relationship between longevity and cell proliferation potential (Röhme, 1981). Uncorrected for body size, the correlation coefficient was 0.95 for eight species of mammals, with $p < 0.001$. Partialling out the effects of body size reduces the correlation coefficient to 0.88 and the *p*-value increases to 0.009. Although still significant, the relationship now is highly sensitive to the human data point, without which the correlation is marginally significant ($p = 0.05$). Perhaps a more biologically reasonable approach would be to correct for body size in this instance by estimating the number of additional proliferative events required to equalize body mass across species. Miller (1997) performed such a reanalysis on Röhme's (1981) data and also found the level of significance reduced ($r = 0.95$ to $r = 0.91$). The human data point becomes even more critical to this relationship, as omitting it makes the relationship nowhere near significant ($r = 0.37$, $p = 0.46$). More recent work on the survival of primary fibroblasts to a range of chemical stressors found a significant positive relationship between stress resistance and maximum longevity also in a sample of eight mammal species (Kapahi et al., 1999). This relationship remained when phylogeny was controlled for; however, no correction for body size was attempted.

Even though correcting for body size and phylogeny makes previously published research less statistically compelling than the original analyses, the original conclusion, may still be valid. Stress resistance, for instance, has been correlated with extended life within the same species in model organisms (reviewed in Kirkwood & Austad, 2000). However, more comprehensive analyses with more judiciously chosen species must be performed if these cellular correlates are to be convincingly related to organismal aging rate.

The second approach to incorporate the effects of body size into comparative analyses is to choose species differing in the presumed dependent variable (in this case longevity or aging rate). Ogburn et al. (1998) used such an approach to examine whether cellular resistance to oxidative challenge could be related to longevity. Using primary kidney epithelial cells, they found that upon exposure to 95% oxygen, hydrogen peroxide, and paraquat cell survival was significantly greater in three species of long-lived birds compared to a similar-sized mouse. In more recent work, they found that this superior resistance to oxidative stress was also found in embryonic fibroblasts from a long-lived bird species, but not in a short-lived bird (Ogburn et al., unpub. data).

Cellular correlates of retarded aging offer a promising avenue for future research. To the extent that such correlates turn out to be causally involved in the aging process, this approach potentially can offer a convenient method for the study of exceptionally long-lived species and can identify protective mechanisms against aging that may not be found in short-lived model organisms.

REFERENCES

Albert, R. E., Benjamin, S.A., & Shukla, R. (1994). Life span and cancer mortality in the beagle dog and humans. *Mechanisms of Ageing & Development, 74,* 149–159.

Allman, J., Kumar, R., & Hasenstaub, A. (1998). Parenting and survival in anthropoid primates: Caretakers live longer. *Proceedings of the National Academy of Sciences, USA, 95,* 6866–6869.

Austad, S. N. (1993). Retarded senescence in an insular population of opossums. *Journal of Zoology, 229,* 695–708.

Austad, S. N., & Fischer, K. E. (1992). Primate longevity: Its place in the mammalian scheme. *Journal of Primatology, 28,* 251–261.

Austad, S. N., & Fischer, K. E. (1991). Mammalian aging, metabolism, and ecology: Evidence from the bats and marsupials. *Journal of Gerontology, 46,* B47–B53.

Austad, S. N., & Holmes, D. J. (1999). Evolutionary approaches to probing aging mechanisms. In B. P. Yu (Ed.), *Methods in aging research* (pp. 437–452). Boca Raton, FL: CRC Press.

Bacon, F. (1638). *The historie of life and death.* London: Humphrey Mosley.

Barclay, R. M. R., & Harder, L. D. (in press). The life histories of bats: Life in the slow lane. In T. H. Kunz & B. Fenton (Eds.), *Ecology of bats.* Chicago: University of Chicago Press.

Bell, G. (1984). Evolutionary and nonevolutionary theories of senescence. *American Naturalist, 124,* 600–603.

Bronson, R. T. (1982). Variation in age at death of dogs of difference sexes and breeds. *American Journal of Veterinary Research, 43,* 2057–2059.

Bulmer, M. (1988). Sex ratio in lemmings. *Heredity, 61,* 231–233.

Calder, W. A. III. (1984). *Size, function, and life history.* Cambridge, MA: Harvard University Press.

Carey, J. R., Liedo, P., Orozco, D., Tatar, M., & Vaupel, J. W. (1995). A male–female longevity paradox in Medfly cohorts. *Journal of Animal Ecology, 64,* 107–116.

Christensen, K., Kristiansen, M., Hagen-Larsen, H., Skytthe, A., Bathum, L., Jeune, B., Andersen-Ranberg, K., Vaupel, J. W., & Orstavik, K. H. (2000). X-linked genetic factors regulate hematopoietic stem-cell kinetics in females. *Blood, 97,* 2449–2451.

Clutton-Brock, T. H. (Ed.). (1988). *Reproductive success.* Chicago: University of Chicago Press.

Clutton-Brock, T. H., Albon, S. D., & Guinness, F. E. (1988). Reproductive success in male and female red deer. In T. H. Clutton-Brock (Ed.), *Reproductive success* (pp. 325–343). Chicago: University of Chicago Press.

Comfort, A. (1979). *The biology of senescence,* 3rd ed. Edinburgh, Scotland: Churchill Livingston.

Committee on Animal Models for Research on Aging. (1981). *Mammalian models for research on aging.* Washington, DC: National Academy Press.

Coschigano, K. T., Clemmons, D., Bellush, L. L., & Kopchick, J. J. (2000). Assessment of growth parameters and life span of GHR/BP gene-disrupted mice. *Endocrinology, 141,* 2608–2613.

Cutler, R. G. (1978). Evolutionary biology of senescence. In J. A. Behnke, C. E. Finch, & G. B. Moment (Eds.), *The biology of aging* (pp. 311-360). New York: Plenum Press.

Davey, S. G., Hart, C., Upton, M., Hole, D., Gillis, C., Watt, G., & Hawthorne, V. (2000). Height and risk of death among men and women: Aetiological implications of associations with cardiorespiratory disease and cancer mortality. *Journal of Epidemiology and Community Health, 54,* 97–103.

Deeb, B., & Wolf, N. (1994). Studying longevity and mortality in giant and small breeds of dogs. *Veterinary Medicine* (Suppl.) *89,* 702–713.

Dittus, W. (1975). Population dynamics of the toque monkey, *Macaca sinica.* In R. H. Tuttle (Ed.), *Socioecology and psychology of primates* (pp. 125–151). The Hague, Netherlands: Mouton Press.

Dunbar, R. I. M. (1988). Demography and reproduction. In B. B. Smuts, D. L. Cheney, R. M. Seyfarth, R. W. Wrangham, & T. T. Struhsaker (Eds.), *Primate societies* (pp. 240–249). Chicago: University of Chicago Press.

Dyke, B., Gage, T. B., Alford, P. L., Swenson, B., & Williams-Blangero, S. (1995). A model life table for captive chimpanzees. *American Journal of Primatology, 37,* 25–55.

Edney, E. B., & Gill, R. W. (1968). Evolution of senescence and specific longevity. *Nature, 220,* 281–282.

Fedigan, L. M., & Zohar, S. (1997). Sex differences in mortality of Japanese macaques: Twenty-one years of data from the Arashiyama West population. *American Journal of Physical Anthropology, 102,* 161–175.

Felsenstein, J. (1985). Phylogenies and the comparative method. *American Naturalist, 125,* 1–15.

Garland, T., Jr., Harvey, P. H., & Ives, A. R. (1992). Procedures for the analysis of comparative data using phylogenetically independent contrasts. *Systematic Biology, 41,* 18–32.

Goodrick, C. L. (1975). Life-span and the inheritance of longevity of inbred mice. *Journal of Gerontology, 30,* 257–263.

Graves, J. A. M. (1996). Mammals that break the rules: Genetics of marsupials and monotremes. *Annual Review of Genetics, 30,* 233–260.

Greenwood, P. J. (1980). Mating systems, philopatry, and dispersal in birds and mammals. *Animal Behaviour, 28,* 1140–1162.

Guarente, L., & Kenyon, C. (2000). Genetic pathways that regulate ageing in model organisms. *Nature, 408,* 255–262.

Halley, M. (1992). Maintenance and captive breeding of the brush-tailed phascogale. *International Zoo Yearbook, 31,* 71–78.

Hamilton, J. B. (1948). The role of testicular secretions as indicated by the effects of castration in man and by studies of pathological conditions and the short lifespan associated with maleness. *Recent Progress in Hormone Research, 3,* 257–322.

Hart, R. W., & Setlow, R. B. (1974). Correlation between deoxyribonucleic acid excision-repair and lifespan in a number of mammalian species. *Proceedings of the National Academy of Sciences, USA, 71,* 2169–2173.

Harvey, P. H., & Pagel, M. D. (1991). *The comparative method in evolutionary biology.* Oxford, UK: Oxford University Press.

Hayflick, L. (2000). The future of ageing. *Nature, 408,* 267–269.

Hazzard, W. R. (1994). The sex differential in longevity. In W. R. Hazzard, E. L. Bierman, J. P. Blass, W. H. Ettinger, Jr., & J. B. Halter (Eds.), *Principles of geriatric medicine and gerontology* (3rd ed., pp. 37–48). New York: McGraw-Hill.

Hillesheim, E., & Stearns, S. C. (1992). Correlated responses in life-history traits to artificial selection for body weight in *Drosophila melanogaster. Evolution, 46,* 745–752.

Hochachka, P. W., & Somero, G. N. (1984). *Biochemical adaptation.* Princeton, NJ: Princeton University Press.

Hofman, M. A. (1983). Energy metabolism, brain size and longevity in mammals. *Quarterly Review of Biology, 58,* 495–512.

Holehan, A. M., & Merry, B. J. (1986). The experimental manipulation of ageing by diet. *Biological Reviews of the Cambridge Philosophical Society, 61,* 329–368.

Holmes, D. J., & Austad, S. N. (1995). Birds as animal models for the comparative biology of aging: A prospectus. *Journals of Gerontology, Series A: Biological Sciences and Medical Sciences, 50A,* B59–B66.

Jones, M. L. (1982). Longevity of captive mammals. *Zoologische Garten, 52,* 113–128.

Jones, M. L. (1993). Longevity of ungulates in captivity. *International Zoo Yearbook, 32,* 159–169.

Judge, D. S., & Carey, J. R. (2000). Postreproductive life predicted by primate patterns. *Journals of Gerontology, Series A: Biological Sciences and Medical Sciences, 55A,* B201–B209.

Kasuya, T., & Marsh, H. (1984). Life history and reproductive biology of the short-finned pilot whale, *Globicephala macrorhynchus*. *Report of the International Whaling Commission* (Special Issue 6), 259–310.

Kapahi, P., Boulton, M. E., & Kirkwood, T. B. L. (1999). Positive correlation between mammalian life span and cellular resistance to stress. *Free Radical Biology & Medicine, 26*, 495–500.

Kari, F. W., Dunn, S. E., French, J. E., & Barrett, J. C. (1999). Roles for insulin-like growth factor-1 in mediating the anti-carcinogenic effects of caloric restriction. *Journal of Nutrition in Health and Aging, 3*, 92–101.

Kirkwood, T. B. L., & Austad, S. N. (2000). Why do we age? *Nature, 408*, 233–238.

Kleiber, M. (1961). *The fire of life: An introduction to animal energetics*. New York: Wiley.

Koizumi, A., Masuda, H., Wada, Y., Tsukada, M., Kawamura, K., Kamiyama, S., & Walford, R. L. (1989). Caloric restriction perturbs the pituitary-ovarian axis and inhibits mouse mammary tumore virus production in a high-spontaneous-mammary-tumor-incidence mouse strain (C3H/SHN). *Mechanisms of Ageing and Development, 49*, 93–104.

Le Boeuf, B. J., & Reiter, J. (1988). Lifetime reproductive success in northern elephant seals. In T. H. Clutton-Brock (Ed.), *Reproductive success* (pp. 344–362). Chicago: University of Chicago Press.

Li, Y., Deeb, B., Pendergrass, W., & Wolf, N. (1996). Cellular proliferative capacity and life span in small and large dogs. *Journal of Gerontology, Series A: Biological Sciences and Medical Sciences, 51A*, B403–B408.

Lindstedt, S. L., & Calder, W. A. (1981). Body size, physiological time, and longevity of homeothermic animals. *Quarterly Review of Biology, 56*, 1–16.

Mallouk, R. S. (1975). Longevity in vertebrates is proportional to relative brain weight. *Federation Proceedings, 34*, 2102–2103.

Martin, G. M., Austad, S. N., & Johnson, T. E. (1996). Genetic analysis of aging: Role of oxidative damage and environmental stresses. *Nature Genetics, 13*, 25–34.

McDonald, I. R., Lee, A. K., Bradley, A. J., & Than, K. A. (1981). Endocrine changes in dasyurid marsupials with differing mortality patterns. *General and Comparative Endocrinology, 44*, 292–301.

McNab, B. K. (1972). On the ecological significance of Bergmann's rule. *Ecology, 52*, 845–854.

Medawar, P. B. (1952) *An unsolved problem in biology*. London: H. K. Lewis.

Miller, R. A. (2001). Genetics of increased longevity and retarded aging in mice. In E. J. Masoro & S. N. Austad (Eds.), *Handbook of the biology of aging* (5th ed., pp. 369–395). San Diego, CA: Academic Press.

Miller, R. A. (1997). When will the biology of aging become useful? Future landmarks in biomedical gerontology. *Journal of the American Geriatrics Society, 45*, 1258–1267.

Myroniuk, P. O., & Seebeck, J. H. (1992). *In situ* and *ex situ* conservation of Leadbeater's possum. *International Zoo Yearbook, 31,* 82–90.

National Center for Biotechnology Information. (2001). Human genome information. *www.ncbi.nlm.nih.gov/genome/guide/human/*

Neel, J. V. (1990). Toward an explanation of the human sex ratio. In M. G. Ory & H. R. Warner (Eds.), *Gender, health, and longevity: Multidisciplinary perspectives* (pp. 57–72). New York: Springer Publishing Co.

Newton, I. (Ed.). (1989). *Lifetime reproduction in birds.* London: Academic Press.

Nishida, T. (1990). *The chimpanzees of the Mahale mountains.* Tokyo: University of Tokyo Press.

Nowak, R. M. (1999). *Walker's mammals of the world* (6th ed.). Baltimore: Johns Hopkins University Press.

Ogburn, C. E., Austad, S. N., Holmes, D. J., Kiklevich, J. V., Gollahon, K., Rabinovitch, P. S., & Martin, G. M. (1998). Cultured renal epithelial cells from birds and mice: Enhanced resistance of avian cells to oxidative stress and DNA damage. *Journal of Gerontology, Series A: Biological Sciences and Medical Sciences, 53A,* B287–B292.

Olesiuk, P. F., Bigg, M. A., & Ellis, G. M. (1990). Life history and population dynamics of resident killer whales (*Orcinus orca*) in the coastal waters of British Columbia and Washington State. *Report of the International Whaling Commission,* (Special Issue 12), 209–243.

Ottinger, M. A., Nisbet, I. C. T., & Finch, C. E. (1995). Aging and reproduction: Comparative endocrinology of the common tern and Japanese quail. *American Zoologist, 35,* 299–306.

Packer, C., Herbst, L., Pusey, A. E., Bygott, D., Hanby, J. P., Cairns, S. J., & Mulder, M. B. (1988). Reproductive success of lions. In T. H. Clutton-Brock (Ed.), *Reproductive success* (pp. 363–383). Chicago: University of Chicago Press.

Pero, T. W., Holmgren, K., & Persson, L. (1985). Irradiation induced ADP-ribosyl transferase activity and mammalian longevity. *Mutation Research, 142,* 69–73.

Promislow, D. E. L. (1994). DNA repair and the evolution of longevity: A critical analysis. *Journal of Theoretical Biology, 7,* 291–300.

Promislow, D. E. L. (1991). Senescence in natural populations of mammals: A comparative study. *Evolution, 45,* 1869–1887.

Ricklefs, R. E. (1998). Evolutionary theories of aging: Confirmation of a fundamental prediction, with implications for the genetic basis and evolution of life span. *American Naturalist, 152,* 24–44.

Ricklefs, R. E., & Starck, J. M. (1996). Applications of phylogenetically independent contrasts: A mixed progress report. *Oikos, 77,* 1–9.

Robinson, R. (1973). Relationship between litter size and weight of dam in the dog. *Veterinary Record, 92,* 221–223.

Röhme, D. (1981). Evidence for a relationship between longevity of mammalian species and lifespans of normal fibroblasts in vitro and erythrocytes in vivo. *Proceedings of the National Academy of Sciences, USA, 78,* 5009–5013.

Rood, J. P. (1972). Ecological and behavioral comparisons of three genera of Argentine cavies. *Animal Behaviour Monographs, 5,* 1–83.

Rose, M. R. (1991). *Evolutionary biology of aging.* Oxford, UK: Oxford University Press.

Sacher, G. A. (1959). Relation of lifespan to brain weight and body weight in mammals. *Ciba Foundation Colloquia, 5,* 115–141.

Samaras, T. T., & Elrick, H. (1999). Height, body size, and longevity. *Acta Medica Okayama, 53,* 149–169.

Sgró, C. M., & Partridge, L. (1999). A delayed wave of death from reproduction in *Drosophila. Science, 286,* 2421–2524.

Smith, D. W. E. (1993). *Human longevity.* Oxford, UK: Oxford University Press.

Smith, D. W. E., & Warner, H. R. (1990). Overview of biomedical perspectives: Possible relationships between genes on the sex chromosomes and longevity. In M. G. Ory & H. R. Warner (Eds.), *Gender, health, and longevity: Multidisciplinary perspectives* (pp. 41–55). New York: Springer Publishing Co.

Sonntag, W. E., Lynch, C. D., Cefalu, W. T., Ingram, R. L., Bennett, S. A., Thornton, P. L., & Khan, A. S. (1999). Pleiotropic effects of growth hormone and insulin-like growth factor (IGF)-1 on biological aging: Inferences from moderate caloric-restricted animals. *Journals of Gerontology, Series A: Biological Sciences and Medical Sciences 54A,* B521–B538.

Stahl, W. R. (1962). Similarity and dimensional methods in biology. *Science, 137,* 205–212.

Stearns, S. C., Ackermann, M., Doebeli, M., & Kaiser, M. (2000). Experimental evolution of aging, growth, and reproduction in fruitflies. *Proceedings of the National Academy of Sciences, USA, 97,* 3309–3313.

Teleki, G., Hunt, E. E., & Pfifferling, J. H. (1976). Demographic observations (1963-1973) on the chimpanzees of Gombe National Park, Tanzania. *Journal of Human Evolution, 5,* 559–596.

Tolmasoff, J. M., Ono, R., & Cutler, R. G. (1980). Superoxide dismutase: Correlation with life span and specific metabolic rate in primate species. *Proceedings of the National Academy of Sciences, USA, 77,* 2777–2781.

Turturro, A., Witt, W. W., Lewis, S., Hass, B. S., Lipman, R. D., & Hart, R. W. (1999). Growth curves and survival characteristics of the animals used in the biomarkers of aging program. *Journals of Gerontology, Series A: Biological Science and Medical Sciences, 54A,* B492–B501.

United Nations. (1990). *Demographic yearbook, 1988*. New York: United Nations, Department of International Economic and Social Affairs, Statistics Office.

Van Voorheis, W. A., & Ward, S. (1999). Genetic and environmental conditions that increase longevity in *Caenorhabditis elegans* decrease metabolic rate. *Proceedings of the National Academy of Sciences, USA, 95,* 11399–11403.

Waser, P. M., & Jones, W.T. (1991). Survival and reproductive effort in baner-tailed kangaroo rats. *Ecology, 72,* 771–777.

Waser, P. M., Austad, S. N., & Keane, B. (1986). When should animals tolerate inbreeding? *American Naturalist, 128,* 529–537.

Waters, D. J., Shen, S., & Glickman, L. T. (2000). Life expectancy, antagonistic pleiotropy, and the testis of dogs and men. *Prostate, 43,* 272–277.

Western, D. (1979). Size, life history, and ecology in mammals. *African Journal of Ecology, 17,* 185–204.

Williams, G. C. (1957). Pleiotropy, natural selection, and the evolution of senescence. *Evolution, 11,* 398–411.

CHAPTER 3

Why Does Aging Occur?

THOMAS B. L. KIRKWOOD
DEPARTMENT OF GERONTOLOGY
UNIVERSITY OF NEWCASTLE

This chapter describes and discusses the evolutionary basis of aging and longevity and shows how an evolutionary understanding of the aging process can guide our study of the mechanisms that are involved.

AGING IS NOT PROGRAMMED

A commonly held but mistaken view is that aging is driven by an evolved genetic program and that senescence is controlled in broadly the same way as development. The attraction of the program theory is that it conforms to how we tend to think about evolution, namely that new traits emerge because they adapt the genotype in ways that are fitter for survival. In view of the continuing appeal of the program theory, it is important to be explicit about why this view is now thought to be false.

One suggested advantage of aging is that it prevents old and worn-out individuals from competing for resources with their progeny. This argument is plainly circular, as was pointed out by Medawar (1952), and need be considered no further. Another suggestion is that aging helps to prevent overcrowding and so lessens the risk of severe depletion of resources (Wynne-Edwards, 1962). It is conceivable that aging could play such a role, but there are two very strong objections. First, there is little evidence from natural populations that aging is a significant contributor to mortality in the wild (Kirkwood & Austad, 2000). Undoubtedly, an individual that lives long enough to experience senescence becomes more vulnerable to predators and other hazards. However, life tables for wild populations indicate that mortality during the early and middle periods of life is usually so great that few survive long enough for aging to have a measurable impact on the total death toll. This means that aging is not needed to prevent overcrowding, nor is it easy to see how natural selection could have directly brought about the evolution of a trait that is so rarely seen under normal conditions. Some exceptions to the general rule that aging is rare in the wild may arise in the case of the larger animals. However, even in such species only a minority survive to old age, and in any case these species evolved from smaller, more vulnerable ancestors in which it is reasonable to assume that aging was already established. Thus the exceptions cannot help us to account for the origins of aging.

A second objection to the idea that aging evolved to prevent overcrowding is that the advantage, if it exists, is to the population rather than the individual. If aging had evolved as a means to regulate population size, then a mutant in which the aging process was inactivated would enjoy an advantage and the mutant genotype would spread. For aging to be stably maintained in the long term, it is necessary that "group selection" for advantage to the population outweigh the straightforward selection for advantage to the individual. The requirements for group selection to operate successfully against opposing selection at the level of the individual are stringent (Maynard Smith, 1976), and it is extremely unlikely that they apply to aging. Briefly, it is necessary that the species is distributed among fairly isolated groups and that the introduction of a nonaging mutant into a group should rapidly lead to the group's extinction.

These two objections complement each other. Where one applies less strongly, the other is intensified. For example, if aging does generate significant mortality within a population so that it is more plausible that it has some role to play, then the disadvantage of aging to the individual is greater and the group-selection argument is harder to sustain.

One final claim for the program theories is that aging is necessary for, or helps, evolution to occur (e.g., Libertini, 1988). The idea is that since evolution occurs through the operation of natural selection on successive generations, any process that accelerates the turnover of generations may result in the greater ability of a species to adapt to changes in its environment. The chief weaknesses in this argument are as follows. First, the generation time in the wild is determined for the most part not by aging but by environmental hazards. Second, the argument assumes that the long-term advantage of adaptability outweighs the short-term disadvantage of reduced life span. This depends upon the assumed rate of change in the environment, and the argument encounters the same complex difficulties that concern the evolution of sex and the optimal mutation rate (see Maynard Smith, 1978). In fact, elevated recombination and/or mutation rates would be an alternative and more direct way to accelerate evolutionary change.

ORIGINS AND EVOLUTION OF AGING

If aging is not adaptively programmed, then its evolution must be explained through the indirect action of natural selection. The nonadaptive theories of aging are of two types: (1) aging occurs because the power of natural selection declines during the life span; (2) aging occurs as the by-product of selection for some other trait.

Significance of the Age-Related Decline in the Force of Natural Selection

An important property of any life cycle in which there is the opportunity for repeated reproduction between maturation and death is that the force of natural selection (that is, its ability to discriminate between alternative genotypes) weakens with age (Charlesworth, 1980, 1994; Haldane, 1941; Hamilton, 1966; Medawar, 1952; Williams, 1957). The basic point is that because natural selection acts through the differential effects of genes on reproductive fitness, the force of natural selection must decline in proportion to the decline in the remaining fraction of the organism's total lifetime expectation of reproduction. This is true whether or not the species exhibits aging, because even if individuals do not age they are nonetheless susceptible to environmental mortality. If a gene effect is expressed early in life, it will influence the reproductive success of a larger proportion of individuals born bearing that gene than if it is expressed late, when many such individuals will already have died.

The attenuation with age in the force of natural selection inevitably means that there is only loose genetic control over the late portions of the lifespan. Medawar (1952) suggested that this might be sufficient in itself to account for the origin of aging, the *mutation-accumulation* theory. If a gene with an age-specific time of expression arises by mutation, and if it is beneficial, then natural selection can be expected to favor bringing forward its time of expression so that more individuals can benefit from it. Conversely, if the gene is harmful, selection would tend to defer its time of expression so that its deleterious effects would be less damaging. Once a harmful gene has been so far delayed that it is expressed at an age when most individuals in the wild environment would have died already, it is beyond the reach of any further opposing selection and can spread to fixation by random drift. Medawar (1952) suggested that there might thus accumulate over many generations a miscellaneous collection of late-acting deleterious genes. In the normal environment these genes would only rarely have the opportunity to be expressed. However, in a protected environment, survivorship would be greater and a significant fraction of individuals would experience the effects of these genes, that is, senescence.

A second hypothesis is that aging is a by-product of selection for other beneficial traits (Williams, 1957), the *pleiotropic genes* theory, also known as *antagonistic pleiotropy.* This theory supposes the existence of genes that have good effects early in life and bad effects late in life. Natural selection favors retention of the genes on the basis of their early benefits, but defers the time of expression of the deleterious effects to ages when survivorship in the wild environment is low. The decline in the force of natural selection with age ensures that even quite modest early benefits outweigh severe harmful side effects, provided that the latter occur late enough.

AGING THROUGH OPTIMIZING THE INVESTMENT IN MAINTENANCE

A different approach, which leads to more specific predictions about the nature of the genetic processes responsible for aging, is the *disposable soma* theory (Kirkwood, 1977, 1981; Kirkwood & Holliday, 1979). The disposable soma theory is named for its analogy with disposable goods, which are manufactured with limited investment in durability on the principle that they have a short expected duration of use. The term *soma* is used in the sense introduced by Weismann (1891) to describe those parts of the body which are distinct from the "germ-line" that produces the reproductive cells—the sperm and the egg. We consider how an organism capable of reproducing repeatedly during its lifecycle ought best to allocate energy among the different metabolic tasks it needs to perform. Part of the resources must be used for each of a range of activities such as growth, foraging, defense, and maintenance. As all functions ultimately draw from the same total input of resource, there is an inevitable trade-off (direct or indirect) between the investment that is made in any one function and the investment in others.

The disposable soma theory recognizes that the optimum allocation of energy involves a smaller investment in somatic maintenance than would be required for the soma to last indefinitely. Given the continual hazard of accidental death, each individual soma can have only a finite expectation of life. When the soma dies, the resources invested in its maintenance are lost. Too low an investment in the prevention or repair of somatic damage is unsatisfactory because the soma may disintegrate before it can reproduce. However, too high an investment in maintenance is also wasteful because there is no advantage in maintaining the soma better than is necessary for it to survive its expected lifetime in the wild environment in reasonably sound condition. In the latter case, the fitness of the organism in terms of natural selection, that is, its ability to compete reproductively, would be enhanced by reducing the investment in somatic maintenance and channeling the extra resource into more rapid growth or greater reproductive output. Therefore, fitness is maximized at a level of investment in somatic maintenance that is less than would be required for indefinite somatic survival.

The precise optimum investment in maintenance depends on the species' ecological niche. A species subject to high accidental mortality will do better not to invest heavily in each individual soma, but should concentrate instead on more rapid and prolific reproduction. A species that experiences low accidental mortality may profit by doing the reverse. Thus the disposable soma theory not only explains why aging occurs, but also suggests in broad terms how it is caused. As soon as the division between germ-line and soma evolved, the stage was set for the appearance of aging.

WHY DO WE LIVE AS LONG AS WE DO?

As well as explaining the origins of aging, the evolutionary theories must also account for the divergence of species' life spans. The evolution of increased life span in each of the theories just described can readily be understood as a consequence of reducing the extrinsic risk of accidental death. An adaptation resulting in lower accidental mortality will reduce the rate of attenuation in the force of natural selection at older ages. In the mutation accumulation theory, this applies new pressure to postpone the expression of the late deleterious genes. In the pleiotropic genes theory, the balance between the early beneficial and late harmful effects of the pleiotropic genes will be shifted in favor of reducing the late harmful effects. In the disposable soma theory, the optimum investment in somatic maintenance will be increased. The effect of any of these changes will be to reduce the intrinsic rate of aging, resulting in increased longevity.

More explicit predictions about the mechanisms responsible for determining longevity follow from the disposable soma theory, which suggests that the rate of aging is determined by the multiple maintenance and repair systems that protect against accumulation of somatic damage (Kirkwood, 1996; Kirkwood & Austad, 2000).

TESTS OF THE EVOLUTIONARY THEORIES

Model organisms have been the major means of testing the predictions of the evolutionary theories. For practical reasons, most workers have used either the fruitfly *D. melanogaster* or the nematode *C. elegans,* both of which combine advantages of short life span, low maintenance costs, and excellent background genetics. *D. melanogaster* has a 10-day development period from egg to adult and an adult life span of about 30–40 days. The fly is a random-bred, diploid organism. Its populations therefore harbour high levels of standing genetic variation, in which regard it resembles humans. *C. elegans* has a 20-day life span during which it progresses through a series of immature larval stages to adulthood and then reproduces. If population density is high, causing low nutrient levels, the larva enters an alternative developmental pathway that gives rise to a third-instar dauer larva with arrested development and which is resistant to various forms of stress (Riddle, 1988). *C. elegans* mainly reproduces as a self-fertilizing hermaphrodite, which facilitates the creation of stocks with a very high degree of genetic uniformity and enables the recovery of mutations that affect life span.

Genetic variation for rate of aging has been demonstrated in *D. melanogaster,* mainly by the use of artificial selection on age at reproduction. "Young" lines of flies are propagated in each generation from adults that have just emerged from pupae, whereas "old" lines are propagated from adults that have already been reproducing for some time. Compared with the young lines, the old lines are therefore selected for increased life span because in order to contribute to the next generation, they must survive to the time of egg collection. Greater longevity of old lines has consistently been found in these studies (e.g., Luckinbill, Arking, Clare, Cirocco, & Buck, 1984; Partridge & Fowler, 1992; Roper, Pignatelli, & Partridge, 1993; Rose, 1984). In an alternative approach, direct selection for increased lifespan has been accomplished using an experimental design that exploited the effect of temperature on *Drosophila* longevity (Zwaan, Bijlsma, & Hoekstra, 1995). In this experiment, the progeny from each pair of breeding flies were divided into two groups, one of which was maintained at 15°C and the other at 29°C. At 29°C, maximum life span was less than 60 days, whereas at 15°C mean life span was greater than 120 days. This meant that life spans could be measured on the groups maintained at 29°C and the longest-lived families selected, at a time when the sibling groups kept at 15°C were still reproductively viable.

If trade-offs are important in aging, then we would expect the long-lived flies resulting from artificial selection experiments to pay for their late-life advantage at some point in their life history. Indeed, the long-lived flies were shown to have lower fecundity in early adult life (e.g., Luckinbill et al., 1984; Rose, 1984; Zwaan et al., 1995). Several studies have also reported an increase in the duration of the pre-adult period in old lines (e.g., Partridge & Fowler, 1992; Chippindale, Hoang, Service, & Rose, 1994; Chippindale, Chu, & Rose, 1996). However, these findings have not been universal. Indeed, experiments have revealed the crucial importance of both the environment during selection and testing and the exact selection protocol (Chippindale et al., 1994, 1996; Leroie, Chen, & Rose, 1994;

Leroie, Chippindale, & Rose, 1994; Partridge & Fowler, 1992; Roper et al., 1993;). Sgró and Partridge (1999) demonstrated that reduced early fecundity—the most consistently observed feature associated with increased longevity in artificial selection experiments—was causally involved in the retarded aging of their long-lived lines by abolishing reproduction either through irradiation or genetic manipulation and observing that the differences in aging rate between their controls and long-lived selected lines disappeared.

Trade-offs have also been reported in *C. elegans* where a host of long-lived mutants has been identified, although the results are not entirely consistent (Johnson & Hutchinson, 1993; van Voorheis & Ward, 1999). A recent study of the long-lived *age-1* mutant in *C. elegans* showed that the relative fitness effects of mutations can be strongly affected by environment (Walker, McColl, Jenkins, Harris, & Lithgow, 2000). When mutants were reared together with wild-type individuals under standard culture conditions, neither genotype exhibited a competitive advantage. However, when cultures were alternatively fed and starved—mimicking conditions in nature—the wild-type quickly outcompeted the mutant.

Drosophila has also been used to test the contribution of mutation accumulation to aging. One line of evidence has come from experiments where selection of older flies has been relaxed, allowing deleterious mutations to accumulate more easily (Mueller, 1987). Another comes from studying the increase with age in additive genetic variance for survival rates and levels of inbreeding depression (Charlesworth & Hughes, 1996; Hughes & Charlesworth, 1994; Promislow, Tatar, Khazaeli, & Curtsinger, 1996; Tatar, Promislow, Khazaeli, & Curtsinger, 1996). Demonstrating the effects of mutation accumulation is not straightforward and although the initial studies in *Drosophila* (Charlesworth & Hughes, 1996; Hughes & Charlesworth, 1994) seemed to support mutation accumulation, later experiments and further analysis have led to some uncertainty about this conclusion (Promislow et al., 1996; Shaw, Promislow, Tatar, Hughes, & Geyes, 1999).

From the comparative perspective, numerous opportunities exist to test the prediction that in safe environments (those with low extrinsic mortality) aging will evolve to be retarded, whereas aging should evolve to be more rapid in hazardous environments. Adaptations that reduce extrinsic mortality (wings, protective shells, large brain) are generally linked with increased longevity (bats, birds, turtles, humans). Comparing a mainland population of opossums subject to significant predation by mammals with an island population not subject to mammalian predation, field observations found the predicted slower aging in the island population (Austad, 1993). At the molecular and cellular levels, the disposable soma theory predicts that the proportional effort devoted to cellular maintenance and repair processes will vary directly with longevity. Numerous studies support this idea. For instance, the long-lived rodent species *Peromyscus leucopus* exhibits lower generation of the reactive oxygen species (ROS) that are widely seen as a major contributor to the aging process, higher cellular concentrations of some antioxidant enzymes, and overall lower levels of protein oxidative damage than the shorter-lived species *Mus musculus* (Sohal, Ku, & Agarwal, 1993). A direct relation between species longevity and rate of mitochondrial ROS production in captive mammals has also been found (Barja & Herrero, 2000; Ku, Brunk, & Sohal, 1993), as has a similar relationship between mammals and similar-sized but much longer lived birds (Herrero & Barja, 1999). Markers of glycoxidation, the nonenzymatic modification of reducing sugars, are also found to accumulate more slowly in long-lived, as opposed to short-lived, mammals (Sell et al., 1996). DNA repair capacity has been shown to correlate with mammalian life span in numerous comparative studies (Kirkwood, 1989), as has the level of poly(ADP-ribose) polymerase (Grube & Bürkle, 1992), an enzyme that plays an important role in the maintenance of genomic integrity. The quality of maintenance and repair mechanisms may be revealed by the capacity to cope with external stress. Comparisons of the functional capacity of cultured cells to withstand a variety of imposed stressors have shown that cells taken from long-lived species have superior stress resistance to that of cells from shorter-lived species (Kapahi, Bolton, & Kirkwood, 1999; Martin, Austad, & Johnson, 1996; Ogburn et al., 1998). All of these studies support the idea that it is the evolved capacity of somatic cells to carry out effective maintenance and repair that governs the time taken for damage to accumulate to levels where it interferes with the organism's viability and hence regulates longevity.

EVOLUTION OF LIFE HISTORY PLASTICITY

Many organisms live their lives in highly variable environments and this is sometimes reflected in the evolved plasticity of their life histories. One of the most informative examples of life history plasticity is seen in the response to lack of food. Periods of famine often trigger what appear to be metabolic switches that paradoxically extend the normal life span, without sacrificing subsequent reproduction and survival when favorable conditions return (Austad, 1989). An example is the dauer form of *C. elegans*, described previously, in which conditions of high larval density and low food availability result in a larval form that shows extended longevity accompanied by greatly increased resistance to stress. Another widely studied model is the phenomenon of calorie restriction in laboratory rodents (Weindruch & Walford, 1988) which extends lifespan and postpones a wide range of age-associated diseases. Like *C. elegans* dauer larvae, laboratory rodents under calorie restriction show enhanced resistance to a range of stresses (Masoro, 1998), but unlike the invertebrates, no general reduction in mass-specific metabolic rate is required for the effect. Despite the lack of reduced metabolic rate under calorie restriction, Walford and Spindler (1997) have pointed out a number of biochemical similarities between the calorie restriction state and that of mammalian hibernation, which can also extend life span. A recent evolutionary model (Shanley & Kirkwood, 2000) has shown that rodents may well have evolved a response to temporary fluctuations in resource availability, in which energy is diverted from reproduction to maintenance functions in periods of food shortage, thereby enhancing survival and retaining reproductive potential for when conditions improve. Thus, the evolution of life history plasticity may represent a modulation, to take account of varying food supply, of the same energy allocation considerations that underpin the disposable soma theory.

EVOLUTION OF REPRODUCTIVE SENESCENCE

So far, we have not specifically considered aging of the reproductive system, as distinct from generalized aspects of the aging process. Reproductive aging is of particular interest because loss of reproductive function will accelerate the decline in the force of natural selection (Partridge & Barton, 1996). The reverse is also true. In organisms that continue to grow indefinitely and in which reproductive output increases with size, the decline in the force of natural selection is slowed. This may explain the considerable longevity of some species of fish (Comfort, 1979; Finch, 1990). The reason for leaving reproductive aging until now is that a circular argument can arise if aging of the reproductive system is not properly regarded as a feature that logically must follow the origin of aging more generally. Weismann (1891), for example, originally suggested that aging was necessary to rid a population of old and worn-out individuals who had produced their required quota of offspring and were of no further reproductive value (but see Kirkwood & Cremer [1982] for the later development of Weismann's views). Similar confusion can arise if the postreproductive death in semelparous species is not treated as distinct from aging (see Kirkwood [1985]).

After this preamble, it can be seen that although reproductive aging takes its toll on reproductive function rather than on survival, there is nothing particularly special about it. Once the origin of aging has been accounted for within an organism whose life history could otherwise extend indefinitely, reproductive aging can be seen merely as part of the generalized decline in function. However, the special case of the human menopause merits particular attention.

Menopause occurs around the age of 45 to 50 in women everywhere (Gosden, 1985), and the evolutionary puzzle about menopause is why a woman should cease reproducing at an age when she is only about halfway through her biological life span. Assisted fertilization techniques have recently demonstrated that postmenopausal women can successfully bear children without serious complications. Oocyte depletion triggers menopause, but this merely highlights the question of why natural selection has not produced a larger store of oocytes. The idea that oocytes, being formed early in development, have only a finite period of viability, seems unlikely, even though the increased frequency of chromosomal abnormalities among children born to older mothers suggests some deterioration with time. Female elephants and baleen whales remain fertile at ages past that of the human menopause (Crooze, Hillman, & Lang, 1981; Mizrooh, 1981).

Early female reproductive senescence has been reported in other species (for example, chimpanzees, macaques, toothed whales) but is generally less clear-cut, suggesting that if menopause has an evolutionary basis, this may be found in the special circumstances of the human life history. In particular, menopause could be linked with the evolution of human longevity, notably through the effects of increased brain size and sociality (Austad, 1994; Hamilton, 1966; Hawkes, O'Connell, Jones, Alvarez, & Charnov, 1998; Hill & Hurtado, 1996; Kirkwood & Holliday, 1986; Peccei, 1995). Increased neonatal brain size coupled with the constraint on the birth canal imposed by the mechanics of a bipedal gait has made giving birth unusually difficult for human females. The risks of childbearing, particularly in the absence of modern obstetric care, would increase even more steeply with age if fertility were to persist during the later period of the life span. The problem of a large brain size is also reflected in the fact that human infants are born unusually early, relative to other species, with respect to the completion of brain growth and development. Infants remain highly dependent for extended periods and, in the ancestral environment, their survival would have been unlikely if their mothers died in childbirth. There may thus be a fitness advantage in limiting reproduction to ages when it is comparatively safe, thereby increasing the likelihood of the mother's surviving to raise her existing offspring to independence. Additionally, postmenopausal women may contribute to the successful rearing of their grandchildren, by providing assistance to their own adult offspring and thereby increasing their inclusive fitness, that is, their overall genetic contribution to future generations. A recent analysis suggests that a combination of all these factors is required to explain human menopause (Shanley & Kirkwood, 2000), which may account for the lack of evolutionary support for menopause in other species (Packer, Tatar, & Collins, 1998).

Menopause is sometimes cited as support for the program theory, since it suggests that a strict genetic control of aging may exist. The more plausible explanation, however, is that menopause is not a primary feature of aging but a secondary adaptation to lessen its deleterious effects.

CONCLUSIONS

The conclusions we can draw from studying the biological origins of aging have broad implications for the way we perceive the aging process. First, aging needs to be explained in evolutionary terms, as it is not enough to regard it as merely due to the inevitability of wear and tear. Second, the evolution of aging as a programmed process in its own right seems extremely unlikely. Third, the nonadaptive theories in general offer the most plausible explanation for the evolution of aging and longevity, and these theories make predictions that are amenable to experimental tests (Kirkwood & Austad, 2000; Partridge & Barton, 1993). Specifically, the disposable soma theory suggests that the efficiencies of somatic maintenance processes are crucial in determining longevity. Molecular studies using either a comparative approach or transgenic animals may serve to identify which of these processes play the most important roles.

A final word should be said about the way in which studies of the evolutionary origins of aging throw light on the "programming" of the life span. The point of issue between the program and nonadaptive theories is not whether aging is genetically influenced, as obviously it must be, but why and how this is arranged. This distinction is important because the theories determine the types of mechanism of aging we are likely to consider as appropriate subjects for research.

REFERENCES

Austad, S. N. (1989). Life extension by dietary restriction in the bowl and doily spider, *Frontinella pyramitela*. *Experimental Gerontology, 24*, 83–92.

Austad, S. N. (1993). Retarded senescence in an insular population of opossums. *Journal of Zoology, 229*, 695–708.

Austad, S. N. (1994). Menopause: An evolutionary perspective. *Experimental Gerontology, 29*, 255–263.

Barja, G., & Herrero, A. (2000). Oxidative damage to mitochondrial DNA is inversely related to maximum life span in the heart and brain of mammals. *Federation of American Societies of Experimental Biology Journal, 14*, 312–318.

Charlesworth, B. (1980). *Evolution in age-structured populations.* Cambridge, UK: Cambridge University Press.

Charlesworth, B. (1994). *Evolution in age-structured populations* (2nd ed). Cambridge, UK: Cambridge University Press.

Charlesworth, B., & Hughes, K. A. (1996). Age-specific inbreeding depression and components of genetic variance in relation to the evolution of senescence. *Proceedings of the National Academy of Sciences, USA, 93*, 6140–6145.

Chippindale, A. K., Chu, T. J. F., & Rose, M. R. (1996). Complex trade-offs and the evolution of starvation resistance in *Drosophila melanogaster. Evolution, 50*, 753–766.

Chippindale, A. K., Hoang, D. T. P. M., Service, P. M., & Rose, M. R. (1994). The evolution of development in *Drosophila melanogaster* selected for postponed senescence. *Evolution, 48*, 1880–1899.

Comfort, A. (1979). *The biology of senescence* (3rd ed). Edinburgh, Scotland: Churchill Livingstone.

Crooze, H., Hillman, A. K., & Lang, E. M. (1981). Elephants and their habits: How do they tolerate each other? In C. W. Fowler & T. D. Smith (Eds.), *Dynamics of large mammal populations* (pp. 112–134). New York: Wiley.

Finch, C. E. (1990). *Longevity, senescence and the genome.* Chicago: University of Chicago Press.

Gosden, R. G. (1985). *Biology of menopause. The causes and consequences of ovarian aging.* London: Academic Press.

Grube, K., & Bürkle, A. (1992). Poly(ADP-ribose) polymerase activity in mononuclear leukocytes of 13 mammalian species correlates with species-specific life span. *Proceedings of the National Academy of Sciences, USA, 89*, 11759–11763.

Haldane, J. B. S. (1941). *New paths in genetics.* London: Allen & Unwin.

Hamilton, W. D. (1966) The moulding of senescence by natural selection. *Journal of Theoretical Biology, 12*, 12–45.

Hawkes, K., O'Connell, J. F., Jones, N. G. B., Alvarez, H., & Charnov, E. L. (1998). Grandmothering, menopause, and the evolution of human life histories. *Proceedings of the National Academy of Sciences, USA, 95*, 1336–1339.

Herrero, A., & Barja, G. (1999). 8-oxo-deoxyguanosine levels in heart and brain mitochondrial and nuclear DNA of two mammals and three birds in relation to their different rates of aging. *Aging: Clinical and Experimental Research, 11*, 294–300.

Hill, K., & Hurtado, A. M. (1996). *Ache life history: The ecology and demography of a foraging people.* New York: Aldine de Gruyter.

Hughes, K. A., & Charlesworth, B. (1994). A genetic analysis of senescence in *Drosophila. Nature, 367,* 64–66.

Johnson, T. E., & Hutchinson, E. W. (1993). Absence of strong heterosis for life span and other life history traits in *Caenorhabditis elegans. Genetics, 134,* 465–474.

Kapahi, P., Boulton, M. E., & Kirkwood, T. B. L. (1999). Positive correlation between mammalian life span and cellular resistance to stress. *Free Radical Biology and Medicine, 26,* 495–500.

Kirkwood, T. B. L. (1977). Evolution of aging. *Nature, 270,* 301–304.

Kirkwood, T. B. L. (1981). Repair and its evolution: Survival versus reproduction. In C. R. Townsend & P. Calow (Eds.), *Physiological ecology: An evolutionary approach to resource use* (pp. 165–189). Oxford, England: Blackwell Scientific.

Kirkwood, T. B. L. (1985). Comparative and evolutionary aspects of longevity. In C. E. Finch & E. L. Schneider (Eds.), *Handbook of the biology of aging* (2nd ed., pp. 27–44). New York: Van Nostrand Reinhold.

Kirkwood, T. B. L. (1989). DNA, mutations and aging. *Mutation Research, 219,* 1–7.

Kirkwood, T. B. L. (1996). Human senescence. *BioEssays, 18,* 1009–1016.

Kirkwood, T. B. L., & Austad S. N. (2000). Why do we age? *Nature, 408,* 233–238.

Kirkwood, T. B. L., & Cremer, T. (1982). Cytogerontology since 1881: A reappraisal of August Weismann and a review of modem progress. *Human Genetics, 60,* 101–121.

Kirkwood, T. B. L., & Holliday, R. (1979). The evolution of aging and longevity. *Proceedings of the Royal Society of London, Series B, 205,* 531–546.

Kirkwood, T. B. L., & Holliday, R. (1986). Aging as a consequence of natural selection. In A. J. Collins & A. H. Bittles (Eds.), *The biology of human aging* (pp. 1–16). Cambridge: Cambridge University Press.

Ku, H.-H., Brunk, U. T., & Sohal, R. S. (1993). Relationship between mitochondrial superoxide and hydrogen-peroxide production and longevity of mammalian species. *Free Radical Biology and Medicine, 15,* 621–627.

Leroie, A. M., Chen, W. R., & Rose, M. R. (1994). Long-term laboratory evolution of a genetic life-history trade-off in *Drosophila melanogaster.* 2. Stability of genetic correlations. *Evolution, 48,* 1258–1268.

Leroie, A. M., Chippindale, A. K., & Rose, M. R. (1994). Long-term laboratory evolution of a genetic life-history trade-off in *Drosophila melanogaster.* 1. The role of genotype-by-environment interaction. *Evolution, 48,* 1244–1257.

Libertini, G. (1988). An adaptive theory of the increasing mortality with increasing chronological age in populations in the wild. *Journal of Theoretical Biology, 132,* 145–62.

Luckinbill, L. S., Arking, R., Clare, M. J., Cirocco, W. C., & Buck, S. A. (1984). Selection of delayed senescence in *Drosophila melanogaster. Evolution, 38,* 996–1003.

Martin, G. M., Austad, S. N., & Johnson, T. E. (1996). Genetic analysis of aging: Role of oxidative damage and environmental stresses. *Nature Genetics, 13,* 25–34.

Masoro, E. J. (1998). Influence of caloric intake on aging and on the response to stressors. *Journal of Toxicology and Environmental Health. B. Critical Reviews, 1,* 243–257.

Maynard Smith, J. (1976). Group selection. *Quarterly Review of Biology, 51,* 277–283.

Maynard Smith, J. (1978). *The evolution of sex.* Cambridge, UK: Cambridge University Press.

Medawar, P. B. (1952). *An unsolved problem of biology.* London: H. K. Lewis. (Reprinted in *The uniqueness of the individual,* 1957, London: Methuen).

Mizrooh, S. A. (1981). Analyses of some biological parameters in the Antarctic fin whale. *Report of the International Whaling Commission, 31,* 425–434.

Mueller, L. D. (1987). Evolution of accelerated senescence in laboratory populations of *Drosophila. Proceedings of the National Academy of Sciences, USA, 84,* 1974–1977.

Ogburn, C. E., Austad, S. N., Holmes, D. J., Kiklevich, J. V., Gollahon, K., Ravinovitch, P. S., & Martin, G. M. (1998). Cultured renal epithelial cells from birds and mice: Enhanced resistance of avian cells to oxidavtive stress and DNA damage. *Journal of Gerontology Series A, 53:* B287–B292.

Packer, C., Tatar, M., & Collins, A. (1998). Reproductive cessation in female mammals. *Nature, 392,* 807–822.

Partridge, L., & Barton, N. H. (1993). Optimality, mutation and the evolution of aging. *Nature, 362,* 305–311.

Partridge, L., & Barton, N. H. (1996). On measuring the rate of aging. *Proceedings of the Royal Society of London, Series B, 263,* 1365–1371.

Partridge, L., & Fowler, K. (1992). Direct and correlated responses to selection on age at reproduction in *Drosophila melanogaster. Evolution, 46,* 76–91.

Peccei, J. S. (1995). The origin and evolution of menopause: The altriciality-lifespan hypothesis. *Ethology and Sociobiology, 16,* 425–449.

Promislow, D. E. L., Tatar, M., Khazaeli, A. A., & Curtsinger, J. W. (1996). Age-specific patterns of genetic variance in *Drosophila melanogaster.* I. Mortality. *Genetics, 143,* 839–848.

Riddle, D. L. (1988). The dauer larva. In W. B. Wood (Ed.), *The nematode* Caenorhabditis elegans (pp. 393–412). New York: Cold Spring Harbor Laboratory.

Roper, C., Pignatelli, P., & Partridge, L. (1993). Evolutionary effects of selection on age at reproduction in larval and adult *Drosophila melanogaster. Evolution, 47,* 445–455.

Rose, M. R. (1984). Laboratory evolution of postponed senescence in *Drosophila melanogaster. Evolution, 38,* 1004–1010.

Sell, D. R., Lane, M. A., Johnson, W. A., Masoro, E. J., Mock, O. B., Reiser, K. M., Fogarty, J. F., Cutler, R. G., Ingram, D. K., Roth, G. S., & Monnier, V. M. (1996). Longevity and the genetic determination of collagen glycoxidation kinetics in mammalian senescence. *Proceedings of the National Academy of Sciences, 9,* 455–490.

Sgró, C. M., & Partridge, L. (1999). A delayed wave of death from reproduction in *Drosophila. Science, 286,* 2521–2524.

Shanley, D. P., & Kirkwood, T. B. L. (2000). Calorie restriction and aging: A life history analysis. *Evolution, 54,* 740–750.

Shanley, D. P., & Kirkwood, T. B. L. (2001). Evolution of the human menopause. *BioEssays, 23,* 282–287.

Shaw, F. H., Promislow, D. E. L., Tatar, M., Hughes, K. A., & Geyes, C. J. (1999). Toward reconciling inferences concerning genetic variation in *Drosophila melanogaster. Genetics, 152,* 553–566.

Sohal, R. S., Ku, H.-H., & Agarwal, S. (1993). Biochemical correlates of longevity in two closely-related rodent species. *Biochemical and Biophysical Research Communications, 196,* 7–11.

Tatar, M., Promislow, D. E. L., Khazaeli, A. A., & Curtsinger, J. W. (1996). Age-specific patterns of genetic variance in *Drosophila melanogaster.* II. Fecundity and its genetic covariance with age-specific mortality. *Genetics, 143,* 849–858.

Van Voorheis, W. A., & Ward, S. (1999). Genetic and environmental conditions that increase longevity in *Caenorhabditis elegans* decrease metabolic rate. *Proceedings of the National Academy of Sciences, 95,* 11399–11403.

Walford, R. L., & Spindler, S. R. (1997). The response to calorie restriction in mammals shows features also common to hibernation: A cross-adaptation hypothesis. *Journal of Gerontology, 52,* B179–B183.

Walker, D. W., McColl, G., Jenkins, N. L., Harris, J., & Lithgow, G. J. (2000). Evolution of lifespan in *C. elegans. Nature,* 405, 296–297.

Weindruch, R., & Walford, R. L. (1988). *The retardation of aging and disease by dietary restriction.* Springfield, IL: Charles Thomas.

Weismann, A. (1891). *Essays upon heredity and kindred biological problems* (Vol. 1, 2nd ed., pp. 141–142). Oxford, UK: Clarendon Press.

Williams, G. C. (1957). Pleiotropy, natural selection and the evolution of senescence. *Evolution, 11,* 398–411.

Wynne-Edwards, V. C. (1962). *Animal dispersion in relation to social behavior.* Edinburgh, Scotland: Oliver & Boyd.

Zwaan, B. J., Bijlsma, R., & Hoekstra, R. F. (1995). Direct selection of lifespan in *Drosophila melanogaster. Evolution, 49,* 649–659.

CHAPTER 4

A Conceptual Assessment of Age-Associated Physiological Changes in Mammals

EDWARD J. MASORO
DEPARTMENT OF PHYSIOLOGY
UNIVERSITY OF TEXAS HEALTH SCIENCE CENTER
AT SAN ANTONIO

HISTORICAL BACKGROUND

That old people suffer physiological deterioration is obvious to even a casual observer, and this deterioration has been of interest to philosophers and physicians throughout history (Birren, 1996). Aristotle (384–322 B.C.) thought that the old body became cold and dry, ultimately resulting in death. Galen (A.D. 129–199) also believed the body dried out as the individual grew old, which was the view of the Arabic philosopher and physician Avicenna (980–1037) as well. Not surprisingly, Benjamin Franklin (1706–1790) felt that aging involved a loss in body electricity. Although many different opinions have been put forth over the centuries about age changes in human physiology, quantitative measurements of such changes were not attempted until the twentieth century.

That is because physiology as an experimental science essentially did not begin until the nineteenth century. Although the occasional important physiological study appeared before then (for example, that of William Harvey [1578–1657] on the circulatory system), it was Claude Bernard (1813–1878) in France and Hermann von Helmholtz (1824–1894) in Germany who established physiology as an academic scientific discipline. Until the middle of the twentieth century, however, male medical students were used for most of the research on human physiology; thus until recently, physiological knowledge was to a great extent limited to the functional characteristics of young men.

Status of Knowledge Circa 1960

In 1960, Nathan Shock presented a seminar to Duke University's Council of Gerontology on the physiological changes that occur during human aging (Shock, 1962). In his article, Shock illustrated the age changes in human physiology with a graph that showed the percentage of decline in function (he set function as 100% at 30 years of age). Nerve conduction velocity, basal metabolic rate, cardiac index, glomerular filtration rate, vital capacity, renal plasma flow, and maximal breathing rate were all found to decline between ages 30 and 85 in a fairly linear fashion. The extent of the decline varied, depending on the function being assessed (for example, the velocity of nerve conduction declined over that age interval by about 15%, while the maximal breathing capacity declined by about 60%). Although Shock characterized the changes as declines in function, he really was addressing deterioration of function. For example, although he was well aware that an increase in arterial blood pressure with advancing age is a functional deterioration, for the sake of simplicity he chose to graphically illustrate those functions that decrease with age.

Criticisms of Early Studies

Since 1960, research on the physiology of aging has increased a great deal. The information generated by these studies and the gerontological expertise acquired by many investigators have led to criticism of the findings and interpretations of the early studies, including the work presented by Nathan Shock at his 1960 seminar. One major criticism relates to conclusions about age changes that were based on findings from studies using the cross-sectional design without proper evaluation of the potential confounders inherent in such a study design. Another concern is the use of human subjects without adequate assessment of their disease status, and not taking into account the lifestyle and environment of the subjects. Ignoring the heterogeneity of age changes among individuals is also considered a serious failing of the early studies as well as many recent ones.

These criticisms and investigators' responses to them are the subject of this chapter, which brings into focus several major issues that currently confront biological gerontology. This article will concentrate on age changes in human physiology because at the organismic level, such changes have been better studied in humans than in animal models. Of course, animal models enable exploration of the cellular and molecular basis of altered physiology but such considerations are left to the chapters on animal models and on molecular and cellular biology. Before beginning this discussion, it is necessary first to make clear the meaning of the word "aging" in the context of this chapter.

DEFINITION OF AGING

It is important to know how an author defines aging because the word has more than one meaning. For example, Costa and McCrae (1995) define it as what happens to an organism over time. Such a definition encompasses no change (indeed, they stress the importance of assessing stability), beneficial changes (which would predominate during the developmental period of life), and deteriorative changes. This definition is not the one being used in this chapter. Rather, aging is defined here as the deteriorative changes during the adult period of life that underlie an increasing vulnerability to challenges and thereby decrease the ability of the organism to survive: that is, *aging* is used as a synonym for *senescence*. This definition is in line with the concept of biological age, in contrast to chronological age and the search for biomarkers of aging (McClearn, 1997). By this definition, aging refers to the occurrence of deteriorative processes with time and thus, if there is no deterioration over a time interval, aging has not occurred during that interval.

CROSS-SECTIONAL STUDY DESIGN

To study age changes in the physiology of humans is a challenging undertaking because of the long length of life of the subjects (the same as that of the investigators). The cross-sectional study design has been the one most widely used to meet this challenge.

Description

In studies of cross-sectional design, a particular physiological function or functions are measured in subjects of different ages (say, ages 20, 40, 60, and 80) at a given point in time (for example, during the 2000 calendar year). It is called a cross-sectional design because data are collected from a cross-section of the population. This design has been popular because it enables a human study to be accomplished quickly (in less than a calendar year if sufficient resources are available).

Confounders

Although the gerontologist's aim is to study changes in physiology due to aging, the subjects in different age groups of a cross-sectional study may differ in regard to a variety of factors in addition to that of age. It is these other factors that lead to the question of whether a difference between age groups is due to aging. A major source of such confounders is frequently referred to as *cohort effects* (Evans, 1995). For example, when investigating the influence of age on cognition, the fact that the number of years of schooling has increased in the developed countries throughout the twentieth century is a potential confounding cohort effect (Katzman, 1995). That is, it is difficult to know to what extent a difference in the cognitive function between cohorts of 30 and 80 years of age is due to aging or to the cohort level of education.

The other major confounder is called selective mortality (Elahi, Muller, & Rowe, 1996). The older the age of a group, the smaller the number of the birth cohort still alive. Moreover, those individuals with risk factors for diseases, which frequently cause death before old age, are the ones who are preferentially removed from the birth cohort, thus the term selective mortality. For example, those individuals with low levels of high density lipoprotein-cholesterol (HDL-cholesterol) are at greater risk of death due to coronary heart disease (a major cause of mortality) than individuals with high levels of HDL-cholesterol (Crow, Bilato, & Lakatta, 1996). Thus, the finding of higher levels of HDL-cholesterol in a group of 80-year-olds compared to a group of 50-year-olds may be due either to an aging effect or to the fact that those who reached 80 years of age were those in the birth cohort with high HDL-cholesterol levels throughout life.

Addressing the Problem of Confounders

In the longitudinal study design, the same subjects are studied repeatedly over extended periods of time, thus providing data on physiological changes in the same individual with increasing age. Superficially, such a design would seem to avoid the potential of confounders inherent in the cross-sectional study design. However, deeper consideration reveals problems that plague the longitudinal study design, including confounders similar to those occurring in cross-sectional studies. A major problem of the longitudinal study design is the need for a stable experimental structure over an extended period of time. It is to be expected that a fraction of the subjects will stop participating in the study for a variety of reasons, including illness and death. However, maintaining stable analytical methodology is probably the more serious challenge. Turnover of laboratory personnel, the upgrading of instrumentation, and the temptation to use improved analytical procedures, to name a few variants, alter the experimental structure during the course of the study. Another problem is the effect of measurement of a physiological parameter on subsequent measurements of that parameter. For example, it was found that in a longitudinal study in which blood pressure was measured at 2-year intervals, the values obtained in the beginning of the study were higher than those later in the study, presumably because familiarity with the measurement procedure reduced the subjects' anxiety (Kannel & Gordon, 1973).

A study reported by Hershcopf and colleagues (1982) on serum cholesterol levels of participants in the Baltimore Longitudinal Study of Aging shows that longitudinal design studies have a potential for confounders similar to those of the cross-sectional design. They measured the change in serum cholesterol in an 8-year longitudinal study (1963 to 1971) in men of different age groups and found that there was a significant increase in men as they progressed from age 40 to 50 years, a result in agreement with the simultaneous cross-sectional findings obtained with the same groups of men. However, a similar study carried out from 1969 to 1977 on a different group of men showed a significant decrease in serum cholesterol as the men progressed from age 40 to 50. This finding disagreed with the cross-sectional findings of both studies and the 1963 to 1971 longitudinal study. They also noted that the level of serum cholesterol was lower in every age group in the second cross-sectional study than in the first. The most likely conclusion is that aging causes serum cholesterol to increase between 40 and 50 years of age, and that some secular effect caused it to decrease in the second longitudinal study. That secular factor may well have been a decrease in dietary intake of animal fat during the 1969–1977 period because of the publicity at that time regarding the role of animal fat in coronary heart disease. The important point is that in this case, two longitudinal studies and two cross-sectional studies were needed to arrive at the likely correct conclusion about the influence of aging on serum cholesterol levels in men during middle age.

Conclusions About Study Designs

Costa and McCrae (1995) discuss hybrids of longitudinal and cross-sectional design as a way of identifying whether a finding is the result of aging or a confounder. However, no design is foolproof. Ultimately, it is necessary for the investigator to make a judgment call. The cross-sectional design is the one of choice in an initial study of the influence of aging on a physiological process, because such research can be carried out quickly at a relatively low cost. However, the investigators must carefully search for possible confounders and utilize the longitudinal study design and possibly hybrid designs, as needed, in the quest for a definitive answer. It should be obvious that the cross-sectional design is only useful for the study of population aging; the study of the aging of an individual is always a longitudinal study. The early workers should not to be criticized for using the cross-sectional design, but they can be criticized for not paying more attention to the possibility of confounders.

DISEASE STATUS

Many diseases are more prevalent or occur only at advanced ages (Brody & Schneider, 1986). These diseases include coronary heart disease, many types of cancer, type II diabetes, osteoporosis, osteoarthritis, Alzheimer's disease, and Parkinson's disease to name a few. These diseases underlie much age-associated physiological deterioration. Whether to include or exclude subjects with age-associated diseases when studying the physiology of aging is an issue that needs further evaluation.

Criticism of Early Studies

In the early cross-sectional studies, the young subjects were often medical students or university and hospital employees, while the old subjects were frequently patients in long-term-care facilities or even acute care hospitals (Elahi et al., 1996). Such studies have been criticized for relating more to health status than to aging. That criticism is valid insofar as possibly involving subjects with acute diseases. However, it is not at all clear that those with chronic age-associated diseases should be excluded from study when the question is one of how aging influences a physiological system. Before addressing this issue further, it is enlightening to first review how the research community has responded to this criticism.

Response to the Criticism

The response of much of the research community to this criticism has been to select subjects free of discernible disease; this procedure has been referred to as "cleaning up" the physiological data (Rowe, Wang, & Elahi, 1990). There are problems with this approach. First, an increasing fraction of birth cohorts suffers from at least one age-associated disease as the age of the birth cohorts increases; thus a large fraction of the population of advanced age will be excluded from such studies. The prevalence of type II diabetes is about 18% in White Americans and 25% in non-White Americans in the age range of 64 to 74 years (Sinclair & Croxon, 1998); the prevalence of osteoarthritis is about 30% in those over age 75 years and is higher in women than men (Scott, 1998); the prevalence of Alzheimer's disease and related dementia is estimated to be 10% to 15% in older adult Americans (Evans et al., 1989). When this information is coupled with the fact that coronary heart disease, congestive heart failure, osteoporosis, cataracts, Parkinson's disease, many types of cancer, benign prostatic hyperplasia, and other diseases become increasingly prevalent at advanced age, the fraction of the elderly population free of one or more age-associated disease must be very small indeed. In addition, whether a disease is discernible depends on the ability to detect it. For instance, the thallium-stress test has enabled the detection of occult coronary heart disease that was not discernible before, and those with this subclinical disease that was detected by this technology were found to exhibit deterioration in cardiovascular function (Lakatta, 1985). Thus, as technology improves, it is to be expected that an increasing fraction of the population will be excluded from aging studies because of age-associated disease. Then there is the arbitrary question of whether to call a problem a disease or simply a physiological deterioration: For instance, when should bone loss that occurs to some extent with advancing age in all people (Kalu, 1995) be called osteoporosis? Finally, the current view of the evolution of senescence implicates age-associated diseases as an integral part of aging (Rose, 1991), which will be discussed presently.

The Concept of "Normal Aging"

Despite the reasons just discussed for not excluding those with age-associated diseases from studies on physiological processes, the concept of "normal aging" has been, and is, widely applied by those conducting such studies (Shock, 1984). Normal aging is defined as senescence in the absence of disease yet because aging in the absence of one or more age-associated disease processes is clearly uncommon, it seems more appropriate to refer to such research as the study of atypical aging rather than normal aging. Probably the most compelling of reasons to discard the concept of normal aging is that the evolutionary biology of aging makes age-associated disease an almost inevitable component of organismic aging. Senescence occurs because the force of natural selection decreases with increasing age. The suggested genetic mechanisms underlying senescence are (a) genetic mutations with deleterious consequences expressed only in late life; and (b) antagonistic pleiotropic genes, that is, genes with beneficial actions in early life and deleterious ones in late life. Age-associated diseases are the likely consequence of both of these genetic mechanisms.

Conclusions on Age-Associated Diseases and the Study of the Physiology of Aging

If the aim is to learn about physiological changes that occur with aging, then the population to be studied should be comprised of individuals broadly representative of the general population. In cross-sectional studies, this means that the subjects should be selected to include those with particular age-associated disease in proportion to its frequency in individuals of that age in the general population. Although this ideal is probably impossible to achieve, studies should be designed that will approach it. This does not mean that it is not valuable to conduct studies in which the subjects are free of discernible disease. Indeed, the reductionist approach has been a powerful tool in biology and as such, studies with disease-free subjects will continue to provide important information. However, these studies should be designated by what they aim to accomplish rather than being referred to misleadingly as normal aging.

LIFESTYLE AND ENVIRONMENTAL FACTORS

The classic view is that aging is an intrinsic phenomenon (Strehler, 1977). This concept must be reconciled with the robust and reproducible findings that restriction of caloric intake by rats and mice markedly extends their life span by slowing the aging processes (Masoro, 2000). Moreover, there is increasing evidence that environmental factors play a major role in human aging (Rowe & Kahn, 1998).

The Concept of Primary and Secondary Aging

Busse (1969) recognized this dilemma long ago and tried to resolve the problem by proposing the concept of primary and secondary aging. He defined primary aging as the universal changes occurring with age within a species or population, changes not caused by disease or environmental influences. Secondary aging was defined as changes involving interactions of primary aging with environmental influences and disease processes.

Criticism of the Concept of Primary and Secondary Aging

The usefulness of the concept of primary and secondary aging is challenged by recent developments in biological gerontology. The research of Vieira and colleagues (2000) clearly shows that the effect of genes on life span and aging in *Drosophila melanogaster* is dependent on environmental interactions. In addition, in general terms senescence is viewed by many as the result of the long-term accumulation of unrepaired damage, the specific nature and site of the damage relating to the genetic characteristics and environmental circumstances of the individual and species (Martin, Austad, & Johnson, 1996; Masoro, 1999). If this view is correct, then damage due to intrinsic living processes, the environment as well as lifestyle, and their interactions are all causes of aging. Because environmental and lifestyle factors cause damage by affecting the molecular structure of the organism, such damage could be viewed as intrinsic. However, such a broad view would be counterproductive because it would deemphasize the importance of environmental factors in aging. Moreover, recent evidence increasingly indicates the major role of environment and lifestyle in the physiological deteriorations that occur in aging; it is significant that such factors can potentially be modified to slow the rate of aging (Rowe & Kahn, 1998). Thus, in the view of this author, the concept of primary and secondary aging serves to confuse rather than enlighten.

HETEROGENEITY AMONG PEOPLE IN PHYSIOLOGICAL AGE CHANGES

When assessing age changes in a physiological function observed in cross-sectional studies, gerontologists have focused on average differences among age groups. As a result, the differences among individuals in age-associated change have largely been ignored.

Individual Differences in Physiological Age Changes

There are great individual differences in age-associated changes in physiological processes. The age change in glomerular filtration provides a particularly striking example. In a cross-sectional study conducted by Rowe, Andres, Tobin, Norris, and Shock (1976), the glomerular filtration rate was found to decline from about 140 ml/min/1.73 m^2 body surface in men in the age range of 25–34 years to about 97 ml/min/1.73 m^2 in the age range of 75–84 years. Other investigators have reported similar findings. However, a longitudinal study carried out on 446 participants of the Baltimore Longitudinal Study of Aging revealed marked individual differences in the age change in glomerular filtration rate with one third of the subjects not showing any age change; the average change was strikingly similar to those observed in the earlier cross-sectional studies (Lindeman, Tobin, & Shock, 1985). Thus, even a marked average decline in a physiological process in a population does not mean that nearly everyone will show a decline in that function.

The Concepts of "Usual Aging" and "Successful Aging"

In a *Science* article, Rowe and Kahn (1987) developed a conceptual framework for considering the differences among individuals in the changes with age in physiological processes. They introduced the concept that the disease-free population can be classified as undergoing, for a given physiological function, either "usual aging" or "successful aging."

More recently, Rowe and Kahn (1998) published *Successful Aging,* a book for laypersons that expanded these concepts. Usual aging refers to older adults who are functioning well yet who are at risk for disease or disability. Many in this group will have modest increases in systolic blood pressure, abdominal fat, and blood sugar, as well as deterioration in the function of one or more physiological systems. Indeed, individuals in the usual-aging subgroup are at significant risk for disease, disability, and premature death. Successful aging refers to the much smaller subgroup of disease-free older adults who exhibit three key characteristics: low risk of disease and disability, high level of mental and physical function, and active engagement in life.

Factors Underlying "Successful Aging"

Rowe and Kahn (1998) focus on environment and lifestyle as major determinants of successful aging. Adequate physical exercise, appropriate diet, good personal habits (not smoking or using illegal drugs or indulging in an immoderate intake of alcoholic beverages), and a good psychosocial environment all play an important role in successful aging. Surprisingly, the authors barely mention the likely importance of an individual's genetic constitution.

Concerns About the Concept of "Successful Aging"

This popular concept requires critical evaluation, and three questions are of particular concern. (1) What fraction of the population currently fits in the category of successful aging and what are future projections in this regard? (2) Is it valid to imply that a very advanced age can be reached without significant physiological deterioration? And, probably most important, (3) Is the concept useful or misleading?

As discussed previously, an increasing fraction of a birth cohort suffers from age-associated diseases as the age of the cohort increases. By the eighth decade of life, only a small fraction will be free of one or more age-associated diseases. Thus, by that time the successful aging subgroup—a small number of the disease-free population—must be a vanishing fraction of the living members of that birth cohort. Of course, it is possible that in the future many will adopt the lifestyle that Rowe and Kahn feel underlies successful aging, and by doing so the number of people in that subgroup will be increased substantially. Of course, such a projection assumes that genetic constitution has little or no role in achieving successful aging.

Rowe and Kahn do not mention how the successful aging subgroup functions as chronological age increases. Do they live to a very old age and die without experiencing appreciable physiological deterioration? Or do they undergo marked physiological deterioration before death at an advanced age? If the latter, what does the concept of successful aging provide other than the well-known fact that individuals age at different rates, with some aging very slowly indeed. In fact, the concept of biological age as distinct from chronological age was proposed some time ago (Borkan & Norris, 1980).

A paper surveying American and European studies of centenarians by Forette (1997) shows that the majority of centenarians are seriously disabled. About half of centenarians in a Hungarian study were found to be demented. In a French study, one third needed help to eat and one half for toileting; two thirds were not able to walk 500 meters and 80% could not climb stairs. It seems reasonable to assume that when these centenarians were in their eighth decade, most were in the successful aging subgroup and that they subsequently underwent marked physiological deterioration.

Research on animal models leads to a similar conclusion. Strong evidence is emerging that molecular damage due to living processes, such as the oxidative stress accompanying fuel utilization, plays a major role in aging (Sohal & Weindruch, 1996). Although modifying environment and lifestyle may slow the rate of such accumulative damage, it is not likely to eliminate it. The findings of studies carried out on caloric restriction in rats in my laboratory are in accord with this. Reducing the caloric intake of the rats by 40% increased both the median and the maximum length of life and markedly slowed the rate of physiological deterioration (Masoro, 2000). At ages where the rats on the higher caloric intake had already died, those on the low caloric intake were healthy and vigorous. Of course, ultimately the rats on the low caloric intake died, with cancer as the major disease process involved. To determine how long the rats on both levels of caloric intake lived in a deteriorated state, the duration of the terminal loss of weight (an invariable occurrence before death from natural causes) was measured. The duration was the same for both groups of rats. Thus, although caloric restriction slows the rate of aging, it does not shorten the period of senescent deterioration.

Therefore, "slowing the rate of aging" would be the more appropriate term when referring to the beneficial effects of the lifestyle and environment described by Rowe and Kahn (1998). It should be noted that the concept of successful aging tends to mislead because it implies that physiological deterioration due to aging can be avoided rather than merely slowed. It leads to the view held by some in the public policy arena that an appropriate lifestyle, with an emphasis on diet, weight control, and exercise, can enable people to reach very old age without the disabilities that are so costly in societal resources. In fact, by increasing the length of life, such a lifestyle may well have just the opposite effect. There has been an emergence of centenarians during the past century, and there is reason to believe they may become commonplace during the twenty-first century (Jeune & Kannisto, 1997). If so, lifestyle may be an important factor in this projected increase. However, as discussed earlier, most centenarians are so deteriorated physiologically that they require a great deal of societal assistance. It is important that those in public policy realize we do not know what the societal impact will be of adopting a lifestyle that slows aging and extends length of life. It may well not be what one would expect from the term successful aging.

SUMMARY

The cross-sectional design has been used in most studies of physiological changes that occur as humans age. These investigations indicate that physiological processes deteriorate with increasing age. It is recognized that the possibility of confounders that can cloud gerontologic interpretation of the findings is inherent in the cross-sectional design. To uncover such confounders, studies of the longitudinal design and hybrids of the cross-sectional and longitudinal designs have been used. Ultimately, however, the investigator has to make a judgment call regarding the possibility that the conclusions about aging are compromised because of one or more confounders.

Age-associated diseases influence the age changes in physiology. Because of this, many investigators choose to use subjects free of such diseases in what they call the study of normal aging. The concept of normal aging is questionable because most individuals at advanced ages suffer from one or more chronic age-associated diseases, which the evolutionary theory of aging indicates are an inherent aspect of aging. Studies using subjects free of age-associated disease are valuable as a reductionist approach to the study of aging; however, they do not provide a valid assessment of physiological change that commonly occurs with increasing age.

Environmental factors and lifestyle markedly influence age changes in physiological processes. The concept of primary and secondary aging suggests that aging is an intrinsic process that is modified by environment and lifestyle. However, based on our current understanding of the biology of aging, it is more appropriate to view intrinsic living processes and extrinsic factors both as direct causes of aging and its accompanying physiological deterioration.

There are marked individual differences in the length of time and extent of physiological deterioration with advancing age. Individuals who show little physiological deterioration in the seventh, eighth, or even ninth decade of life are said to be undergoing successful aging, a concept that tends to be misleading. A more accurate view would be that the rate of physiological deterioration with age differs among individuals, with some showing an extremely slow rate of deterioration.

REFERENCES

Birren, J. E. (1996). History of gerontology. In J. E. Birren (Ed.), *Encyclopedia of gerontology* (Vol. 1, pp. 655–665). San Diego: Academic Press.

Borkan, G. A., & Norris, A. H. (1980). Assessment of biological age using a profile of physical parameters. *Journal of Gerontology, 35,* 177–184.

Brody, J. A., & Schneider, E. L. (1986). Diseases and disorders of aging: A hypothesis. *Journal of Chronic Diseases, 39,* 871–876.

Busse, E. W. (1969). Theories of aging. In E. W. Busse & E. Pfeiffer (Eds.), *Behavior and adaptation in adult life* (pp. 11–32). Boston: Little, Brown.

Costa, P. T., Jr., & McCrae, R. R. (1995). Design and analysis of aging studies. In E. J. Masoro (Ed.), *Handbook of physiology, Section 11, Aging* (pp. 25–36). New York: Oxford University Press.

Crow, M. T., Bilato, C., & Lakatta, E. G. (1996). Atherosclerosis. In J. E. Birren (Ed.), *Encyclopedia of gerontology* (Vol. 1, pp. 123–129). San Diego: Academic Press.

Elahi, D., Muller, D. C., & Rowe, J. W. (1996). Design, conduct, and analysis of human aging research. In E. L. Schneider & J. W. Rowe (Eds.), *Handbook of the biology of aging* (4th ed., pp. 24–36). San Diego: Academic Press.

Evans, D. A. (1995). Human studies. In E. J. Masoro (Ed.), *Handbook of physiology, Section 11, Aging* (pp. 83–92). New York: Oxford University Press.

Evans, D. A., Funkenstein, H. H., Albert, M. S., Scherr, P. A., Cook, N. R., Chown, M. J., Hebert, L. E., Hennekens, C. H., & Taylor, J. O. (1989). Prevalence of Alzheimer's disease in a community population of older persons: Higher than previously reported. *Journal of the American Medical Association, 262,* 2551–2556.

Forette, B. (1997). Centenarians: Health and frailty. In J.-M. Robine, J. W. Vaupel, B. Jeune, & M. Allard (Eds.), *Longevity: To the limits and beyond* (pp. 105–112). Berlin, Germany: Springer-Verlag.

Hershcopf, R. J., Elahi, D., Andres, R., Baldwin, H. L., Raizes, G. S., Schocken, D. D., & Tobin, J. D. (1982). Longitudinal changes of serum cholesterol in man: An epidemiological search for etiology. *Journal of Chronic Diseases, 35,* 101–114.

Jeune, B., & Kannisto, V. (1997). Emergence of centenarians and supercentenarians. In J.-M. Robine, J. W. Vaupel, B. Jeune, & M. Allard (Eds.), *Longevity: To the limits and beyond* (pp. 77–89). Berlin, Germany: Springer-Verlag.

Kalu, D. N. (1995). Bone. In E. J. Masoro (Ed.), *Handbook of physiology, Section 11, Aging* (pp. 395–412). New York: Oxford University Press.

Kannel, W. B., & Gordon, T. (1974). *The Framingham study: An epidemiological investigation of cardiovascular disease.* Washington, DC: Department of Health, Education, and Welfare.

Katzman, R. (1995). Human nervous system. In E. J. Masoro (Ed.), *Handbook of physiology, Section 11, Aging* (pp. 325–344). New York: Oxford University Press.

Lakatta, E. G. (1985). Health, disease, and cardiovascular aging. In Committee on an Aging Society, Institute of Medicine and National Research Council, *America's aging—Health in an older society* (pp. 73–104). Washington, DC: National Academy Press.

Lindeman, R. D., Tobin, J. D., & Shock, N. W. (1985). Longitudinal studies on the rate of decline in renal function with age. *Journal of the American Geriatrics Society, 33,* 278–285.

Martin, G. M., Austad, S. M., & Johnson, T. E. (1996). Genetic analysis of ageing: Role of oxidative damage and environmental stresses. *Nature Genetics, 13,* 25–34.

Masoro, E. J. (1999). *Challenges of biological aging.* New York: Springer Publishing Co.

Masoro, E. J. (2000) Caloric restriction and aging: An update. *Experimental Gerontology, 35,* 299–305.

McClearn, G. E. (1997). Biomarkers of age and aging. *Experimental Gerontology, 32,* 87–94.

Rose, M. R. (1991). *Evolutionary biology of aging.* New York: Oxford University Press.

Rowe, J. W., & Kahn, R. L. (1987). Human aging: Usual and successful. *Science, 237,* 137–149.

Rowe, J. W., & Kahn, R. L. (1998). *Successful aging.* New York: Pantheon.

Rowe, J. W., Andres, R., Tobin, J. D., Norris, A. H., & Shock, N. W. (1976). The effect of age on creatinine clearance in men: A cross sectional and longitudinal study. *Journal of Gerontology, 31,* 155–163.

Rowe, J. W., Wang, S. Y., & Elahi, D. (1990). Design, conduct, and analysis of human aging research. In E. L. Schneider & J. W. Rowe (Eds.), *Handbook of the biology of aging* (3rd ed., pp. 63–71). San Diego: Academic Press.

Scott, D. L. (1998). Arthritis in the elderly. In R. Tallis, H. Fillit, & J. C. Brocklehurst (Eds.), *Brocklehurst's textbook of geriatric medicine and gerontology* (5th ed., pp. 1155–1178). London: Churchill Livingston.

Shock, N. W. (1962). The science of gerontology. In B. C. Jeffers (Ed.), *Proceedings of seminars 1959–1961* (pp. 123–140). Durham, NC: Duke University Press.

Shock, N. W. (Ed.) (1984). *Normal human aging: The Baltimore Longitudinal Study of Aging* (NIH Publ. 84-2450). Washington, DC: U.S. Government Printing Office.

Sinclair A. J., & Croxson, S. C. M. (1998). Diabetes mellitus in the older adult. In R. Tallis, H. Fillit, & J. C. Brocklehurst (Eds.), *Brocklehurst's textbook of geriatric medicine and gerontology* (5th ed., pp. 1051–1071). London: Churchill Livingstone.

Sohal, R. S., & Weindruch, R. (1996). Oxidative stress, caloric restriction, and aging. *Science, 273,* 59–63.

Strehler, B. L. (1977). *Time, cells, and aging.* New York: Academic Press.

Vieira, C., Pasyukova, E. G., Zeng, Z. B., Hackett, J. B., Lyman, R. F., & Mackay, T. (2000). Genotype-environment interaction for quantitative trait loci affecting life span in *Drosophila melanogaster. Genetics, 154,* 213–227.

CHAPTER 5

Cellular Aging

R. G. ALLEN, ARTHUR K. BALIN,
AND VINCENT J. CRISTOFALO
LANKENAU INSTITUTE FOR MEDICAL RESEARCH
WYNNEWOOD, PA

Most types of mammalian cells exhibit a limited proliferative capacity when placed in a culture environment. The cessation of mitotic activity following a fixed number of divisions is usually referred to as replicative senescence or aging in vitro. The senescence phenomenon has also been observed in the cells of non-mammalian species (Goldstein, 1974). Interestingly, although cell culture models were studied intensely during much of the twentieth century, clear evidence that cellular senescence even existed was not presented until 1961 (Hayflick & Moorhead, 1961). Prior to that it was generally believed that individual cells were potentially immortal, in the same way that bacteria and most protozoa are considered immortal, when separated from organisms and placed in a culture environment (Carrel & Burrows, 1910a, 1910b, 1911; Carrel & Ebling, 1921). This view was based on studies with chick cells, and the apparent immortality may actually have resulted from repeated contamination of tissue culture components with fresh chick embryo cells (Hayflick, 1970, 1977).

It is now known that after migration of cells from tissue into the culture environment, there is an initial phase of rapid proliferation, during which cell cultures can be subcultivated frequently. This initial phase is followed by one of declining proliferative capacity, which ultimately culminates in a total loss of mitotic activity (Hayflick & Moorhead, 1961; Matsumura, Zerrudo, & Hayflick, 1979). During this later phase the cells change in size and morphology, become granular, and accumulate debris. As populations of cells divide successive times, the generation time of the culture increases; there is also failure of an increasing fraction of the population to replicate at all (reviewed in Cristofalo & Pignolo, 1995). It has been shown that substantial heterogeneity develops in populations of cells as they proliferate with some members of the population exhibiting a high proliferative capacity while others are capable of only a small number of divisions (Smith & Whitney, 1980). A limited proliferative life span has been described for a variety of cell types, including fibroblasts (Hayflick & Moorhead, 1961; Rohme, 1981), glial cells (Ponten, 1973), keratinocytes (Rheinwald & Green, 1975), vascular smooth muscle cells (Bierman, 1978), lens cells (Tassin, Malaise, & Courtois, 1979), endothelial cells (Mueller, Rosen, & Levine, 1980), lymphocytes (Tice, Schneider, Kram, & Thorne, 1979), and melanocytes (Medrano et al., 1994). While the proliferative life span differs between various types of cells, the proliferative capacity tends to be relatively constant for any given cell type.

Senescence-dependent cessation of growth is not identical to the G_0 growth arrest that occurs in early passage cells that exhibit contact-inhibited growth or that are serum starved. Several lines of evidence suggest that senescent cells are blocked in an aberrant phase of the cell cycle with many characteristics of late G_1. For example, thymidine kinase usually appears at the G_1/S boundary and is not detected in G_0. Thymidine kinase activity is expressed in cultures of proliferatively young and senescent WI-38 cells (Cristofalo, 1973; Olashaw, Kress, & Cristofalo, 1983). Thymidine triphosphate synthesis, which normally occurs in late G_1, is unimpaired in senescent cells (Olashaw et al., 1983). Furthermore, the nuclear fluorescence pattern of senescent cells stained with quinacrine dihydrochloride is also typical of cells blocked in late G_1 or at the G_1/S boundary (Gorman & Cristofalo, 1985; Pignolo, Martin, Horton, Kalbach, & Cristofalo, 1998). Rittling, Brooks, Cristofalo, and Baserga (1986) demonstrated that 11 genes expressed between early G_1 and the G_1/S boundary are mitogen-inducible in both young and senescent cells; however, growth-regulated genes such as *cdc2, cycA,* and *cycB,* which are expressed in G_1, are repressed in senescent cells (Stein, Drullinger, Robetorye, Pereira-Smith, & Smith, 1991). These observations suggest the possibility that senescent cells are irreversibly arrested in a unique state different from the normal stages of the cell cycle.

COMPONENTS OF SENESCENCE

Although the tendency of various types of nontransformed cells to senesce is established, the underlying causes of the phenomenon are far less clear. Through many different experiments it has been shown that the inability of cell cultures to proliferate indefinitely cannot be ascribed to inadequate nutrition, pH variation, toxic metabolic products, microcontaminants, or to depletion by serial dilution of some essential metabolite (Cristofalo & Pignolo, 1993; Hayflick, 1977). Both environmental and genetic factors appear to influence the proliferative life span of fibroblasts from normal individuals (Cristofalo, Palazzo, & Charpentier, 1980; Cristofalo, Phillips, Sorger, & Gerhard, 1989; Cristofalo & Pignolo, 1993). The extent to which the tissue culture environment is a determinant of proliferative potential has been an intensely debated topic for some time. Rubin suggested that the limited replicative life span of cells in culture might be an artifact resulting from the failure of the cells to adapt to the trauma of dissociation and the differences between the culture and in vivo environments (Rubin, 1997). Similarly, several recent studies have questioned whether the limited proliferative life of cells in culture is an inherent cellular property or an artifact of the culture environment (Mathon, Malcolm, Harrisingh, Cheng, & Lloyd, 2001; Sherr & DePinho, 2000; Tang, Tokumoto, Apperly, Lloyd, & Raff, 2001).

The steady loss of replicative potential is accompanied by a greater heterogeneity of cell sizes, as well as a shift to much larger cell sizes. Characteristic morphological alterations accompany the changes in cell size seen with senescence in culture. An increase in nuclear size, in nucleolar size, and in the number of multinucleated cells (Matsumura et al., 1979) parallels the increase in cell size seen in slowly replicating or nonreplicating cultures. Prominent Golgi apparati, evacuated endoplasmic reticula, increased numbers of cytoplasmic microfilaments, vacuolated cytoplasm, and large lysosomal bodies have been observed in senescent human fibroblasts (see Cristofalo & Pignolo, 1995). Late-passage cultures display a reduced harvest density and a lowered saturation density at the plateau phase of growth (Cristofalo, 1988). At the end of their life span in vitro, substantial cell death occurs; however, a stable population emerges that can exist in a viable, nonproliferative state for many months (Pignolo, Rotenberg, & Cristofalo, 1994). This stable population is capable of maintaining only an extremely low saturation density, equivalent to less than 5% of that reached by early-passage cultures. The observed decrease in saturation densities probably reflects an increased sensitivity to intercellular contact, rather than increased numbers of larger cells (Pignolo et al., 1994). Changes at the level of extracellular matrix (ECM), specific secretory proteins not connected with the ECM, and membrane-associated molecules occur in late passage cells, but it is unclear whether they account for alterations in the nature of cell contact among these cells (Ferber et al., 1993; Frederich, Phillips, & Cristofalo, 1992; Goldstein, Moerman, Jones, & Baxter, 1991; Kleinsek, 1989; Kumar, Millis, & Baglioni, 1992; Mann, McKeown-Longo, & Millis, 1988; Millis, Hoyle, McCue, & Martini, 1992; Millis, Sottile, Hoyle, Mann, & Diemer, 1989; Mueller et al., 1980; Pereira-Smith, Fisher, & Smith, 1985; Pignolo, Cristofalo, & Rotenberg, 193; Sottile, Hoyle, & Millis, 1988; Sottile, Mann, Diemer, & Millis, 1989; Stein & Atkins, 1986; West, Shay, Wright, & Linskens, 1996).

It has been suggested repeatedly that cellular aging may result from some form of differentiation (Bell et al., 1979; Bell et al., 1978; Cristofalo, 1972; Martin, Sprague, Norwood, & Pendergrass, 1974), which would presumably be driven by the culture environment. In fact, morphology differences at different points along a putative differentiation path have been identified (Bayreuther, Francz, Gogol, Maier, & Meinrath, 1991; Bayreuther et al., 1988; Kontermann & Bayreuther, 1979). Stronger support for the hypothesis was recently presented using cultures of rodent tissue. It was demonstrated that rat oligodendrocyte precursor cells grew indefinitely when they were prevented from differentiating by adjusting the composition of their culture medium. Oligodendrocyte precursor cells placed in serum-free medium that contains both platelet-derived growth factor (PDGF) and thyroid hormone (TH) are able to divide only a small number of times before reaching a senescent phase in which they are incapable of any further growth. If the TH is excluded from the medium, the cells can be grown indefinitely with no apparent sign of senescence (Tang et al., 2001). Whether other types of cells exhibit a limited proliferative capacity as a result of differentiation has not been established. Thus far, significant extensions of culture life span have been possible only in nonhuman cells. Nevertheless, it is noteworthy that most of the morphological changes associated with the senescence of human fibroblasts can be prevented by the addition of carnosine to the culture medium (McFarland & Holliday, 1994).

Although the culture environment may have a significant impact on the proliferative capacity of cultures, there is also a genetic component to senescence. Skin fibroblasts from pairs of monozygotic twins show no significant difference in replicative life span within each pair but do exhibit such differences among pairs (Ryan, Ostrow, Breakefield, Gershon, & Upchurch, 1981). Experiments that evaluated the ability of transformed cell lines to complement recessive defects responsible for an immortalized phenotype reportedly identified at least four complementation groups (Pereira-Smith & Smith, 1983, 1988). In these experiments, the fusion of two immortalized cell lines resulted in hybrids that either exhibited indefinite cell division (indicating the same genetic defect; same complementation group) or finite cell division (indicating different genetic defects; different complementation group). These results suggest that there is a limited number of genes or sets of genes that may be responsible for "escape" from senescence. The interpretation of these results has become more complicated, because other laboratories failed to confirm these results. Specifically, it has been reported that fusions of infinite life-span cells of different complementation groups failed to exhibit finite life spans (Ryan, Maher, & McCormick, 1994) and that the fusion of cells within the same complementation group resulted in hybrids with limited life spans (Duncan,

Whitaker, Moy, & Reddel, 1993; Whitaker, Kidston, & Reddel, 1992). Of course, the possibility remains that escape from senescence may not be regulated by the same steps that regulate senescence.

Heterokaryons, formed from the fusion of senescent cells with early-passage proliferative cells or immortalized cells exhibit a nonproliferative phenotype indicating dominance of the senescent phenotype. However, the fusion of senescent cells with immortalized variants having high levels of DNA polymerase α (DNA pol α) or those transformed by DNA tumor viruses results in heterokaryons that proliferate (Norwood, Smith, & Stein, 1990; Pendergrass, Angello, Saulewicz, & Norwood, 1991; Pereira-Smith & Smith, 1982; Stein, Yanishevsky, Gordon, & Beeson, 1982). Consistent with these observations are numerous reports documenting the presence of inhibitors of DNA synthesis in senescent cells (Burmer, Zeigler, & Norwood, 1982; Drescher-Lincoln & Smith, 1984; Noda, Ning, Venable, Periera-Smith, & Smith, 1994; Pereira-Smith et al., 1985; Stein & Atkins, 1986). Poly A^+ RNA extracted from senescent fibroblasts and microinjected into proliferation-competent cells inhibits their entry into DNA synthesis (Lumpkin, McClung, Pereira-Smith, & Smith, 1986). The nature of these inhibitors remains poorly understood at the present time.

Evidence that the cessation of proliferation is a programmed phenomenon has also been provided by studies that characterized the apparently reversible escape from cellular senescence using SV40 large T antigen as a mediator of this transition (Radna et al., 1989; Wright, Pereira-Smith, & Shay, 1989). This evidence suggests that senescence confers at least two distinct mortality states. The search for chromosomes carrying senescence-inducing genes has relied on the cytogenetic comparison of hybrids between immortal and normal human diploid fibroblasts for the loss of specific chromosomes and the concomitant potential for unlimited division. These studies have implicated human chromosomes 1, 5, and 6 as putative sites for senescence-related genes (Ning et al., 1991; Ozer et al., 1996; Sugawara, Oshimura, Koi, Annab, & Barrett, 1990).

One senescence marker that has been identified is the protein statin. Although it is not specific to senescent cells, it is specific to a quiescent state and its concentration increases sharply in cells that have reached the end of their proliferative life span (Wang, 1989). Statin is also elevated in nondividing tissues in vivo (Bissonnette, Lee, & Wang, 1990) and increases during differentiation to a postmitotic phenotype (Connolly, Sarabia, Kelvin, & Wang, 1988). Although it is clearly elevated in senescent cells, it is not known whether increased statin contributes to the senescent phenotype or is only a result of the loss of proliferative activity.

It is also known that the expression of several growth-suppressing genes, such as p53, p21 and p16, increases with age (Atadja, Wong, Garkavtsev,

Veillette, & Riabowol, 1995; Hara et al., 1996; Noda et al., 1994). Treatment of normal cells with antisense p53 and retinoblastoma protein (pRB) extend the life span of senescent cells in a cooperative manner (Hara, Tsurui, Shinozaki, Nakada, & Oda, 1991). In normal cells, disruption of tumor/growth suppressor genes such as $p21^{Waf1/Cip1/sdi1}$, a gene controlled by p53, can extend proliferative life span (Brown, Wei, & Sedivy, 1997). Additionally, transfection of human tumor cells that lack p53 with the wild-type gene can induce a senescent phenotype, yet elimination of p53, and hence p21, fails to prevent senescence in human cells (Medcalf, Klein-Szanto, & Cristofalo, 1996). Loss of $p16^{INK4}$, an inhibitor of Cdk 4 and Cdk 6, has also been reported to extend proliferative life span (Noble et al., 1996), while constitutive activation of MEK (a component of the MAP kinase cascade) induces both p53 and p16 and results in permanent growth arrest in primary murine fibroblasts. Overexpression of constitutively active MEK causes uncontrolled mitogenesis and transformation in cells lacking either p53 or $p16^{INK4a}$ (Lin et al., 1998).

The reason that expression of these growth regulators changes during senescence is unknown. Recently, $p16^{INK4a}$ was found to be regulated by the Ets1/Ets2 transcription factors. Ets-mediated transcription of $p^{16INK4a}$ is blocked by interaction with the Id family of helix-loop-helix proteins. Ets2 is up regulated by the Ras-Raf-MEK kinase cascade. Ets2 is abundant in early passage cells but activation of the MAP kinase pathway and Ets2 activity are both strongly diminished in senescent cultures (Ohtani et al., 2001). Id protein abundance also declines in senescent cells (Nehlin, Hara, Kuo, Collins, & Campisi, 1997), which may stimulate a compensatory increase in Ets1 activity (Ohtani et al., 2001). The net effect of these changes is an increase in $p16^{INK4a}$ associated with senescence. Studies conducted in our laboratory show that senescence is associated with a nearly total loss of activated Elk-1 following mitogenic stimuli (Cristofalo, unpublished). It is interesting to note that Elk-1 suppresses the expression of $p16^{INK4a}$, hence the senescence-associated decrease in active Elk-1 may also contribute significantly to that of $p16^{INK4a}$.

TELOMERE SHORTENING

Chronological time appears to be far less important than division events in determining in vitro life span (Cristofalo et al., 1980; Dell, Orco, Mertens, & Kruze, 1974). Thus, in contrast to aging in vivo, senescence is independent of the passage of time. This observation suggests that the clock that controls proliferative life span counts only the number of replications rather than the passage of time. One seemingly plausible mechanism by which cells may tally their mitotic history is through loss of telomeric repeats during replication. The telomeres of human chromosomes are composed of several kilobases of simple repeats $(TTAGGG)_n$. Telomeres protect chromosomes from degradation, rearrangements, end-to-end fusions, and chromosome loss (Feng et al., 1995). During replication DNA polymerases synthesize DNA in a 5′ to 3′ direction; they also require an RNA primer for initiation. The terminal RNA primer required for DNA replication cannot be replaced with DNA, which results in a loss of telomeric sequences with each mitotic cycle (Olovnikov, 1971, 1973, 1996; Watson, 1972). Loss of telomeric repeats during senescence has been demonstrated experimentally and is tightly linked to the cessation of mitotic activity that occurs during cellular senescence (Allsopp et al., 1992; Levy, Allsopp, Futcher, Greider, & Harley, 1992; von Zglinicki, Saretzki, Döcke, & Lotze, 1995; Wright & Shay, 1992). Cells expressing T-antigen are postulated to exhibit an increase in their proliferative life span because they are able to continue proliferating beyond the usual limit imposed by telomere length (Counter et al., 1992). Immortalized and transformed cells exhibit telomerase activity, which compensates for telomere loss by adding repetitive units to the telomeres of chromosomes after mitosis (Blasco, Funk, Villeponteau, & Greider, 1995; Feng et al., 1995; Hiyama et al., 1995; Wainwright, Middleton, & Rees, 1995). Proliferative senescence can be delayed and possibly eliminated by transfection of normal cells with telomerase to prevent telomere loss (Bodnar et al., 1998). It is also interesting to note that other repetitive DNA sequences become shorter during proliferative senescence (Harley, Shmookler-Reis, & Goldstein, 1982; Shmookler-Reis & Goldstein, 1980). Nevertheless, the exact role of telomere shortening in proliferative senescence remains unclear (Shay & Wright, 2001).

Although important, telomere loss does not fully account for cellular senescence. For example, rodent chromosomes contain much longer telomeres than humans, yet the proliferative life span of rodent cells in culture is much shorter than that of human cells (Rudolph et al., 1999; Wright & Shay, 2000). As normal human oral keratinocytes senesce, they lose telomerase activity but exhibit no apparent shortening of telomeres (Kang, Guo, & Park, 1998). Furthermore, telomere-shortening alone cannot account for the morphological changes that appear in senescent cells or the alterations observed in their signal transduction pathways (Cristofalo, Volker, Francis, & Tresini, 1998). As noted above, premature differentiation may limit the life span of cells in culture without a corresponding loss of telomeres (Tang et al., 2001); however, it is presently unclear that this is a factor in limiting the life span of all or even most types of cells in a culture environment.

CELL CULTURE AS A MODEL OF AGING

Following fertilization and initial cell divisions, the cells of embryos differentiate into a potentially "immortal" germ cell lineage and a mortal somatic cell lineage. The limited proliferative capacity of somatic cells in culture has been suggested to indicate that biological aging is the manifest cellular phenomenon in replicative senescence in vitro (Hayflick & Moorhead, 1961). The direct relationship between some species' life spans in vivo and the maximum life spans of their cells in vitro appeared to support this hypothesis (Cristofalo & Pignolo, 1993; Goldstein, 1974; Rohme, 1981). Various disease states of cell donors have been found to significantly influence the proliferative life spans of cells in culture. For example, cell strains established from diabetics (Goldstein, Littlefield, & Soeldner, 1969; Goldstein, Moerman, Soeldner, Gleason, & Barnett, 1978) and Werner's patients (Danes, 1971; Goldstein & Harley, 1979; Martin, 1978; Martin, Sprague, & Epstein, 1970; Oshima, Campisi, Tannock, & Martin, 1995) exhibit a marked attenuation of proliferative capacity. Cultures established from individuals with Hutchinson-Gilford syndrome (Goldstein & Harley, 1979) or Down syndrome (Goldstein & Harley, 1979; Schneider & Epstein, 1972) may also exhibit decreased life span; however, results with these cell lines are more variable (Brown, 1990). Perhaps most important, cultures of normal human cells were observed to exhibit a negative correlation between proliferative life span and the age of the donor from whom the culture was established (Allsopp et al., 1992; Bierman, 1978; Bruce, Deamond, & Ts'o, 1986; Goldstein et al., 1978; Hayflick, 1965; Le Guilly, Simon, Lenoir, & Bourel, 1973; Martin et al., 1970; Schneider & Mitsui, 1976). Additionally, the colony-forming capacity of individual cells has also been reported to decline as a function of donor age (Schneider, 1979; Smith, Pereira-Smith, & Schneider, 1978). While other types of evidence appeared to be consistent with the model, it was the relationship between donor age and proliferative life span that would ultimately be viewed as the evidence lending the strongest support

Unfortunately, these studies were always plagued by large individual variations and relatively low correlations. For example, one large study (Martin, Ogburn, & Sprague, 1981), determined replicative life span in more than 100 cell lines yet obtained a correlation coefficient of only –0.33. Even this low correlation was significant for the sample size examined; however, it was difficult to assess whether the reported negative correlations between donor age and replicative life span were the result of any physiological changes that had occurred in vivo (Martin et al., 1981; Rubin, 1997). Although disease states of the donor were known to affect proliferative life span, only one study evaluated the health of the donors from which the cell lines were established (Goldstein et al., 1978). Other studies include cell lines established from donors that were not screened thoroughly for disease, as well as cell lines derived from cadavers to determine the effects of donor age on proliferative potential in most studies. Undetected diseases as well as variations in the biopsy site have probably influenced the results of most studies.

Studies of rodent skin fibroblasts appear to support the existence of a small, though significant, inverse correlation between donor age and replicative life span (Bruce & Deamond, 1991; Bruce et al., 1986; Pignolo, Masoro, Nichols, Brandt, & Cristofalo, 1992). Furthermore, it has also been observed that treatment of hamster skin fibroblasts with growth promoters can extend the proliferative life of cultures established from young donors but has negligible effects on cultures established from older donors (Deamond & Bruce, 1991). However, even in rodents, the relationship between donor age and proliferative potential is not entirely clear. An examination of hamster skin fibroblast cultures established from the same donors at different ages reveals no age-associated changes in proliferative potential in animals older than 12 months (Bruce & Deamond, 1991).

To address some of these issues, we examined the proliferative potential of 124 human fibroblast cell lines from the Baltimore Longitudinal Study of Aging (BLSA; Cristofalo, Allen, Pignolo, Martin, & Beck, 1998). All of these cell lines were established from donors described as healthy at the time the biopsy was taken, using the criteria of the BLSA. This study revealed no significant change in proliferative potential of cell lines with donor age, nor did we observe a significant difference between fetal and adult-derived cultures (Cristofalo, Allen et al., 1998). In the only other study that determined the health status of the donors, Goldstein and colleagues (Goldstein et al., 1978) also failed to observe a relationship between proliferative life span and donor age in healthy donors, but did observe a relationship with donor age in diabetic donors. In fact, the correlation was so strong in diabetic donors that if they were not screened out of the study, the results were skewed to show an inverse correlation between donor age and proliferative life span in the general population. It has been argued for some time that the relatively low correlations observed between donor age and proliferative life span were the result of large individual variations between the donors examined. It thus seemed reasonable to believe that if cell lines established at different times from the same individual were compared, a stronger correlation between donor age and proliferative capacity could be observed. In order to test this hypothesis, we performed such a longitudinal study by determining the replicative life span of cell lines established from individuals sampled sequentially at different ages. As in the case of the cross-sectional analysis, no relationship between donor age and replicative potential was found in this longitudinal study. Indeed, cell lines established from individuals at older ages frequently exhibited a slightly greater proliferative potential than the cell lines established from the same individuals at younger ages (Cistofalo, Allen et al., 1998).

It is puzzling that no differences existed in proliferative life span in any of the groups compared. In all studies reported to date, the proliferative life span of any given culture is dependent upon the mitotic history of the cells. There is little reason to doubt that at least some of the cells in adults have divided more times than cells in fetal tissues, yet the number of divisions observed in culture in these two groups of cells is similar (Cristofalo, Allen et al., 1998). Large changes occur in skin during aging that leave the aged dermis less cellular, less vascular, its matrix more disorganized, and its collagen content decreased (Bouissou, Pieraggi, & Julian, 1984; Mays, Bishop, & Laurent, 1988; Montagna & Carlisle, 1979; Pieraggi, Julian, & Bouissou, 1984; Shuster, Black, & McVitie, 1975; West, 1994). Yet, cultures established from young and old adults exhibit no difference in growth characteristics or proliferative life span. The probable explanation for this is that the process for establishing cultures results in selection of the most vigorously growing cells. The observed similarity between the proliferative life of cultures derived from young and old adults does not preclude the existence of senescence in vivo, nor does it invalidate senescence as a model of aging (in fact, the use of model was never dependent on the existence of such a relationship). Nevertheless, the discovery is important to understanding the culture model and particularly to interpretation of results obtained with the model. It also demonstrates that the initial selection for vigor when establishing cultures cannot be ignored.

As in most other complex fields of biology, progress in gerontology depends on the thoughtful use and integration of both reductionist models, such as cell culture, and models that test hypotheses in intact tissues, organs, and organisms. The analysis of cell culture systems brings with it some weaknesses, but there are also strengths that complement those studies performed using intact animals and people. The use of diploid cell culture is vital to understanding aging in humans not because the Hayflick system provides an infallible point-by-point analogy to the aging process, but rather because it permits the manipulation of cellular processes (with indisputable involvement in whole animal aging) with a level of control that is impossible with any other model system. Thus, the primary concern with the use of cell culture models, as with any other model system, is to understand and account for limitations of the model when interpreting results.

BIOMARKERS OF CELLULAR AGING IN VITRO AND IN VIVO

A central question to the use of cell culture as an aging model is whether or not senescence occurs in vivo. In addition to the loss of division potential associated with aging in vitro and in vivo, as described earlier, many other significant alterations that occur with senescence in vitro also occur with cellular senescence in vivo. These changes include, but are not limited to, increased ploidy of genetic material, increased cell size, decreased mitogenic response to growth signals (Plisko & Gilchrest, 1983), the decreased expression of genes potentially involved in growth control (Pignolo et al., 1993), the increased expression of genes that help shape the extracellular matrix (Millis et al., 1992), and various changes in cell morphology (Steinhardt, 1985). Early studies by Robbins, Levine, and Eagle (1970) were unable to identify any cells in the skin of older individuals with the fibroblast phenotype, which emerges in vitro. On the other hand, the three-dimensional environment of the cells is obviously different in culture than in vivo and this may have altered the appearance of cells that reached senescence in situ. A comprehensive analysis of senescence in vivo is best performed using specific biochemical or genetic markers of proliferative age rather than reliance on morphological changes. Unfortunately, the discovery of a truly specific marker for senescence (or youth) remains elusive.

One potentially universal marker of aging was reported by Dimri and colleagues (1995) who observed increases in cytochemically detectable β-galactosidase activity (SA β-gal) at pH 6.0 both in cell cultures and in tissue sections obtained from old donors. They also observed that immortal cells exhibited no SA β-gal staining under identical culture conditions (Dimri et al., 1995). Additionally, they interpreted their results as providing a link between replicative senescence and aging in vivo. Their observation appeared to be supported by Pendergrass et al., who reported that SA β-gal positive staining increased as a function of age in rhesus monkeys (Pendergrass et al., 1999). However, the hypothesis remains controversial. Yegorov, Akimov, Hass, Zelenin, and Prudovsky (1998) reported SA β-gal positive cells in quiescent cultures of Swiss 3T3 as well as some types of human cancer cells that were chemically stimulated to differentiate. None of the cell types examined by Yegorov and colleagues (1998) can be classified as senescent. Furthermore, Krishna, Sperker, Fritz, and Klotz (1999) used biochemical analysis to demonstrate that β-gal activity was present at both pH 6.0 and pH 4.5 in a number of different tumor cells. We also examined this phenomenon recently and observed that SA β-gal positive staining was present in subconfluent senescent WI-38 fibroblasts but was essentially absent from subconfluent early passage cells, which supported the conclusion of Dimri et al. (1995). Conversely, we were unable to detect any correlation with donor age either in tissue sections or in skin fibroblast cultures established from donors of different ages. The source of these discrepancies cannot be entirely elucidated; however, it is clear that this type of staining cannot be used as a marker for all types of aging under all conditions and that it is not documented in vivo.

We recently found that EPC-1, a protein that declines with proliferative aging, is present in a mosaic pattern in skin sections. Furthermore, the average length of telomeres, which decreases progressively with increasing numbers of mitoses (Levy et al., 1992) exhibits large variations in multiple subclones established from one individual (Allsopp & Harley, 1995). Both of these observations suggest that loss of proliferative potential in vivo occurs in a mosaic pattern and that both long- and short-lived cells may lie in close proximity in tissues. When cells are placed in a culture environment, the majority of population is derived from the cells in vivo that retain the greatest growth capacity. Hence, the selection during the procedure to establish cultures probably obscures differences in proliferative capacity that exist in vivo.

CELL CULTURE AS A MODEL OF DEVELOPMENT

Although there is no clear relationship between donor age and proliferative life span, a comparison of cell cultures established from fetal and adult tissue reveals that a number of developmental differences are maintained in the culture environment (Allen & Balin, 1988, 1989; Allen et al., 1995; Allen et al., 1997; Furth, Allen, Tresini, Keogh, & Cristofalo, 1997; Keogh et al., 1996). Many of the known differences are related to antioxidant defense. This is interesting because changes in cellular redox environment have been shown to influence pathways important to development and very large changes in redox state are associated with differentiation in a number of cell types (Allen & Balin, 1989; Allen & Tresini, 2000). A number of differences unrelated to antioxidant defenses also exist in fetal and adult tissue (Furth et al., 1997; Karlsson & Paulsson, 1994; Wharton, 1984). For example, both transformed cells and fetal cells produce an autocrine migratory factor that permits invasion of the collagen lattice, but this factor is not produced by adult fibroblasts (Schor, Schor, Grey, & Rushton, 1988; Schor, Schor, Rushton, & Smith, 1985). At present, no systematic comparison of fetal and adult traits retained in cell cultures has been made. Nevertheless, it is clear that some development-associated differences are maintained after the cells are placed in a culture environment.

At least some analogous similarities exist between senescence in fetal fibroblasts and developmental changes that occur in vivo. The expression of the antioxidant enzyme superoxide dismutase (SOD-2) is dramatically higher in adult tissues than in fetal cells, in vivo and this difference is maintained in a culture environment. SOD-2 increases during proliferative senescence of fetal foreskin fibroblasts (Linskens et al., 1995) but no change is observed in fibroblast cultures established from fetal lung (Allen, Tresini, Keogh, Doggett, & Cristofalo, 1999; Linskens et al., 1995). Other antioxidant defenses also exhibit senescence-related changes that parallel differences observed between fetal and adult cells. For example, fetal cells exhibit a large increase in GSH in response to changes in ambient oxygen tension, while the response of early passage adult cells is much smaller (Balin, unpublished). Senescent fetal cells exhibited a diminished GSH response to increased oxidative stress (Allen et al., 1999). It has been observed that addition of PDGF-BB stimulated an increase in mRNA abundance of the transcript encoding PDGF-A chain in fetal and newborn cells; however, the response was greatly diminished in adult cells. The senescence of newborn fibroblasts appears to result in the acquisition of the adult phenotype with diminished responsiveness to PDGF-BB (Karlsson & Paulsson, 1994). The migratory characteristics and growth factor requirements for migration differ between fetal and postnatal cells (Kondo & Yonezawa, 1995; Slayback, Cheung, & Geyer, 1977); fibroblasts from newborns have an intermediate phenotype for production of growth factors and competence factor (Clemmons, 1983; Kondo & Yonezawa, 1995). Some of these differences remain disparate even as these cultures become senescent. As discussed earlier, certain types of fetal cells may be forced to differentiate when placed in a culture environment; however, cells in culture are deprived of the normal signals that direct the sequence of activation of developmental pathways. Differentiation, if it does occur under these conditions, is probably to an aberrant state never observed in vivo.

SUMMARY

Cell cultures have been and continue to be used as heuristic models to examine numerous processes. Through the use of the culture model, cells may be isolated from interference from homeostatic perturbations from other types of cells. This allows isolation of the specific reaction or process of interest. Of course, it may also prevent interactions that maintain a normal phenotype in vivo. It has been known for several decades that "normal" cells placed in a culture environment exhibit a limited capacity to proliferate. The cause of the cessation of division in later-passage cultures is unknown, but environmental as well as genetic factors are believed to play a role in this senescence process. The loss of chromosomal telomeric repeats is believed to be very important to aging in vitro, and overexpression of telomerase has been observed to immortalize cells. The existence of a relationship between donor age and life span has frequently been cited as one justification for use of cellular senescence in aging studies; however, it has been demonstrated that this relationship does not exist when cultures are established from healthy donors. Although this discovery does not invalidate the model, it does alter the way in which data obtained from a senescence model should be interpreted. An understanding of the processes that lead to senescence-associated changes in human cells may aid in understanding the forces that govern human aging. The question of whether senescence actually occurs in vivo has been difficult to address because there are no specific markers for senescence. Some recent advances have been made that suggest the possibility that senescence occurs in a mosaic pattern in vivo. Developmental traits of fetal cells differ from adults in many cases; these differences are maintained when cells are placed in a culture environment.

REFERENCES

Allen, R. G., & Balin, A. K. (1988). Developmental changes in the superoxide dismutase activity of human skin fibroblasts are maintained in vitro and are not caused by oxygen. *Journal of Clinical Investigation, 82,* 731–734.

Allen, R. G., & Balin, A. K. (1989). Oxidative influence on development and differentiation: An overview of a free radical theory of development. *Free Radical Biology and Medicine, 6,* 631–661.

Allen, R. G., Keogh, B. P., Gerhard, G., Pignolo, R., Horton, J., & Cristofalo, V. J. (1995). Expression and regulation of SOD activity in human skin fibroblasts from donors of different ages. *Journal of Cellular Physiology, 165,* 576–587.

Allen, R. G., Keogh, B. P., Tresini, M., Gerhard, G. S., Volker, C., Pignolo, R. J., Horton, J., & Cristofalo, V. J. (1997). Development and age-associated differences in electron transport potential and consequences for oxidant generation. *Journal of Biological Chemistry, 272,* 24805–24812.

Allen, R. G., & Tresini, M. (2000). Oxidative stress and gene regulation. *Free Radical Biology and Medicine, 28,* 463–499.

Allen, R. G., Tresini, M., Keogh, B. P., Doggett, D. L., & Cristofalo, V. J. (1999). Differences in electron transport potential antioxidant defenses and oxidant generation in young and senescent fetal lung fibroblasts (WI-38). *Journal of Cellular Physiology, 180,* 114–122.

Allsopp, R. C., & Harley, C. B. (1995). Evidence for a critical telomere length in senescent human fibroblasts. *Experimental Cell Research, 219,* 130–136.

Allsopp, R. C., Vaziri, H., Patterson, C., Goldstein, S., Younglai, E. V., Futcher, A. B., Greider, C. W., & Harley, C. B. (1992). Telomere length predicts replicative capacity of human fibroblasts. *Proceedings of the National Academy of Sciences, USA, 89,* 10114–10118.

Atadja, P., Wong, H., Garkavtsev, I., Veillette, C., & Riabowol, K. (1995). Increased activity of p53 in senescing fibroblasts. *Proceedings of the National Academy of Sciences, USA, 92,* 8348–8352.

Bayreuther, K., Francz, P. I., Gogol, J., Maier, M., & Meinrath, G. (1991). Differentiation of primary and secondary fibroblasts in cell culture systems. *Mutation Research, 256,* 233–242.

Bayreuther, K., Rodemann, H. P., Hommel, R., Dittamann, K., Albiez, M., & Francz, P. I. (1988). Human skin fibroblasts in vitro differentiate along a terminal cell lineage. *Proceedings of the National Academy of Sciences, USA, 85,* 5112–5116.

Bell, E., Marek, L., Sher, S., Merrill, C., Levinstone, D., & Young, I. (1979). Do diploid fibroblasts in culture age? *International Review of Cytology* (Suppl. 10), 1–9.

Bell, E., Marek, L. F., Levinstone, D. S., Merril, C., Sher, S., & Eden, M. (1978). Loss of division potential in vitro: Aging or differentiation? *Science, 202,* 1158–1163.

Bierman, E. L. (1978). The effects of donor age on the in vitro life span of cultured human arterial smooth-muscle cells. *In Vitro Cellular and Developmental Biology, 14,* 951–955.

Bissonnette, R., Lee, M. J., & Wang, E. (1990). The differentiation process of intestinal epithelial cells is associated with the appearance of statin, a non-proliferation-specific nuclear protein. *Journal of Cell Science, 95* (Pt. 2), 247–254.

Blasco, M. A., Funk, W., Villeponteau, B., & Greider, C. W. (1995). Functional characterization and developmental regulation of mouse telomerase RNA. *Science, 269,* 1267–1270.

Bodnar, A. G., Ouellette, M., Frolkis, M., Holt, S. E., Chiu, C.-P., Morin, G. B., Harley, C. B., Shay, J. W., Lichtsteiner, S., & Wright, W. E. (1998). Extension of life-span by introduction of telomerase into normal human cells. *Science, 279,* 349–352.

Bouissou, H., Pieraggi, M. T., & Julian, M. (1984). Dermis aging. *Pathology Research Practices, 178,* 515–517.

Brown, J. P., Wei, W., & Sedivy, J. M. (1997). Bypass of senescence after disruption of $p^{21CIP/WAF1}$ gene in normal diploid human fibroblasts. *Science, 277,* 831–834.

Brown, W. T. (1990). Genetic diseases of premature aging as models of senescence. In V. J. Cristofalo & M. P. Lawton (Eds.), *Annual Review of Gerontology and Geriatrics* (Vol. 10, pp. 23–52). New York: Springer.

Bruce, S. A., & Deamond, S. F. (1991). Longitudinal study of in vivo wound repair and in vitro cellular senescence of dermal fibroblasts. *Experimental Gerontology, 26,* 17–27.

Bruce, S. A., Deamond, S. F., & Ts'o, P. O. P. (1986). In vitro senescence of Syrian hamster mesenchymal cells of fetal to aged adult origin, inverse relationship between in vivo donor age and in vitro proliferative capacity. *Mechanisms of Ageing and Development, 34,* 151–173.

Burmer, G. C., Zeigler, C. J., & Norwood, T. H. (1982). Evidence for endogenous polypeptide-mediated inhibition of cell-cycle transit in human diploid cells. *Journal of Cell Biology, 94,* 187–192.

Carrel, A., & Burrows, M. T. (1910a). Cultivation of adult tissues and organs outside of the body. *Journal of the American Medical Association, 55,* 1379–1381.

Carrel, A., & Burrows, M. T. (1910b). Cultivation of sarcoma outside of the body. *Journal of the American Medical Association, 55,* 1554.

Carrel, A., & Burrows, M. T. (1911). On the physiochemical regulation of the growth of tissues. *Journal of Experimental Medicine, 13,* 562–570.

Carrel, A., & Ebling, A. H. (1921). Age and multiplication of fibroblasts. *Journal of Experimental Medicine, 34,* 499–523.

Clemmons, D. R. (1983). Age-dependent production of a competent factor by human fibroblasts. *Journal of Cellular Physiology, 114,* 61–67.

Connolly, J. A., Sarabia, V. E., Kelvin, D. J., & Wang, E. (1988). The disappearance of a cyclin-like protein and the appearance of statin is correlated with the onset of differentiation during myogenesis in vitro. *Experimental Cell Research, 174,* 461–471.

Counter, C. M., Avilion, A. A., LeFeuvre, C. E., Stewart, N. G., Greider, C. W., Harley, C. B., & Bacchetti, S. (1992). Telomere shortening associated with chromosome instability is arrested in immortal cells which express telomerase activity. *EMBO Journal, 11,* 1921–1929.

Cristofalo, V. J. (1972). Animal cell cultures as a model for the study of aging. In B. L. Strehler (Ed.), *Advances in gerontological research* (pp. 45–79). New York: Academic Press.

Cristofalo, V. J. (1973). Cellular senescence, factors modulating cell proliferation in vitro. In F. Bourliere, Y. Courtois, A. Maciera-Coelho, & L. Robert (Eds.), *INSERM* (pp. 65–92). Paris: INSERM.

Cristofalo, V. J. (1988). Cellular biomarkers of aging. *Experimental Gerontology, 23,* 297–307.

Cristofalo, V. J., Allen, R. G., Pignolo, R. P., Martin, B. M., & Beck, J. C. (1998). Relationship between donor age and the replicative life spans of human cells in culture: A re-evaluation. *Proceedings of the National Academy of Sciences, USA, 95,* 10614–10619.

Cristofalo, V. J., Palazzo, R., & Charpentier, R. (1980). Limited life span of human diploid fibroblasts in vitro: Metabolic time or replications? In R. C. Adelman, J. Roberts, G. T. Baker, S. I. Baskin, & V. J. Cristofalo

(Eds.), *Neural regulatory mechanisms during aging* (pp. 203–206). New York: Alan Liss.

Cristofalo, V. J., Phillips, P. D., Sorger, T., & Gerhard, G. (1989). Alterations in the responsiveness of senescent cells to growth factors. *Journal of Gerontology, 44,* 55–62.

Cristofalo, V. J., & Pignolo, R. J. (1993). Replicative senescence of human fibroblast-like cells in culture. *Physiological Reviews, 73,* 617–638.

Cristofalo, V. J., & Pignolo, R. J. (1995). Cell culture as a model. In E. J. Masoro (Ed.), *Handbook of physiology—aging* (Vol. 4, pp. 53–82). New York: Oxford University Press.

Cristofalo, V. J., Volker, C., Francis, M. K., & Tresini, M. (1998). Age-dependent modifications of gene expression in human fibroblasts. *Critical Reviews in Eukaryotic Gene Expression, 8,* 43–80.

Danes, B. S. (1971). Progeria: A cell culture study on aging. *Journal of Clinical Investigation, 50,* 2000–2003.

Deamond, S. F., & Bruce, S. A. (1991). Age-related differences in the promoter-induced extension of in vitro proliferative life span of Syrian hamster fibroblasts. *Mechanisms of Ageing and Development, 60,* 143–152.

Dell'Orco, R. T., Mertens, G. B., & Kruze, P. F. (1974). Doubling potential and calendar time of human diploid cells in culture. *Experimental Cell Research, 84,* 363–366.

Dimri, G. P., Lee, X., Basile, G., Acosta, M., Scott, G., Roskelley, C., Medrano, E. E., Linskens, M., Rubelj, I., Pereira-Smith, O., Peacocke, M., & Campisi, J. (1995). A biomarker that identifies senescent human cells in culture and in aging skin in vivo. *Proceedings of the National Academy of Sciences, USA, 92,* 9363–9367.

Drescher-Lincoln, C. K., & Smith, J. R. (1984). Inhibition of DNA synthesis in senescent-proliferating human cybrids is mediated by endogenous proteins. *Experimental Cell Research, 153*(1), 208–217.

Duncan, E. L., Whitaker, N. J., Moy, E. L., & Reddel, R. R. (1993). Assignment of SV40-immortalized cells to more than one complementation group for immortalization. *Experimental Cell Research, 205,* 337–344.

Feng, J., Funk, W. D., Wang, S.-S., Weinrich, S. L., Avilion, A. A., Chiu, C.-C., Adams, R. R., Chang, E., Allsopp, R. C., Yu, J., Le, S., West, M. D., Harley, C. B., Andrews, W. H., Greider, C. W., & Villeponteau, B. (1995). The RNA component of human telomerase. *Science, 269,* 1236–1241.

Ferber, A., Chang, C., Sell, C., Ptasznik, A., Cristofalo, V. J., Hubbard, K., Ozer, H. L., Adamo, M., Roberts, C. T., Jr., & LeRoith, D. (1993). Failure of senescent human fibroblasts to express the insulin-like growth factor-1 gene. *Journal of Biological Chemistry, 268,* 17883–17888.

Frederich, K. B., Phillips, P. D., & Cristofalo, V. J. (1992). Stimulation of

DNA synthesis in senescent human cells following incubation with plasma membranes. *Experimental Cell Research, 202,* 386–390.

Furth, J. J., Allen, R. G., Tresini, M., Keogh, B., & Cristofalo, V. J. (1997). Abundance of a1(I) and a1(III) procollagen and p21 mRNAs in fibroblasts cultured from fetal and postnatal donors. *Mechanisms of Ageing and Development, 97,* 131–142.

Goldstein, S. (1974). Aging in vitro. Growth of cultured cells from the Galapagos tortoise. *Experimental Cell Research, 83,* 297–302.

Goldstein, S., & Harley, C. B. (1979). In vitro studies of age-associated diseases. *Federation Proceedings, 38,* 1862–1867.

Goldstein, S., Littlefield, J. W., & Soeldner, J. S. (1969). Diabetes mellitus and aging: Diminished plating efficiency of cultured human fibroblasts. *Proceedings of the National Academy of Sciences, USA, 64,* 155–160.

Goldstein, S., Moerman, E. J., Jones, R. A., & Baxter, R. C. (1991). Insulin-like growth factor binding protein 3 accumulates to high levels in culture medium of senescent and quiescent human fibroblasts. *Proceedings of the National Academy of Sciences, USA, 88,* 9680–9684.

Goldstein, S., Moerman, E. J., Soeldner, J. S., Gleason, R. E., & Barnett, D. M. (1978). Chronologic and physiologic age affect replicative life-span of fibroblasts from diabetic, prediabetic, and normal donors. *Science, 199,* 781–782.

Gorman, S. D., & Cristofalo, V. J. (1985). Reinitiation of cellular DNA synthesis in BrdU-selected nondividing senescent WI-38 cells by simian virus 40 infection. *Journal of Cellular Physiology, 125,* 122–126.

Hara, E., Smith, R., Parry, D., Tahara, H., Stone, S., & Peters, G. (1996). Regulation of $p16^{CDKN2}$ expression and its implications for cell immortalization and senescence. *Molecular and Cellular Biology, 16,* 859–867.

Hara, E., Tsurui, H., Shinozaki, A., Nakada, S., & Oda, K. (1991). Cooperative effect of antisense-Rb and antisense-p53 oligomers on the extension of life span in human diploid fibroblasts, TIG-1. *Biochemical and Biophysical Research Communications, 179,* 528–534.

Harley, C. B., Shmookler Reis, R. J., & Goldstein, S. (1982). Loss of repetitious DNA in proliferating somatic cells may be due to unequal recombination. *Journal of Theoretical Biology, 94,* 1–12.

Hayflick, L. (1965). The limited in vitro lifetime of human diploid strains. *Experimental Cell Research, 37,* 614–636.

Hayflick, L. (1970). Aging under glass. *Experimental Gerontology, 5,* 291–303.

Hayflick, L. (1977). The cellular basis for biological aging. In C. E. Finch & L. Hayflick (Eds.), *Handbook of the biology of aging* (pp. 159–186). New York: van Nostrand Reinhold.

Hayflick, L., & Moorhead, P. S. (1961). The serial cultivation of human diploid cell strains. *Experimental Cell Research, 25,* 585–621.

Hiyama, K., Ishioka, S., Shirotani, Y., Inai, K., Hiyama, E., Murakami, I.,

Isobe, T., Inamizu, T., & Yamakido, M. (1995). Alterations in telomeric repeat length in lung cancer are associated with loss of heterozygosity in p53 and Rb. *Oncogene, 10,* 937–944.

Kang, M. K., Guo, W., & Park, N. H. (1998). Replicative senescence of normal human oral keratinocytes is associated with the loss of telomerase activity without shortening of telomeres. *Cell Growth and Differentiation, 9,* 85–95.

Karlsson, C., & Paulsson, Y. (1994). Age-related induction of platelet-derived growth factor A-chain mRNA in normal human fibroblasts. *Journal of Cellular Physiology, 158,* 256–262.

Keogh, B. P., Allen, R. G., Pignolo, R., Horton, J., Tresini, M., & Cristofalo, V. J. (1996). Expression of hydrogen peroxide and glutathione metabolizing enzymes in human skin fibroblasts derived from donors of different ages. *Journal of Cellular Physiology, 167,* 512–522.

Kleinsek, D. A. (1989). Selection of mRNAs expressed during cellular senescence in vitro. *Age, 12,* 55–60.

Kondo, H., & Yonezawa, Y. (1995). Fetal-adult phenotype transition, in terms of the serum dependency and growth factor requirements, of human skin fibroblast migration. *Experimental Cell Research, 220,* 501–504.

Kontermann, K., & Bayreuther, K. (1979). The cellular aging of rat fibroblasts in vitro is a differentiation process. *Gerontology, 25,* 261–274.

Krishna, D. R., Sperker, B., Fritz, P., & Klotz, U. (1999). Does pH 6 β-galactosidase activity indicate cell senescence? *Mechanisms of Ageing and Development, 109,* 113–123.

Kumar, S., Millis, A. J. T., & Baglioni, C. (1992). Expression of interleukin 1-inducible genes and production of interleukin 1 by aging human fibroblasts. *Proceedings of the National Academy of Sciences, USA, 89,* 4683–4687.

Le Guilly, Y. L., Simon, M., Lenoir, P., & Bourel, M. (1973). Long-term culture of human adult liver cells: Morphological changes related to in vitro senescence and effect of donor's age on growth potential. *Gerontoglia (Basel), 19,* 303–313.

Levy, M. Z., Allsopp, R. C., Futcher, A. B., Greider, C. W., & Harley, C. B. (1992). Telomere end-replication problem and cell aging. *Journal of Molecular Biology, 225,* 951–960.

Lin, A. W., Barradas, M., Stone, J. C., van Aelst, L., Serrano, M., & Lowe, S. W. (1998). Premature senescence involving p53 and p16 is activated in response to constitutive MEK/MAPK mitogenic signaling. *Genes and Development, 12,* 3008–3019.

Linskens, M. H. K., Fseng, J., Andrews, W. H., Enlow, B. E., Saati, S. M., Tonkin, L. A., Funk, W. D., & Villeponteau, B. (1995). Cataloging altered gene expression in young and senescent cells using enhanced differential display. *Nucleic Acids Research, 23,* 3244–3251.

Lumpkin, C. K., Jr., McClung, J. K., Pereira-Smith, O. M., & Smith, J. R. (1986). Existence of high abundance antiproliferative mRNA's in senescent human diploid fibroblasts. *Science, 232*, 393–395.

Mann, D. M., McKeown-Longo, P. J., & Millis, A. J. (1988). Binding of soluble fibronectin and its subsequent incorporation into the extracellular matrix by early- and late-passage human skin fibroblasts. *Journal of Biological Chemistry, 263*, 2756–2760.

Martin, G. M. (1978). Genetic syndromes in man with potential relevance to pathobiology of aging. In D. Bergsma & D. E. Harrison (Eds.), *Genetic effects on aging* (pp. 5–39). New York: Alan Liss.

Martin, G. M., Ogburn, C. E., & Sprague, C. A. (1981). Effects of age on cell division capacity. In D. Danon, N. W. Shock, & M. Marios (Eds.), *Aging: A challenge to science and society* (Vol. 1, pp. 124–135). Oxford, UK: Oxford University Press.

Martin, G. M., Sprague, C. A., & Epstein, C. J. (1970). Replicative life span of cultivated human cells. *Laboratory Investigation, 23*, 86–92.

Martin, G. M., Sprague, C. A., Norwood, T. H., & Pendergrass, W. R. (1974). Clonal selection, attenuation and differentiation in an in vitro model of hyperplasia. *American Journal of Pathology, 74*, 137–154.

Mathon, N. F., Malcolm, D. S., Harrisingh, M. C., Cheng, L., & Lloyd, A. C. (2001). Lack of replicative senescence in normal rodent glia. *Science, 291*, 872–875.

Matsumura, T., Zerrudo, Z., & Hayflick, L. (1979). Senescent human diploid cells in culture: Survival, DNA synthesis and morphology. *Journal of Gerontology, 34*, 328–334.

Mays, P. K., Bishop, J. E., & Laurent, G. J. (1988). Age-related changes in the proportion of types I and III collagen. *Mechanisms of Ageing and Development, 45*, 203–212.

McFarland, G. A., & Holliday, R. (1994). Retardation of the senescence of cultured human diploid fibroblasts by carnosine. *Experimental Cell Research, 212*, 167–175.

Medcalf, A. S. C., Klein-Szanto, A. J. P., & Cristofalo, V. J. (1996). Expression of ^{P21} is not required for senescence of human fibroblasts. *Cancer Research, 56*, 4582–4585.

Medrano, E. E., Yang, F., Boissy, R., Farooqui, J., Shah, V., Matsumoto, K., Nordlund, J. J., & Park, H. Y. (1994). Terminal differentiation and senescence in the human melanocyte: Repression of tyrosine-phosphorylation of the extracellular signal-regulated kinase 2 selectively defines the two phenotypes. *Molecular Biology of the Cell, 5*, 497–509.

Millis, A. J., Hoyle, M., McCue, H. M., & Martini, H. (1992). Differential expression of metalloproteinase and tissue inhibitor of metalloproteinase genes in aged human fibroblasts. *Experimental Cell Research, 201*, 373–379.

Millis, A. J. T., Sottile, J., Hoyle, M., Mann, D. M., & Diemer, V. (1989). Collagenase production by early- and late-passage cultures of human fibroblasts. *Experimental Gerontology, 24,* 559–575.

Montagna, W., & Carlisle, K. (1979). Structural changes in aging human skin. *Journal of Investigative Dermatology, 73,* 47–53.

Mueller, S. N., Rosen, E. M., & Levine, E. M. (1980). Cellular senescence in a cloned strain of bovine fetal aortic endothelial cells. *Science, 207,* 889–891.

Nehlin, J. O., Hara, E., Kuo, W.-L., Collins, C., & Campisi, J. (1997). Genomic organization, sequence, and chromosome localization of the human helix-loop-helix Id1 gene. *Biochemical and Biophysical Research Communications, 231,* 628–634.

Ning, Y., Weber, J. L., Killary, A. M., Ledbetter, D. H., Smith, J. R., & Pereira-Smith, O. M. (1991). Genetic analysis of indefinite division in human cells: Evidence for a cell senescence-related gene(s) on human chromosome 4. *Proceedings of the National Academy of Sciences, USA, 88,* 5635–5639.

Noble, J. R., Rogan, E. M., Neumann, A. A., Maclean, K., Bryan, T. M., & Reddel, R. R. (1996). Association of extended in vitro proliferative potential with loss of $p16^{INK4}$ expression. *Oncogene, 13,* 1259–1268.

Noda, A., Ning, Y., Venable, S. F., Periera-Smith, O. M., & Smith, J. R. (1994). Cloning of senescent cell-derived inhibitors of DNA synthesis using an expression screen. *Experimental Cell Research, 211,* 90–98.

Norwood, J., Smith, T. M., & Stein, D. S. (1990). Famotidine and hyperpyrexia [letter]. *Annals of Internal Medicine, 112,* 632.

Ohtani, N., Zebedee, Z., Huot, T. J. G., Stinson, J. A., Sugimoto, M., Ohashi, Y., Sharrocks, A. D., Peters, G., & Hara, E. (2001). Opposing effects of Ets and Id proteins on $p16^{INK4a}$ expression during cellular senescence. *Nature, 409,* 1067–1070.

Olashaw, N. E., Kress, E. D., & Cristofalo, V. J. (1983). Thymidine triphosphate synthesis in senescent WI38 cells. Relationship to loss of replicative capacity. *Experimental Cell Research, 149,* 547–554.

Olovnikov, A. M. (1973). A theory of marginotomy. The incomplete copying of template margin in enzymic synthesis of polynucleotides and biological significance of the phenomenon. *Journal of Theoretical Biology, 41,* 181–190.

Olovnikov, A. M. (1996). Telomeres, telomerase, and aging: Origin of the theory. *Experimental Gerontology, 31,* 443–448.

Oshima, J., Campisi, J., Tannock, C. A., & Martin, G. M. (1995). Regulation of *c-fos* expression in senescing Werner syndrome fibroblasts differs from that observed in senescing fibroblasts from normal donors. *Journal of Cellular Physiology, 162,* 277–283.

Ozer, H. L., Banga, S. S., Dasgupta, T., Houghton, J., Hubbard, K., Jha, K.

K., Kim, S. H., Lenahan, M., Pang, Z., Pardinas, J. R., & Patsalis, P. C. (1996). SV40-mediated immortalization of human fibroblasts. *Experimental Gerontology, 31*, 303–310.

Pendergrass, W. R., Angello, J. C., Saulewicz, A. C., & Norwood, T. H. (1991). DNA polymerase alpha and the regulation of entry into S phase in heterokaryons. *Experimental Cell Research, 192*, 426–432.

Pendergrass, W. R., Lane, M. A., Bodkin, N. L., Hansen, B. C., Ingram, D. K., Roth, G. S., Yi, L., Bin, H., & Wolf, N. S. (1999). Cellular proliferation potential during aging and caloric restriction in rhesus monkeys *(Macaca mulatta). Journal of Cellular Physiology, 180*, 123–130.

Pereira-Smith, O. M., Fisher, S. F., & Smith, J. R. (1985). Senescent and quiescent cell inhibitors of DNA synthesis. Membrane-associated proteins. *Experimental Cell Research, 160*, 297–306.

Pereira-Smith, O. M., & Smith, J. R. (1982). Phenotype of low proliferative potential is dominant in hybrids of normal human fibroblasts. *Somatic Cell Genetics, 8*, 731–742.

Pereira-Smith, O. M., & Smith, J. R. (1983). Evidence for the recessive nature of cellular immortality. *Science, 221*, 964–966.

Pereira-Smith, O. M., & Smith, J. R. (1988). Genetic analysis of indefinite division in human cells: Identification of four complementation groups. *Proceedings of the National Academy of Sciences, USA, 85*, 6042–6046.

Pieraggi, M. T., Julian, M., & Bouissou, H. (1984). Fibroblast changes in cutaneous aging. *Virchows Archiv. A. Pathological Anatomy and Histology, 402*, 275–287.

Pignolo, R. J., Cristofalo, V. J., & Rotenberg, M. O. (1993). Senescent WI-38 cells fail to express *EPC-1*, a gene induced by young cells upon entry into the G_0 state. *Journal of Biological Chemistry, 268*, 8949–8957.

Pignolo, R. J., Martin, B. G., Horton, J. H., Kalbach, A. N., & Cristofalo, V. J. (1998). The pathway of cell senescence: WI-38 cells arrest in late G_1 and are unable to traverse the cell cycle from a true G_0 state. *Experimental Gerontology, 33*, 67–80.

Pignolo, R. J., Masoro, E. J., Nichols, W. W., Brandt, C. I., & Cristofalo, V. J. (1992). Skin fibroblasts from aged Fischer 344 rats undergo similar changes in replicative life span but not immortalization with caloric restriction of donors. *Experimental Cell Research, 201*, 16–22.

Pignolo, R. J., Rotenberg, M. O., & Cristofalo, V. J. (1994). Alterations in contact and density-dependent arrest state in senescent WI-38 cells. *In Vitro Cellular and Developmental Biology, 30A*, 471–476.

Plisko, A., & Gilchrest, B. A. (1983). Growth factor responsiveness of cultured human fibroblasts declines with age. *Journal of Gerontology, 38*, 513–518.

Ponten, J. (1973). Aging properties of glia. In F. Bourliere, Y. Courtois,

A. Macieira-Coelho, & L. Robert (Eds.), *INSERM* (pp. 53–64). Paris: INSERM.

Radna, R. L., Caton, Y., Jha, K. K., Kaplan, P., Li, G., Traganos, F., & Ozer, H. L. (1989). Growth of immortal simian virus 40 tsA-transformed human fibroblasts is temperature dependent. *Molecular and Cellular Biology, 9*, 3093–3096.

Rheinwald, J. G., & Green, H. (1975). Serial cultivation of strains of human epidermal keratinocytes: The formation of keratinizing colonies from single cells. *Cell, 6*, 331–343.

Rittling, S. R., Brooks, K. M., Cristofalo, V. J., & Baserga, R. (1986). Expression of cell cycle-dependent genes in young and senescent WI-38 fibroblasts. *Proceedings of the National Academy of Sciences, USA, 83*, 3316–3320.

Robbins, E., Levine, E. M., & Eagle, H. (1970). Morphologic changes accompanying senescence of cultured human diploid cells. *Journal of Experimental Medicine, 131*, 1211–1222.

Rohme, D. (1981). Evidence for a relationship between longevity of mammalian species and life spans of normal fibroblasts in vitro and erythrocytes in vivo. *Proceedings of the National Academy of Sciences, USA, 78*, 5009–5013.

Rubin, H. (1997). Cell aging in vivo and in vitro. *Mechanisms of Ageing and Development, 98*, 1–35.

Rudolph, K. L., Chang, S., Lee, H. W., Blasco, M., Gottlieb, G. J., Greider, C., & DePinho, R. A. (1999). Longevity, stress response, and cancer in aging telomerase-deficient mice. *Cell, 96*, 701–712.

Ryan, J. M., Ostrow, D. G., Breakefield, X. O., Gershon, E. S., & Upchurch, L. (1981). A comparison of the proliferative and replicative life span kinetics of cell cultures derived from monozygotic twins. *In Vitro, 17*, 20–27.

Ryan, P. A., Maher, V. M., & McCormick, J. J. (1994). Failure of infinite life span human cells from different immortality complementation groups to yield finite life span hybrids. *Journal of Cellular Physiology, 159*, 151–160.

Schneider, E. L. (1979). Cell replication and aging: In vitro and in vivo studies. *Federation Proceedings, 38*, 1857–1861.

Schneider, E. L., & Epstein, C. J. (1972). Replication rate and life span of cultured fibroblasts in Down's syndrome. *Proceedings of the Society for Experimental Biology and Medicine, 141*, 1092–1094.

Schneider, E. L., & Mitsui, Y. (1976). The relationship between in vitro cellular aging and in vivo human age. *Proceedings of the National Academy of Sciences, USA, 73*, 3584–3588.

Schor, S. L., Schor, A. M., Grey, A. M., & Rushton, G. (1988). Foetal and cancer patient fibroblasts produce an autocrine migration-stimulating factor not made by normal adult cells. *Journal of Cell Science, 90,* 391–399.

Schor, S. L., Schor, A. M., Rushton, G., & Smith, L. (1985). Adult, foetal and transformed fibroblasts display different migratory phenotypes on collagen gels: Evidence for an isoformic transition during foetal development. *Journal of Cell Science, 73,* 221–234.

Shay, J. W., & Wright, W. E. (2001). Telomeres and telomerase: Implications for cancer and aging. *Radiation Research, 155,* 188–193.

Sherr, C. J., & DePinho, R. A. (2000). Cellular senescence: Mitotic clock or culture shock? *Cell, 102,* 407–410.

Shmookler Reis, R. J., & Goldstein, S. (1980). Loss of reiterated DNA sequences during serial passage of human diploid fibroblasts. *Cell, 21,* 739–749.

Shuster, S., Black, M. M., & McVitie, E. (1975). The influence of age and sex on skin thickness, skin collagen and density. *British Journal of Dermatology, 93,* 639–643.

Slayback, J. R., Cheung, L. W., & Geyer, R. P. (1977). Comparative effects of human platelet growth factor on the growth and morphology of human fetal and adult diploid fibroblasts. *Experimental Cell Research, 110,* 462–466.

Smith, J. R., Pereira-Smith, O. M., & Schneider, E. L. (1978). Colony-size distribution as a measure of in vivo and in vitro aging. *Proceedings of the National Academy of Sciences, USA, 75,* 1353–1356.

Smith, J. R., & Whitney, R. G. (1980). Intraclonal variation in the proliferative potential of human diploid fibroblasts: Stochastic mechanisms for cellular aging. *Science, 207,* 82–84.

Sottile, J., Hoyle, M., & Millis, A. J. (1988). Differential response of early and late passage fibroblasts to collagenase stimulatory factor in conditioned media. *Collagen and Related Research, 8,* 361–374.

Sottile, J., Mann, D. M., Diemer, V., & Millis, A. J. (1989). Regulation of collagenase and collagenase mRNA production in early- and late-passage human diploid fibroblasts. *Journal of Cellular Physiology, 138,* 281–290.

Stein, G. H., & Atkins, L. (1986). Membrane-associated inhibitor of DNA synthesis in senescent human diploid fibroblasts: Characterization and comparison to quiescent cell inhibitor. *Proceedings of the National Academy of Sciences, USA, 83,* 9030–9034.

Stein, G. H., Drullinger, L. F., Robetorye, R. S., Pereira-Smith, O. M., & Smith, J. R. (1991). Senescent cells fail to express *cdc2, cycA,* and *cycB* in response to mitogen stimulation. *Proceedings of the National Academy of Sciences, USA, 88,* 11012–11016.

Stein, G. H., Yanishevsky, R. M., Gordon, L., & Beeson, M. (1982). Carcinogen-transformed human cells are inhibited from entry into S phase by fusion to senescent cells but cells transformed by DNA tumor viruses overcome the inhibition. *Proceedings of the National Academy of Sciences, USA, 79,* 5287–5291.

Steinhardt, M. (1985). Effect of donor age on clonal differentiation of human skin fibroblasts in vitro. *Gerontology, 31,* 27–38.

Sugawara, O., Oshimura, M., Koi, M., Annab, L. A., & Barrett, J. C. (1990). Induction of cellular senescence in immortalized cells by human chromosome 1. *Science, 247,* 707–710.

Tang, D. G., Tokumoto, Y. M., Apperly, J. A., Lloyd, A. C., & Raff, M. C. (2001). Lack of replicative senescence in cultured rat oligodendrocyte precursor cells. *Science, 291,* 868–871.

Tassin, J., Malaise, E., & Courtois, Y. (1979). Human lens cells have an in vitro proliferative capacity inversely proportional to the donor age. *Experimental Cell Research, 123,* 388–392.

Tice, R. R., Schneider, E. L., Kram, D., & Thorne, P. (1979). Cytokinetic analysis of impaired proliferative response of peripheral lymphocytes from aged humans to phytohemagglutinin. *Journal of Experimental Medicine, 149,* 1029–1041.

von Zglinicki, T., Saretzki, G., Döcke, W., & Lotze, C. (1995). Mild hyperoxia shortens telomeres and inhibits proliferation of fibroblasts: A model for senescence? *Experimental Cell Research, 220,* 186–192.

Wainwright, L. J., Middleton, P. G., & Rees, J. L. (1995). Changes in mean telomere length in basal cell carcinomas of the skin. *Genes, Chromosomes and Cancer, 12,* 45–49.

Wang, E. (1989). Statin, a nonproliferation-specific protein, is associated with the nuclear envelope and is heterogeneously distributed in cells leaving quiescent state. *Journal of Cellular Physiology, 140,* 418–426.

Watson, J. D. (1972). Origin of concatemeric T7 DNA. *Nature-New Biology, 239,* 197–201.

West, M. D. (1994). The cellular and molecular biology of skin aging. *Archives of Dermatology, 130,* 87–95.

West, M. D., Shay, J. W., Wright, W. E., & Linskens, M. H. K. (1996). Altered expression of plasminogen activator and plasminogen activator inhibitor during cellular senescence. *Experimental Gerontology, 31,* 175–193.

Wharton, W. (1984). Newborn human skin fibroblasts senesce in vitro without acquiring adult growth factor requirements. *Experimental Cell Research, 154,* 310–314.

Whitaker, N. J., Kidston, E. L., & Reddel, R. R. (1992). Finite life span of hybrids formed by fusion of different simian virus 40-immortalized human cell lines. *Journal of Virology, 66,* 1202–1206.

Wright, W. E., Pereira-Smith, O. M., & Shay, J. W. (1989). Reversible cellular senescence: Implications for immortalization of normal human diploid fibroblasts. *Molecular and Cellular Biology, 9,* 3088–3092.

Wright, W. E., & Shay, J. W. (1992). Telomere positional effects and the regulation of cellular senescence. *Trends in Genetics, 8,* 193–197.

Wright, W. E., & Shay, J. W. (2000). Telomere dynamics in cancer progression and prevention: Fundamental differences in human and mouse telomere biology. *Nature Medicine, 6,* 849–851.

Yegorov, Y. E., Akimov, S. S., Hass, R., Zelenin, A. V., & Prudovsky, I. A. (1998). Endogenous β-galactosidase activity in continuously nonproliferating cells. *Experimental Cell Research, 243,* 207–211.

CHAPTER 6

Cell Death in Aging

ZAHRA ZAKERI
DEPARTMENT OF BIOLOGY
QUEENS COLLEGE AND GRADUATE CENTER
OF THE CITY UNIVERSITY OF NEW YORK

RICHARD A. LOCKSHIN
DEPARTMENT OF BIOLOGICAL SCIENCES
ST. JOHN'S UNIVERSITY

Since the discovery, promulgation, and acceptance of the ideas of programmed cell death and apoptosis, there has been considerable excitement concerning their roles in aging and senescence. Some of this enthusiasm has been misplaced, in the sense that many researchers and clinicians expected to find defects with age in the machinery of cell death. This is generally not the case. Even in the most spectacular instances of cancer, the implementation of death is not altered; what does change is the regulation of that implementation, or the threshold at which the cell-death machinery is activated. This new understanding makes the subject much more intriguing, as we also now recognize that most cell deaths are suicides and that the balance between commitment to life and induction of death is delicate and subject to both internal and social influences. During aging, loss of cells or failure of regulation of loss of cells results in deterioration of immune responsiveness and many forms of neurodegeneration including Alzheimer's disease. In acute circulatory failures including heart attacks and stroke, death of the infarcted cells is neither immediate nor inevitable: appropriate interventions may stave off cell suicide and reduce the amount of damage. Often in viral infections, the virus strives to prevent the death of its host cell while the host cell tries to commit suicide. The balance of these struggles determines whether or not the virus is contained in apoptotic cells and destroyed and whether (as in AIDS) cell suicide itself becomes a serious problem. Finally, some cancers result from reduced cell death rather than increased cell division, whereas others may be attacked by specifically targeting them and invoking the cell-suicide machinery that they possess. As yet unexplored is the possibility that the osteoblast/osteoclast ratio might be maintained by attempting to regulate cell deaths (Manolagas, 2000). Even at the cosmetic level, loss or proliferation of melanocytes (graying and age spots, respectively) may involve questions of cell death (Cline, 1988; Lerner, 1971; Ortonne, 1990; Tobin, Hagen, Botchkareu, & Paus, 1998). Balding is generally considered to be a result of quiescence (telogen phase) rather than the death of hair follicles, but there is considerable apoptosis during the catagen phase (Lindner et al., 1997; Paul, 1998). Thus for all of the major concerns in biological aging cell death is involved, and intervention to adjust for disregulation becomes a part of our therapeutic armamentarium.

TYPES OF CELL DEATH

There are several categories of cell death, identified by different criteria: necrosis or oncosis, programmed cell death, apoptosis (type I apoptosis), and autophagic cell death (type II apoptosis) (Bursch, Ellinger, Gerner, Froehwein, & Schulte-Hermann, 2000; Bursch, Hochegger, Torak, Marian, Ellinger, & Hermann, 2000; Zakeri, Bursch, Tenniswood, & Lockshin, 1995; Zakeri, Quaglino, Latham, & Lockshin, 1993). They were initially distinguished on the basis of morphological criteria, essentially, that some cells swelled and burst while others shrank or fragmented (Kerr, Wyllie, & Curry, 1972; Wyllie, 1993) and the observation that some types of cell death required, surprisingly, synthesis of new proteins (Lockshin, 1969; Tata, 1966). Later, several lines of research documented the relevance of these distinctions by describing biochemical and molecular characteristics of specific types of death. At the same time, recognition that the biochemical and molecular characteristics were not universal gave rise to subclassification of types of cell death. The first category, necrosis, is essentially uncontrolled and will occur if a cell acutely depletes its ATP or is severely physically injured. If it is not already ruptured, calcium enters the cell, which accumulates lactic acid (the result of glycolysis) and osmotically lyses (Trump & Berezesky, 1995, 1998). Its disorganized contents are spilled into the surrounding tissues, provoking an inflammatory response. In contrast to this necrosis, the other types are biologically controlled and may be described as cell suicides.

Necrosis or *oncosis* is a disorganized affair, resulting from acute injury to the cell. It is recognized as a swelling and rounding of the cell and its organelles, especially mitochondria; appearance of calcium deposits in mitochondria; aggregation and precipitation of chromatin in the swollen nucleus; lysis of the cell and other membranes; and production of a hyperemic, inflammatory reaction in the surrounding tissue. The mechanism by which this occurs is effective depletion of energy resources or ability to use ATP, failure of ion pumps, entry of Ca^{++} into mitochondria, and imbibition of water because of the increased oncotic pressure from accumulation of lactic acid (Trump & Berezesky, 1995, 1998). This situation can arise through infarct, toxicity of reactive oxygen species, cytotoxins, severe alterations in pH, or other causes. A cell becomes necrotic without specific synthesis or activation of enzymes. Although it appears in most situations disorganized, there are some situations that suggest a degree of regulation of this type of cell death. As presented for the mutation mec-4 by Driscoll in *C. elegans* (Driscoll, 1992) there may be intermediate types of cell death.

The term *programmed cell death* was originally applied to developmental situations (Lockshin & Williams, 1964, 1965a, 1965b, 1965c, 1965d) and led to the recognition that, at least in development, initiation of death was under genetic control (Ellis, Yuan & Horvitz, 1991). It may take many forms, including both apoptosis and autophagic cell death. In many situations other than development, the machinery for cell death is preestablished in the cell, residing in an inhibited state until released by any of several inducing mechanisms. In embryos or developing animals, cell death is often programmed, in that it requires synthesis of still unidentified proteins, but this is not the case for nondevelopmental situations. The term programmed implies active genetic control of the death. In some instances in embryos and metamorphosing animals, the genetic control is exerted shortly before the cell dies (Wadewitz & Lockshin, 1988). In other instances and frequently in adult organisms, the genetic control is the preconfiguration of the cell such that it is inhibited from activating its death mechanisms, and release from this configuration is an epigenetic affair.

Classical *apoptosis* is a constellation of morphological, biochemical, and molecular changes resulting in a stereotyped death including many of the following: cell shrinkage, condensation, and blebbing; condensation of chromatin, frequently along the nuclear membrane (margination); hydrolysis of DNA between nucleosomes but no further, resulting in fragments differing in size by 180 base pairs, identifiable by electrophoresis in agarose as a "ladder" of fragments (Arends, Morris, & Wyllie, 1990); frequently, depolarization of mitochondria and leakage of some components, including cytochrome c, into the cytoplasm (Ferri, Jacotot, Blanco, Este, & Kroemer, 2000); frequently, activation of specific selective proteases, caspases (so named because they contain the amino acid cysteine at their active site and they cleave proteins only at specific sequences of four amino acids terminating in aspartic acid: *c*ysteinyl *asp*artic acid proteases [Cryns & Yuan, 1998]); exteriorization of a component of the inner side of the cell membrane, phosphatidyl serine, to the external side of the cell membrane

(Fadok et al., 2000; Savill & Fadok, 2000; Schlegel, Callahan, & Williamson, 2000); and recognition of the phosphatidyl serine by phagocytes and phagocytosis of the apoptotic fragments (Hengartner, 2000). This constellation is quite common, though individual components may not be easily detectable, since apoptosis typically occurs in single cells rather than in a large group of cells affected by the same stress, as in necrosis. Furthermore, an individual apoptosis may be carried to completion within an hour or two and, unlike mitosis, there is currently no means of recognizing the past occurrence of an incident of apoptosis. Our understanding of its importance comes heavily from laboratory experiments and our observation of spontaneous or other mutations in members of the apoptosis pathways.

Autophagic cell death may include some of these components but displays far more prominently the formation of autophagic vesicles or regions of cytoplasm sequestered within isolation membranes before fusion with lysosomes and digestion within the cell (Beaulaton & Lockshin, 1977, 1982). Cells with massive cytoplasm, such as mammary epithelium and neurons, frequently display this type of death, with the markers of apoptosis appearing at later stages. Variants of this process have been reported several times (Bursch et al., 2000; Sperandio, DeBelle, & Bredesen, 2000; Xue, Fletcher, & Tolkovsky, 1999; Zakeri et al., 1995). Both apoptosis and autophagic cell death require energy, are under the control of the affected cell and occasionally under the command of other cells, and avoid inflammation. These distinctions are summarized in Table 6.1. The reader should appreciate that these classifications do not have firm borders, as many cell deaths span more than one type. For instance, a cell may initiate apoptosis but fail to complete it and finally lyse in a necrotic fashion. In situations of acute toxicity, the initial cell deaths may be necrotic while later, gravely injured cells undergo apoptosis (Columbano, 1995; Ledda-Columbano et al., 1991). A cell with substantial cytoplasm may start an autophagic cell death and later, when much of the cytoplasm has been destroyed, it will revert to a more apoptotic morphology (Zakeri, Quaglino, Latham, & Lockshin, 1993).

MECHANISMS OF CELL DEATH

What happens during aging and during therapeutic responses to limit damage involves both the implementation of cell death and its control. In the most acute situations (infarct), the primary goal is to prevent the implementation of cell death. In more chronic situations, the control or regulation mechanisms are of greater interest. For all of these, it is necessary to understand how cell death is invoked and effected. The best understood sequences of events have been studied in classical apoptosis

TABLE 6.1 Characteristics of Different Types of Cell Death

Description	Necrosis	Apoptosis	Autophagic
Cell size and shape	Swells, lyses	Shrinks, condenses, blebs	Shrinks, eventually blebs
Chromatin	Disorganized	Condenses along nuclear membrane	Condenses late
DNA	Degrades as smear	Degrades as ladder	No degradation until late, then as ladder
Mitochondria	Depolarize and lyse	Depolarize, leak cyt c and other materials into cytoplasm	Autophagocytosed
Caspases	Not activated	Activated	Not activated?
Phosphatidyl serine	Not exteriorized	Exteriorized	Exteriorized?
Phagocytosis	As inflammatory response	Apoptotic blebs phagocytosed	Fragments phagocytosed at very end

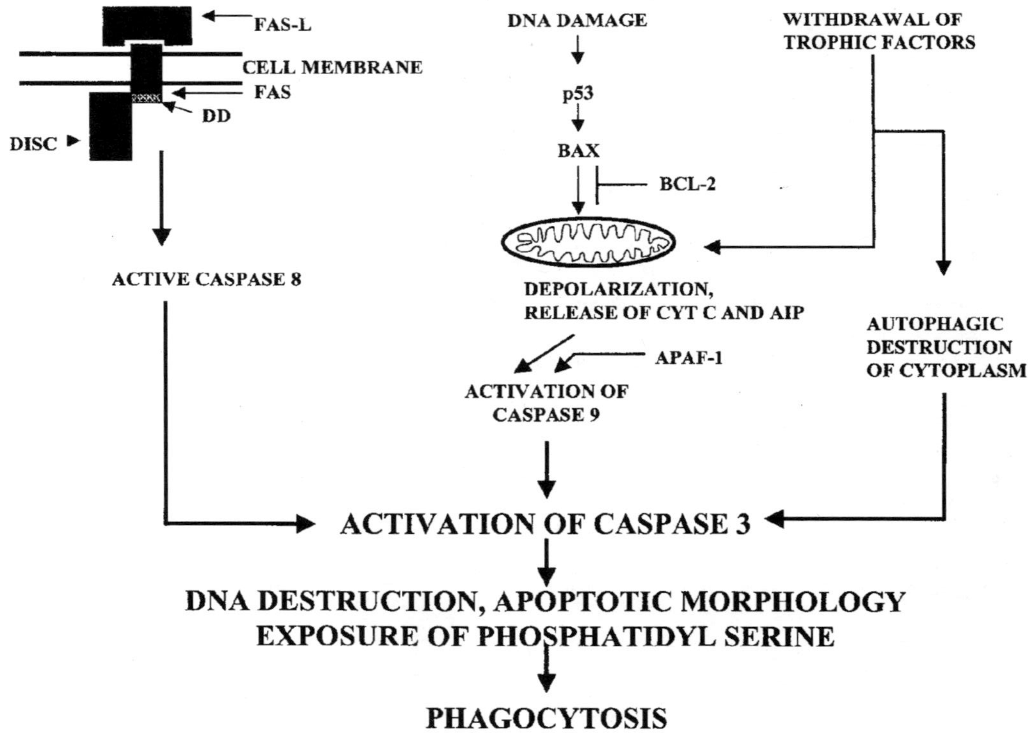

FIGURE 6.1 Major known pathways of apoptosis. Ligands interacting with cell-surface receptors typically activate caspase 8, which in turn activates caspase 3. DNA damage, withdrawal of trophic factors, and other stresses lead to depolarization of mitochondria, release from the mitochondria of cytochrome c, and activation of caspase 9. Caspase 9 activates caspase 3. There are other routes, including caspase-independent routes, which are however poorly understood. DD = death domain, DISC = death-inducing signaling complex, APAF-1 = apoptosis-activating factor 1, AIP = apoptosis-inducing protein or factor.

and are illustrated in Figure 6.1. The reader should appreciate that at the beginning of 2001 there were approximately 30,000 papers on the subject and that the schemes illustrated vastly oversimplify the processes. Many of the steps involve protein complexes of five or more components, and many of the components interact elsewhere in the sequence, resulting in an intricate web of feedback inhibitions, stimulations, and activations. An individual cell may not possess all pathways, and its death will be limited to those available. If one pathway is disrupted, the cell may die by another (Matsumura et al., 2000).

Death Receptors

Particularly in the immune system, in which regulation of populations of different types of cells is a delicate and exquisite affair, cell death can be regulated by the interaction of a cell-surface receptor protein with a ligand either soluble and circulating or attached to another cell. These receptors are structurally similar and are described as members of the tumor necrosis factor (TNF) family (Marsters, Pitti, Sheridan, & Ashkenazi, 1999; Schneider & Tschopp, 2000; Sperandio et al., 2000; Wang & Watanabe, 1999; Wyllie & Golstein, 2001). The ligands include many types of molecules, including some growth factors. Typically, attachment of the ligand to the receptor causes the receptors to aggregate within the cell membrane, allowing activation of a complex attached to the cytoplasmic (usually C-terminal) end of the membrane protein; an example would be Fas.

Fas is a member of a group or family of cell-surface receptor proteins—the death receptor proteins (a subset of the tumor necrosis factor receptor [TNF-R] family)—all of which contain, on the cytoplasmic side, a small sequence of amino acids to which the DISC (death-inducing signaling complex) binds. This sequence, called the death domain, is essential for the transduction of the apoptotic signal (Golstein, 1997; Golstein, Marguet, & DePraetere, 1995a, 1995b; Krammer, 2000; Nagata & Golstein, 1995). The members of this family signal apoptosis by the sequence of ligand binding, trimerization of the receptor and assembly of the DISC, binding of FADD (Fas-associated death domain protein) to the complex, and association of an initiator protease described in the discussion of capsases further on.

The Role of Mitochondria

Several years ago a series of daring experiments, in which nuclei from healthy cells were combined with cytoplasm from apoptotic cells (Lazebnik, Cole, Cooke, Nelson, & Earnshaw, 1993), led to the search for cytoplasmic activators and effectors of apoptosis and eventually to the conclusion that mitochondria played a major role in apoptosis. This conclusion was consistent with other, more directly biological, evidence: Neurons are extremely sensitive to derangements in their energetics or overstimulation (excitotoxicity) (Beal, 1992; Bowling, Schultz, Brown, & Beal, 1993; Parker, Filley, & Parks, 1990; Schapira et al., 1990). Mitochondria are the source of most free radical and reactive oxygen species (ROS) generation, and ROS are known to be destructive to cells through several mechanisms. Apoptosis involves a defense system to prevent ROS from forming (Petit, Susin, Zamzami, Mignotte, & Kroemer, 1996; Skulachev, 1996; Yakes & Van Houten, 1997). Swelling of the mitochondria also releases an apoptosis-inducing protein (possibly a protease) that is normally sequestered in the intermembrane space (Skulachev, 1996). A critical target for ROS seems to be mtDNA (Yakes & Van Houten, 1997). Mutations in mitochondrial DNA-derived cytochrome c oxidase are associated with an increase in late-onset Alzheimer's disease (Wallace, 1992). There is, however, an even more direct role. Mitochondrial involvement is detected even prior to nuclear apoptosis (chromatin condensation and DNA fragmentation) by the loss of the inner mitochondrial transmembrane potential ($\Delta\psi_m$), mediated by the opening of the mitochondrial permeability transition (PT) pores (Hirsch, Marzo, & Kroemer, 1997; Marchetti et al., 1996; Zamzami et al., 1996). Opening of these pores allows the escape of reactive oxygen species, matrix calcium and glutathione, cytochrome c, and several other proteins that affect apoptosis (Ferri et al., 2000; Hirsch et al., 1997). The escape to the cytoplasm of cytochrome c is particularly interesting, as cytoplasmic cytochrome c can activate further steps of apoptosis, as will be discussed in the next section.

There is suggestion that alteration of mitochondria occurs during aging. Mutations in mtDNA are implicated in several neurodegenerative diseases (Alzheimer's disease, for example) (Yakes & Van Houten, 1997). Oxidative stress and damage is postulated to be a major causal factor in the gradual loss of function during aging (Agarwal & Sohal, 1994). Oxidants generated by mitochondria seem to be a major source of the oxidative lesions that accumulate with age. There are several mitochondrial functions that decline with age: (a) Intrinsic rate of proton leakage across the inner mitochondrial membrane; (b) membrane fluidity; (c) decreased level and function of cardiolipin, which supports the function of the proteins in the inner mitochondrial membrane. All of these decrements have been linked to antioxidant defenses, in that free radical and peroxide quenchers can block the decrement, and inhibition of the antioxidant enzymes SOD, catalase, and GSH peroxidase can block mitosis and lead to cell death (Leibovitz & Siegel, 1980; Remacle, Michiels, & Raes, 1992). In summary, there is substantial evidence that apoptosis and several apoptosis-mediated decrements in aging are mediated by the mitochondria and in particular by the mishandling of ROS. Incidental data from several sources suggest that adjustment of antioxidants may help to correct this situation.

Caspases

The field of apoptosis took a giant step forward when one of the genes critical for apoptosis in the nematode worm *Caenorhabditis,* ced-3, was sequenced and proved to be similar to that for the protease interleukin-converting enzyme (ICE) (Yuan, Shaham, Ledoux, Ellis, & Horwitz, 1993). This discovery led to a rapid search among mammalian cells and the discovery of a family of highly specific proteases (the caspase family as defined earlier) that proved to be very important for apoptosis. In many types of apoptosis, several of the morphological changes—and the final commitment to death—are coincident with the activation of caspase 3, which is usually activated as a result of one of two separate cascades involving other caspases. In situations in which apoptosis is induced by interaction of a cell membrane receptor and its ligand, the pathway usually involves the activation of caspase 8, which then activates caspase 3. When initiation of death is brought about by an early depolarization of mitochondria, cytochrome c in the cytoplasm competes with and displaces an Apoptosis Activating Factor (APAF-1) from a sequestering complex, allowing the activation of caspase 9, which then activates caspase 3. Inhibition of caspase 3 can usually block the appearance of apoptotic morphology and, in acute and transient situations, even preserve the cell. For reviews, see Matsumura et al. (2000) and Nicholson (2000). Of course, if the cell is restricted in other fashion, for instance, chronic deprivation of essential trophic factors, it will still die but will not look apoptotic. The appearance of such "zombie" cells has occasionally misled researchers and created false hope of treatments or cures.

Signals for Phagocytosis

At first interpretation, it is not intuitive that a cell should ask to be eaten, yet this appears to be the case. The biological function of apoptosis of damaged cells is that they should be eliminated without inflammation. Thus apoptotic cells (as opposed to necrotic cells) expose an "eat-me" signal that is recognized by phagocytes. The cell membrane is asymmetric, with some molecules exposed only on the cytoplasmic side and others only on the extracellular side. The lipid phosphatidylserine (PS) is normally found only on the cytoplasmic side (Schlegel et al., 2000). At some point during the conversion to apoptotic morphology (the timing is not yet certain) the cell activates a "flipase" and invests energy in exteriorizing PS and perhaps other components. This PS and the other components are readily recognized by phagocytes, which quickly engulf the apoptotic cell or apoptotic fragments (Chung, Gumienny, Hengartner, & Driscoll, 2000; Fadok et al., 2000; Savill & Fadok, 2000; Schlegel et al., 2000). Necrotic cells, which expose far less or no PS, are not nearly so efficiently phagocytosed. The remnants of cells dying by autophagic cell death are phagocytosed, but the exteriorization of PS has not been evaluated in this circumstance (Hengartner, 2000).

CELL DEATH IN AGING

The Immune System

The immune system is born and lives on a constant seesaw of proliferation and death. At its origin in the developing fetus, cells potentially capable of recognizing and reacting to both non-self and self antigens are created by splicing and recombination of their DNA; decisions must be made as to which cells will recognize probable antigens and should be preserved, which recognize self and should be eliminated, and which are probably useless or, at most, excess baggage. Accordingly, the lives of the precursors of both B cells (which make antibodies) and T cells (which defend against altered cells, including those infected with viruses and those mutated and potentially cancerous) are tightly regulated (Budd, 1998; Newell, Haughn, Maroun, & Julius, 1990; Osborne, 1996, 1998). Those that recognize the massive presence of antigens coming presumptively from the host organism (self) are rapidly and aggressively destroyed (negative selection); those that are slightly stimulated and are likely to be useful in the future are preserved (positive selection); and those that do not recognize anything at all are allowed to die (death by neglect). Negative selection operates through the Fas-FasL mechanism, while death by neglect uses routes typified by growth factor withdrawal. In adult life, infections lead to a rapid increase in the number of effector cells (clonal expansion of antibody-producing cells or cytotoxic T cells), but at the resolution of the challenge these cells must be eliminated. Activated T cells are more susceptible to killing than are quiescent T cells. Disruption of the cell-death mechanism leads to disease: Loss of the Fas-FasL mechanism produces autoimmune lymphoproliferative syndrome in humans and lupus-like diseases in mice, while overactivation of bcl-2 produces follicular lymphomas (bcl-B-cell lymphoma). (These cells remain capable of undergoing apoptosis but their threshold for activation of the apoptosis response is considerably raised.) Thus the population of immunocompetent cells remains throughout life the result of competing stimuli for reproduction and apoptosis (Osborne, 1996, 1998).

A number of immune functions decline with age, and there is compelling evidence that cell death plays an important role. Many immune problems develop or increase in frequency with age, including autoimmune disorders (Ginaldi et al., 2000) and increase in CD4+ T cells (Ishimaru et al., 2000) and changes in cell surface recognition molecules (Itzhaki et al., 2000). Changes during aging in apoptosis of polymorphonuclear granulocytes could play a role in the increased incidence of certain immune system–related pathologies of aging such as cancer, infections, and autoimmune disorders. There is less proliferation and also altered frequency of apoptosis in elderly mice, resulting in different ratios of circulating cells and altered responses to challenge (Ginaldi et al., 2000). Increased apoptosis of bone marrow pre-B cells in old mice may contribute to this decline (Kirman et al., 1998). Hyperstimulation increases CD8 T cell apoptosis and decreases apoptosis induced by agonist withdrawal in mice (Telford & Miller, 1999) and humans (Aggarwal, Gollapudi, & Gupta, 1999; Spaulding, Guo, & Effros, 1999a). The time courses are changed, but the intrinsic mechanisms are not (Tortorella, Piazzolla, Spaccavento, Jirillo, & Antonaci, 1999). Caspase 3 and 8 activities are increased (Aggarwal & Gupta, 1999), but some authors attribute T-cell senescence to defective Fas-induced apoptosis (Burgess et al., 1999). In general, cells in older adults are more sluggish in response and more fragile or susceptible to apoptosis. There is a decline in growth factors (Burgess et al., 1999), which is known in cell culture situations to increase susceptibility to apoptosis. An increased expression of functional Fas receptors is associated with increased susceptibility to apoptosis of T lymphocytes in older adult humans (Phelouzat et al., 1997). Overall, there is evidence for decreased proliferation and responsiveness and increased fragility throughout the immune system. Such changes in the dynamics may lead to a state in which an older individual is little better protected than someone with advanced AIDS.

The immediate consequences are a severely increased risk of infection and a higher risk of cancer, both significant problems among the aged population. Changes in susceptibility to apoptosis are part of this situation and are potentially an area for treatment. Lymphoproliferation (lpr) mice that bear a mutation in Fas (present on T lymphocytes) produce excess T lymphocytes, develop autoimmune disease, and are short-lived (Zhou et al., 1995). That caloric restriction extends the life of these mice argues for the involvement of T lymphocyte death in the life span. In normal mice, T cell count and Fas expression decrease with age (Zhou et al., 1995).

Central Nervous System

The central nervous system is defined and sculpted by cell death. The embryo's solution to the problem of how to correctly wire the CNS and the targets of the sensory and motor neurons appears to be to overproduce neurons and allow them to compete for appropriate targets, the latter of which will provide necessary trophic factors or other support. Those that fail to attain these targets—up to half of the neurons in some regions—die. Thus neurons from their origin are heavily dependent on extracellular supports.

Neurons are continually lost throughout life at variable rates. For instance, dopamine neurons in the substantia nigra are lost at 0.5–1% per year (Naoi & Maruyama, 1999). These cells are not typically replaceable, but the impact is often minor. A sufficient loss of cells in the substantia nigra, however, can lead to Parkinson's disease (Forno, 1980). Other examples include the loss of striatal neurons in Huntington's disease (Coyle & Schwarcz, 1976) and motor neurons in amyotrophic lateral sclerosis (ALS, Lou Gehrig's disease). In Alzheimer's disease, neurons are lost from the hippocampus and basal forebrain. They are also lost from this region in epilepsy and stroke (Pulsinelli, 1992; Van Hoesen, Hyman, & Damasio, 1986). Recent findings concerning Alzheimer's disease and the related deteriorations seen in Down's syndrome (Sawa, 1999) indicate an important concept that may be applicable to many other situations in the CNS. Cells in Alzheimer's and Down's syndrome die by apoptosis, with the death showing high regional specificity (West, Kawas, Martin, & Troncoso, 2000) but their apoptosis machinery is not at fault (Yuan & Yankner, 2000). Rather, the neurons are subject to severe stress, including loss of trophic factors (Putcha, Deshmukh, & Johnson, 2000) and accumulation of beta amyloid (Shoji et al., 2000), which may be neurotoxic (Tanzi, 1990). The toxicity of beta amyloid is paralleled by toxicity of other abnormal protein structures in other neurodegenerative diseases: tau in frontotemporal dementia; huntington in Huntington's disease, and alpha-synuclein in Parkinson's disease (Yuan & Yankner, 1999, 2000). In all of these situations the affected neurons agonize, apparently for extended times, before committing to apoptosis. Here, appropriate therapeutic interventions would be to recognize signs of cell stress and to relieve the stress by both removing or inhibiting the toxic element if possible and supporting the stressed cell with neurotrophins or other means of repressing activation of the death domain. For instance, beta amyloid binds to several neuronal receptors as well as to microglia. This interaction triggers signal transduction cascades, from which free radicals are generated, caspases are activated, and calcium enters the cell. The entering calcium can activate other proteases such as calpain. (The generation of free radicals is considered toxic in other neurodegenerative diseases such as ALS.) Efforts are under way to attack each of these several steps, with the goal of ultimately preventing the cell death. The therapeutic requirement will be to target that prevention to the specific cells, avoiding disregulation of apoptosis elsewhere in the body.

Neuronal loss is normally assumed not to be a major part of healthy human aging, though it certainly is in many pathologies. Neuronal loss is perhaps signaled by environmental or other, unknown factors. This loss of significant numbers of neurons leads to dementia. It appears that in the neurodegenerative diseases, cells are placed under stress and activate their cell-death programs. Clinicians would like to identify the signals of cell stress that lead to apoptosis in order to intervene, either to relieve that stress or to fortify the cell to withstand the stress.

An entirely different consideration in neurological disease is the acute situation of ischemia, most often caused by infarct, blood loss, or cardiac insufficiency or failure, all considerations in older adults. In the acute situation, cells are not instantly killed but rather temporize for periods up to a few hours, during which time they can be rescued if the initiation of apoptosis is prevented (Lockshin, Facey, & Zakeri, 2001). Here, immediate intervention at a late and determinative step—the activation of caspase 3—is warranted, with the goal of preventing apoptosis until more favorable conditions can be restored. In experimental models, the approach has been to administer caspase 3 inhibitors, and the results have been dramatic: a 50% decrease in infarct volume in heart and brain, with correspondingly decreased loss of physiological function and increased survival of the experimental animal (Nicholson, 2000) Such experiments suggest that the initial circulatory disaster is not permanently destructive and that there is considerable opportunity during the early stages to reduce the amount of damage. Since this is an acute, urgent, and temporary intervention, there is less concern about disrupting apoptosis elsewhere in the body. Approaches such as these are so promising that they are being moved rapidly to clinical trials.

Cancer

The frequency of many cancers increases with age, ultimately resulting in approximately 30% of deaths in older adults. Although most people consider cancer a disease in which cell division runs amok, it is often a disease of cell death as well. The rate of progression of many tumors correlates inversely with the rate of apoptosis more tightly than it correlates with the rate of mitosis (Thompson, 1995), and indeed, healthy homeostasis requires a precise balance between cell loss and mitosis. Loss of function of proapoptotic genes and gain of function of antiapoptotic genes have both been associated with cancers (Amati, Littlewood, Evan, & Land, 1993; Hermeking & Eick, 1994; Saenz Robles, Symonds, Chen, & Van Dyke, 1994), as will be described.

All humans probably generate one to a few potentially cancerous cells per day, and it is the responsibility of the T cells to recognize and destroy them. Thus many cancers probably arise because a deteriorating immune system shows a lapse in immune surveillance. At the next level, all cells in mammals are designed to immediately initiate apoptosis if they lose either growth factors or other factors associated with intimate contact with appropriate partners. Cancer cells lose this dependency and therefore fail to self-destruct (Benson, Mitchell, & Dix, 1996). Third, some cancers, particularly in the lymphatic system, are in reality population expansions brought about by decreased cell death. In B cell lymphoma, the antiapoptotic factor bcl-2 is constitutively on, and the cells do not die on schedule. Presumably other tumors have similar origins. More generally, several years ago molecular analysis identified a gene coding for a 53 kiloDalton protein, p53, that was mutated in up to 50% of cancers (Hollstein, Sidransky, Vogelstein, & Harris, 1991; Vogelstein & Kinzler, 1992). It was considered a checkpoint protein activated by damaged DNA. If there was sufficient damage (single- or double-strand breaks), p53 would prevent the cell from beginning mitosis. The cell would then have time to repair the damage before dividing and would not replicate defective DNA. Later it became apparent that p53 had a further role. If DNA was damaged in a cell that had already begun to divide, intact p53 could force that cell to undergo apoptosis (Lowe et al., 1994; Lowe, Jacks, Housman, & Ruley, 1994; Lowe & Ruley, 1996). The significance of p53 mutations was not that cells with mutated or lost p53 would not be able to delay mitosis, but that cells with damaged DNA would not be destroyed. They would then pass on the damaged DNA and would contribute to the substantial karyotype variability typical of highly malignant cells. As in other cases, the cells with mutated p53 can still undergo apoptosis, but they cannot respond to the primary signaling mechanism resulting from damaged DNA. Thus failure of apoptosis signaling is a major mechanism for the survival of tumor progenitor cells. As yet there is no evidence that any cancers are caused by direct loss of apoptosis machinery such as caspases. However, better control of apoptosis does appear to be influential. Chronic dietary restriction increases the rate of apoptotic cell death in hepatocytes in middle-aged mice; this increase is associated with a significant decrease in the subsequent development of spontaneous hepatoma in the susceptible B6C3F1 strain and an increased life span potential (Muskhelishvili, Hart, Turturro, & James, 1995; James, Muskhelishvili, Gaylor, Turturro, & Hart, 1998).

Another cancer-associated gene associated with cell death is the retinoblastoma gene Rb (many cases of retinoblastoma derive from a mutation of this gene). Disruption of genes related to Rb leads to loss of G_1 control (Sage et al., 2000). The interaction of p53 and Rb can regulate cell proliferation, cell senescence, and apoptosis in human vascular smooth muscle cells (Muskhelishvili et al., 1995; Bennett, MacDonald, Chan, Boyle, & Weissberg, 1998).

The issue of signaling mechanisms is important for the propagation of cells with abnormal DNA, but it is also a therapeutic consideration. Most therapies for cancer, such as radiation and chemotherapy, are horribly toxic. They act as antimitotics and antimetabolites, damaging any cell with a high mitotic rate or metabolism. These toxicities result in hair loss, nausea and diarrhea, decreased immunological resistance, and neural problems that limit radiation and chemotherapy. Physicians therefore try combined methods, targeting tumors in a cross fire of radiation or using combined therapies, each of which is toxic to the tumor as well as to other organs individually. The goal of the combined therapy is to create a summed toxicity to the tumor while reducing the damage to other organs. A far better approach would be to resuscitate the dormant ability of tumor cells to undergo apoptosis. Such experiments are currently under way. They include efforts to use antibodies or other molecules that are capable of identifying the tumor cells. These would serve as the targeting mechanisms, with linked molecules used to bind, for instance, to Fas and thus activate the apoptosis pathway. Other efforts include studying the biology of the tumor to look for requirements such as growth factors that could be blocked, leading to activation of apoptosis. Currently, this approach is among the most exciting directions for chemotherapy.

Other Evidence for Cell Death in Aging

Similar arguments can be made for other tissues and organs is which regulation of cell death is known to be affected by aging. The rate of proliferation from intestinal crypt cells does not change with age, yet the number of cells in the crypt decreases, suggesting that the rate of apoptosis increases. There is also evidence that the expansion of atherosclerotic plaques results from decreased apoptosis (Bennett et al., 1998). Morphological changes in gingival tissue may be associated with the increase of periodontal disease in aging individuals. There is a significant increase in the number of TUNEL-positive cells in the submucosal connective tissue of the gingival epithelium in mice over 40 weeks old. An increase in the number of TUNEL-positive cells was also found in the submucosal connective tissue of the junctional epithelium in mice over 20 weeks old. This increase in apoptosis explains the decrease in the cellular component of the submucosal connective tissue. However, there are no changes in the epithelial layers of the gingival epithelium or the junctional epithelium (Sakai et al., 1999). Another example of cellular decline with age as a result of apoptosis is reported for the submandibular acinar cells (Liu, Denny, & Denny, 2000). These reports argue that apoptosis occurs normally during aging and that it can also explain the loss of cells.

In the case of insults as part of disease or cellular response to insults, many studies show either increased or decreased sensitivity to cell death depending on the organ, tissue, cell type, and stimulus. For example, after castration there is less cell death in all four lobes of the prostate in old compared to young rats (Banerjee, Banerjee, & Brown, 2000; Liu et al., 2000). By contrast, when mouse hearts are exposed to ischemia followed by reperfusion, the size of infarct is greater in older mice than in younger mice. There are also higher levels of myofiber tears, DNA fragmentation, and mitochondrial disruption (Azhar, Gao, Liu, & Wei, 1999). This and other reports argue for differential regulation of cell sensitivity to the activation of cell death.

Finally, in the most general sense, dietary restriction, which is known to increase longevity, maintains cell turnover and apoptosis at juvenile levels (James et al., 1998).

CELL DEATH IN SENESCENT CELLS

Human diploid fibroblasts have a finite replication capacity in vitro (Hayflick, 1965). This situation has rendered WI-38 and other cell lines a model system for the study of human aging (see chapter 5 in this book for a discussion of the significance of cell senescence to aging). One of the areas of investigation has been the comparison of cell death between senescent cells and their younger counterparts. However, the number of studies is limited.

Cell senescence—a terminal differentiation and ultimate death of cultured cells so that they fail to replicate indefinitely—is a phenomenon distinct from apoptosis. Cell senescence is considered by many to relate to aging, in spite of the fact that with the possible occasional exception of the immune system, most older subjects have not exhausted the replicative potential of those cells that are capable of undergoing mitosis. Cell senescence may limit the potential of cells to grow tumors (Campisi, 2000) and anticancer agents induce growth arrest and a senescent phenotype (Wang, 1997). Several authors consider senescent cells resistant to apoptosis or that they enter a state of antiapoptosis, a hypothesis consistent with their generally depressed metabolic activity (Wang, 1995; Spaulding, Guo, & Effros, 1999b). However, as is the case in the in vivo aging, this does not always hold and is dependent on the analysis and the insult imposed on the cell.

When there is an active cell division in young cells we find also a 2% to 5% cell death during normal culturing. Pignolo and colleagues reported that there is a 50% cell loss at the end of replicative life span or "phase-out."

They attribute this to the fact that the senescent cells have become postmitotic. Furthermore they show that forced increase in the density of senescent cells results in an attrition to the density attained during spontaneous phase-out. This behavior of the cells results in the maintenance of a specific cell density (Pignolo, Rotenberg, & Cristofalo, 1994). That these cells can die indicates that the machinery of cell death is intact and operative in these cells. In several reports, the insult to induce cell death is deprivation (from 10% to 0 or 1%) of serum for several weeks, an artificial situation that an in vivo cell may never see. (Interstitial fluid, the normal environment of a cell not in the vascular system, contains approximately 20% of the protein of plasma. For reticuloendothelial cells that frequently cross from circulation into tissues, the normal environment is less certain. Cells are typically cultured in 10% serum.) We find that with serum deprivation, young and old WI-38 cells lose equivalent numbers of cells for up to 5 days, after which time the old cells sustain higher losses, although a subset of cells remains for up to 4 weeks in both populations. There is also a dramatic loss of mitochondrial potential in old cells as compared to young cells without serum and in old cells even when they are supplemented with serum. However, the cells recover after 72 hours and the levels of mitochondrial function reach that of young and control cells (Davis & Zakeri, in preparation). It appears in this situation that mitochondrial function is not directly correlated with cell death because we see a higher level of cell death after 5 days. However, the transient depolarization of the mitochondria could have contributed to this later cell death. That serum deprivation affects mitochondrial function differentially between young and old cells suggests that the senescent cells have altered their response.

In addition to serum deprivation, we have also found that senescent WI-38 cells are more sensitive than young cells to cell-death inducers such as cycloheximide and tumor necrosis factor, but they manifest sensitivity similar to that of young cells when ceramide and ethanol are used. Furthermore, in all these situations, the old cells die by apoptosis as measured by several markers of apoptosis (Davis & Zakeri, in preparation). Although we find this sensitivity in old WI-38 cells, there are other stresses in which we see no difference in cell death between young and old. For instance, Spaulding and colleagues have reported that when subjected to stress, CD8+ T cells that have reached replicative senescence show reduction of apoptosis in response to stimuli when compared to quiescent early-passage cultures from the same donor (Spaulding et al., 1999b).

These results argue for the hypothesis that senescent cells have the capability to die and in many instances they may be more or less sensitive than their younger counterparts. The fact that they behave differently from the young cells suggests the conclusion that the control of the cell-death machinery rather than the machinery itself has been affected by senescence.

CONCLUSIONS

Cell death is a highly regulated and delicately balanced process. The decision of any cell to die can be grossly estimated in culture, but is in fact a consensus based on many factors in the history and immediate context of the cell. The bulk of evidence to date suggests that in aging the physical machinery of cell death remains intact, but the threshold at which the cell responds to stimuli changes, perhaps because of extrinsic factors such as changes in growth factors or other components of the environment. Since apoptosis is a very important factor in senescence, it behooves us to understand its control and structure. Only then will we be able to adjust the response for therapeutic goals.

ACKNOWLEDGMENTS

This work was supported by grants from the National Institute on Aging, the National Institute for General Medical Sciences, and an IMSD grant to St. John's University from the National Institutes of Health.

REFERENCES

Aggarwal, S., Gollapudi, S., & Gupta, S. (1999). Increased TNF-alpha-induced apoptosis in lymphocytes from aged humans: Changes in TNF-alpha receptor expression and activation of caspases. *Journal of Immunology, 162,* 2154–2161.

Aggarwal, S., & Gupta, S. (1999). Increased activity of caspase 3 and caspase 8 in anti-Fas-induced apoptosis in lymphocytes from ageing humans. *Clinical and Experimental Immunology, 117,* 285–290.

Aggarwal, S., & Sohal, R. S. (1994). DNA oxidative damage and life expectancy in houseflies. *Proceedings of the National Academy of Sciences, USA, 91,* 12332–12335.

Amati, B., Littlewood, T. D., Evan, G. I., & Land, H. (1993). The c-Myc protein induces cell cycle progression and apoptosis through dimerization with Max. *EMBO Journal, 12,* 5083–5087.

Arends, M. J., Morris, R. G., & Wyllie, A. H. (1990). Apoptosis: The role of the endonuclease. *American Journal of Pathology, 136,* 593–608.

Azhar, G., Gao, W., Liu, L., & Wei, J. Y. (1999). Ischemia-reperfusion in the adult mouse heart influence of age. *Experimental Gerontology, 34,* 699–714.

Banerjee, S., Banerjee, P. P., & Brown, T. R. (2000). Castration-induced apoptotic cell death in the Brown Norway rat prostate decreases as a function of age. *Endocrinology, 141,* 821–832.

Beal, M. F. (1992). Does impairment of energy metabolism result in excitotoxic neuronal death in neurodegenerative illnesses? *Annals of Neurology, 31,* 119–130.

Beaulaton, J., & Lockshin, R. A. (1977). Ultrastructural study of the normal degeneration of the intersegmental muscles of *Antheraea polyphemus* and *Manduca sexta* (Insecta, Lepidoptera) with particular reference to cellular autophagy. *Journal of Morphology, 154,* 39–58.

Beaulaton, J., & Lockshin, R. A. (1982). The relation of programmed cell death to development and reproduction: Comparative studies and an attempt at classification. *International Review of Cytology, 29,* 215–235.

Bennett, M. R., MacDonald, K., Chan, S. W., Boyle, J. J., & Weissberg, P. L. (1998). Cooperative interactions between RB and p53 regulate cell proliferation, cell senescence, and apoptosis in human vascular smooth muscle cells from atherosclerotic plaques. *Circulation Research, 82,* 704–712.

Benson, D., Mitchell, N., & Dix, D. (1996). On the role of aging in carcinogenesis. *Mutation Research, 356,* 209–216.

Bowling, A. C., Schulz, J. B., Brown, R. H., Jr., & Beal, M. F. (1993). Superoxide dismutase activity, oxidative damage, and mitochondrial energy metabolism in familial and sporadic amyotrophic lateral sclerosis. *Journal of Neurochemistry, 61,* 2322–2325.

Budd, R. C. (1998). Autoimmunity—A disorder of apoptosis? In R. A. Lockshin, Z. Zakeri, & J. L. Tilly, (Eds.), *When cells die: A comprehensive evaluation of apoptosis and programmed cell death* (pp. 279–288). New York: Wiley-Liss.

Burgess, W., Liu, Q., Zhou, J., Tang, Q., Ozawa, A., Vanhoy, R., Arkins, S., Dantzer, R., & Kelley, K. W. (1999). The immune-endocrine loop during aging: Role of growth hormone and insulin-like growth factor-I. *Neuroimmunomodulation, 6,* 56–68.

Bursch, W., Ellinger, A., Gerner, C., Froehwein, U., & Schulte-Hermann, R. (2000). Programmed cell death (PCD): Apoptosis, autophagic PCD, or others? In Z. Zakeri, R. A. Lockshin, & A. C. Martinez (Eds.), *Mechanisms of cell death II* (pp. 1–12). New York: New York Academy of Sciences.

Bursch, W., Hochegger, K., Torok, L., Marian, B., Ellinger, A., & Hermann, R. S. (2000). Autophagic and apoptotic types of programmed cell death exhibit different fates of cytoskeletal filaments. *Journal of Cell Science, 113* (Pt 7), 1189–1198.

Campisi, J. (2000). Cancer, aging and cellular senescence. *In Vivo, 14,* 183–188.

Chung, S., Gumienny, T. L., Hengartner, M. O., & Driscoll, M. (2000). A common set of engulfment genes mediates removal of both apoptotic and necrotic cell corpses in *C. elegans. Nature Cell Biology, 2,* 931–937.

Cline, D. J. (1988). Changes in hair color. *Dermatologic Clinics, 6,* 295–303.

Columbano, A. (1995). Cell death: Current difficulties in discriminating apoptosis from necrosis in the context of pathological processes in vivo. *Journal of Cellular Biochemistry, 58,* 181–190.

Coyle, J. T., & Schwarcz, R. (1976). Lesion of striatal neurones with kainic acid provides a model for Huntington's chorea. *Nature, 263,* 244–246.

Cryns, V. L., & Yuan, J. Y. (1998). The cutting edge: Caspases in apoptosis and disease. In R. A. Lockshin, Z. Zakeri, & J. L. Tilly (Eds.), *When cells die: A comprehensive evaluation of apoptosis and programmed cell death* (pp. 117–210). New York: Wiley-Liss.

Driscoll, M. (1992). Molecular genetics of cell death in the nematode *Caenorhabditis elegans. Journal of Neurobiology, 23,* 1327–1351.

Ellis, R. E., Yuan, J., & Horvitz, H. R. (1991). Mechanisms and functions of cell death. *Annual Review of Cell Biology, 7,* 663–698.

Fadok, V. A., Bratton, D. L., Rose, D. M., Pearson, A., Ezekewitz, R., A., & Henson, P. M. (2000). A receptor for phosphatidylserine-specific clearance of apoptotic cells. *Nature, 405,* 85–90.

Ferri, K. F., Jacotot, E., Blanco, J., Este, J. A., & Kroemer, G. (2000). Mitochondrial control of cell death induced by HIV-1-encoded proteins. In Z. Zakeri, R. A. Lockshin, & A. C. Martinez (Eds.) *Mechanisms of cell death II* (pp. 149–164). New York: New York Academy of Sciences.

Forno, L. S. (1980). Pathology of Parkinson's disease. In C. D. Marsden & S. Fahn (Eds.), *Movement disorders* (pp. 25–40). London: Butterworths.

Ginaldi, L., De Martinis, M., DiOstilio, A., Marini, L., Loreto, M. F., Corsi, M. P., & Quaglino, D. (2000). Cell proliferation and apoptosis in the immune system in the elderly. *Immunologic Research, 21,* 31–38.

Golstein, P. (1997). Cell death: TRAIL and its receptors. *Current Biology, 7,* R750–R753.

Golstein, P., Marguet, D., & DePraetere, V. (1995a). Fas bridging cell death and cytotoxicity: The reaper connection. *Immunological Reviews, 146,* 45–56.

Golstein, P., Marguet, D., & DePraetere, V. (1995b). Homology between reaper and the cell death domains of Fas and TNFR1. *Cell, 81,* 185–186.

Hayflick, L. (1965). The limited in vitro lifetime of human diploid cell strains. *Experimental Cell Research, 37,* 614–636.

Hengartner, M. O. (2000). The biochemistry of apoptosis. *Nature, 407,* 770–776.

Hermeking, H., & Eick, D. (1994). Mediation of c-Myc-induced apoptosis by p53. *Science, 265,* 2091–2093.

Hirsch, T., Marzo, I., & Kroemer, G. (1997). Role of the mitochondrial permeability transition pore in apoptosis. *Bioscience Reports, 17,* 67–76.

Hollstein, M., Sidransky, D., Vogelstein, B., & Harris, C. C. (1991). p53 mutations in human cancers. *Science, 253,* 49–53.

Ishimaru, N., Yoneda, T., Saegusa, K., Yanagi, K., Haneji, N., Moriyama, K., Saito, I., & Hayashi, Y. (2000). Severe destructive autoimmune lesions with aging in murine Sjogren's syndrome through Fas-mediated apoptosis. *American Journal of Pathology, 156*, 1557–1564.

Itzhaki, O., Skutelsky, E., Kaptzan, T., Siegal, A., Michowitz, M., Sinai, J., Huszar, M., Nafar, S., & Leibovici, J. (2000). Macrophage-recognized molecules of apoptotic cells are expressed at higher levels in AKR lymphoma of aged as compared to young mice. *Advances in Experimental Medicine and Biology, 479*, 251–262.

James, S. J., Muskhelishvili, L., Gaylor, D. W., Turturro, A., & Hart, R. (1998). Upregulation of apoptosis with dietary restriction: Implications for carcinogenesis and aging. *Environmental Health Perspective, 106* (Suppl. 1), 307–312.

Kerr, J. F. R., Wyllie, A. H., & Currie, A. R. (1972). Apoptosis: A basic biological phenomenon with wide-ranging implications in tissue kinetics. *British Journal of Cancer, 26*, 239–257.

Kirman, I., Zhao, K., Wang, Y., Szabo, P., Telford, W., & Weksler, M. E. (1998). Increased apoptosis of bone marrow pre-B cells in old mice associated with their low number. *International Immunology, 10*, 1385–1392.

Krammer, P. H. (2000). CD95's deadly mission in the immune system. *Nature, 407*, 789–795.

Lazebnik, Y. A., Cole, S., Cooke, C. A., Nelson, W. G., & Earnshaw, W. C. (1993). Nuclear events of apoptosis in vitro in cell-free mitotic extracts: A model system for analysis of the active phase of apoptosis. *Journal of Cell Biology, 123*, 7–22.

Ledda-Columbano, G. M., Coni, P., Curto, M., Giacomini, L., Faa, G., Oliverio, S., Piacentini, M., & Columbano, A. (1991). Induction of two different modes of cell death, apoptosis and necrosis, in rat liver after a single dose of thioacetamide. *American Journal of Pathology, 139*, 1099–1109.

Leibovitz, B. E., & Siegel, B. V. (1980). Aspects of free radical reactions in biological systems: Aging. *Journal of Gerontology, 35*, 45–56.

Lerner, A. B. (1971). On the etiology of vitiligo and gray hair. *American Journal of Medicine, 51*, 141–147.

Lindner, G., Botchkarev, V. A., Botchkareva, N. V., Ling, G., Van der Veen, C., & Paus, R. (1997). Analysis of apoptosis during hair follicle regression (catagen). *American Journal of Pathology, 151*, 1601–1617.

Liu, P., Denny, P. A., & Denny, P. (2000). The effect of ageing on parenchymal cell populations in adult female mouse submandibular gland. *Archives of Oral Biology, 45*, 585–592.

Lockshin, R. A. (1969). Programmed cell death. Activation of lysis of a mechanism involving the synthesis of protein. *Journal of Insect Physiology, 15*, 1505–1516.

Lockshin, R. A., Facey, C. O. B., & Zakeri, Z. (2001). Cell death in the heart. *Cardiology Clinics, 19,* 1–12.

Lockshin, R. A., & Williams, C. M. (1964). Programmed cell death. II. Endocrine potentiation of the breakdown of the intersegmental muscles of silkmoths. *Journal of Insect Physiology, 10,* 643–649.

Lockshin, R. A., & Williams, C. M. (1965a). Programmed cell death. V. Cytolytic enzymes in relation to the breakdown of the intersegmental muscles of silkmoths. *Journal of Insect Physiology, 11,* 831–844.

Lockshin, R. A., & Williams, C. M. (1965b). Programmed cell death. IV. The influence of drugs on the breakdown of the intersegmental muscles of silkmoths. *Journal of Insect Physiology, 11,* 803–809.

Lockshin, R. A., & Williams, C. M. (1965c). Programmed cell death. I. Cytology of the degeneration of the intersegmental muscles of the Pernyi silkmoth. *Journal of Insect Physiology, 11,* 123–133.

Lockshin, R. A., & Williams, C. M. (1965d). Programmed cell death. III. Neural control of the breakdown of the intersegmental muscles. *Journal Insect Physiology, 11,* 605–610.

Lowe, S. W., Bodis, S., Bardeesy, N., McClatchey, A., Remington, L., Ruley, H. E., Fisher, D. E., Jacks, T., Pelletier, J., & Housman, D. E. (1994). Apoptosis and the prognostic significance of p53 mutation. *Cold Spring Harbor Symposia on Quantitative Biology, 59,* 419–426.

Lowe, S. W., Jacks, T., Housman, D. E., Ruley, H. E. (1994). Abrogation of oncogene-associated apoptosis allows transformation of p53-deficient cells. *Proceedings of the National Academy of Sciences, USA, 91,* 2026–2030.

Lowe, S. W., & Ruley, H. E. (1996). p53-dependent apoptosis in tumor progression and cancer therapy. In N. J. Holbrook, G. R. Martin, & R. A. Lockshin (Eds.), *Cellular aging and cell death* (pp. 209–234). New York: Wiley-Liss.

Manolagas, S. C. (2000). Birth and death of bone cells: Basic regulatory mechanisms and implications for the pathogenesis and treatment of osteoporosis. *Endocrinology Reviews, 21,* 115–137.

Marchetti, P., Castedo, M., Susin, S. A., Zamzami, N., Hirsch, T., Macho, A., Haeffner, A., Hirsch, F., Geuskens, M., & Kroemer, G. (1996). Mitochondrial permeability transition is a central coordinating event of apoptosis. *Journal of Experimental Medicine, 184,* 1155–1160.

Marsters, S. A., Pitti, R. A., Sheridan, J. P., & Ashkenazi, A. (1999). Control of apoptosis signaling by Apo2 ligand. *Recent Progress in Hormone Research, 54,* 225–234.

Matsumura, H., Shimizu, Y., Ohsawa, Y., Kawahara, A., Uchiyama, Y., & Nagata, S. (2000). Necrotic death pathway in fas receptor signaling. *Journal of Cell Biology, 151,* 1247–1256.

Muskhelishvili, L., Hart, R. W., Turturro, A., & James, S. J. (1995). Age-related changes in the intrinsic rate of apoptosis in livers of diet-restricted and ad libitum-fed B6C3F1 mice. *American Journal of Pathology, 147,* 20–24.

Nagata, S., & Golstein, P. (1995). The Fas death factor. *Science, 267,* 1449–1456.

Naoi, M., & Maruyama, W. (1999). Cell death of dopamine neurons in aging and Parkinson's disease. *Mechanisms of Ageing and Development, 111,* 175–188.

Newell, M. K., Haughn, L. J., Maroun, C. R., & Julius, M. H. (1990). Death of mature T cells by separate ligation of CD4 and the T-cell receptor for antigen. *Nature, 347,* 286–289.

Nicholson, D. W. (2000). From bench to clinic with apoptosis-based therapeutic agents. *Nature, 407,* 810–816.

Ortonne, J. P. (1990). Pigmentary changes of the ageing skin. *British Journal of Dermatology, 11,* (Suppl) 35, 21–28.

Osborne, B. A. (1996). Apoptosis and the maintenance of homoeostasis in the immune system. *Current Opinions in Immunology, 8,* 245–254.

Osborne, B. A. (1998). Apoptotic signaling in lymphocytes. In R. A. Lockshin, Z. Zakeri, & J. L. Tilly (Eds.), *When cells die: A comprehensive evaluation of apoptosis and programmed cell death* (pp. 245–166). New York: Wiley-Liss.

Parker, W. D., Jr., Filley, C. M., & Parks, J. K. (1990). Cytochrome oxidase deficiency in Alzheimer's disease. *Neurology, 40,* 1302–1303.

Pau, R. (1998). Principles of hair cycle control. *Journal of Dermatology, 25,* 793–802.

Petit, P. X., Susin, S. A., Zamzami, N., Mignotte, B., & Kroemer, G. (1996). Mitochondria and programmed cell death: Back to the future. *FEBS Letters, 396,* 7–13.

Phelouzat, M. A., LaForge, T., Arbogast, A., Quadri, R. A., Boutet, S., & Proust, J. J. (1997). Susceptibility to apoptosis of T lymphocytes from elderly humans is associated with increased in vivo expression of functional Fas receptors. *Mechanisms of Ageing and Development, 96,* 35–46.

Pignolo, R. J., Rotenberg, M. O., & Cristofalo, V. J. (1994). Alterations in contact and density-dependent arrest state in senescent WI-38 cells. *In Vitro Cellular Development and Biology, 30A,* 471–476.

Pulsinelli, W. (1992). Pathophysiology of acute ischaemic stroke. *Lancet, 339,* 533–536.

Putcha, G. V., Deshmukh, M., & Johnson, E. M., Jr. (2000). Inhibition of apoptotic signaling cascades causes loss of trophic factor dependence during neuronal maturation. *Journal of Cellular Biology, 149,* 1011–1018.

Remacle, J., Michiels, C., & Raes, M. (1992). The importance of antioxidant enzymes in cellular aging and degeneration. *EXS, 62,* 99–108.

Saenz Robles, M. T., Symonds, H., Chen, J., & Van Dyke, T. (1994). Induction versus progression of brain tumor development: Differential functions for the pRB- and p53-targeting domains of simian virus 40 T antigen. *Molecular Cell Biology, 14,* 2686–2698.

Sage, J., Mulligan, G. J., Attardi, L. D., Miller, A., Chen, S., Williams, B., Theodorou, E., & Jacks, T. (2000). Targeted disruption of the three Rb-related genes leads to loss of G(1) control and immortalization. *Genes Development, 14,* 3037–3050.

Sakai, T., Kiyoshima, T., Kobayashi, I., Moroi, R., Ibuki, T., Nagadome, M., Terada, Y., & Sakai, H. (1999). Age-dependent changes in the distribution of BrdU- and TUNEL-positive cells in the murine gingival tissue. *Journal of Periodontology, 70,* 973–981.

Savill, J., & Fadok, V. (2000). Corpse clearance defines the meaning of cell death. *Nature, 407,* 784–788.

Sawa, A. (1999). Neuronal cell death in Down's syndrome. *Journal of Neural Transmission* (Suppl) *57,* 87–97.

Schapira, A. H., Mann, V. M., Cooper, J. M., Dexter, D., Daniel, S. E., Jenner, P., Clark, J. B., & Marsden, C. D. (1990). Anatomic and disease specificity of NADH CoQ1 reductase (complex I) deficiency in Parkinson's disease. *Journal of Neurochemistry , 55,* 2142–2145.

Schlegel, R. A., Callahan, M. K., & Williamson, P. (2000). The central role of phosphatidylserine in the phagocytosis of apoptotic thymocytes. In Z. Zakeri, R. A. Lockshin, & A. C. Martinez. (Eds.), *Mechanisms of cell death II* (pp. 217–225). New York: New York Academy of Sciences.

Schneider, P., & Tschopp, J. (2000). Apoptosis induced by death receptors. *Pharmaceutica Acta Helvetiae, 74* 281–286.

Shoji, M., Kawarabayashi, T., Sato, M., Sasaki, A., Saido, T. C., Matsubara, E., Tomidokoro, Y., Kanai, M., Shizuka, M., Ishiguro, K., Ideda, M., Harigaya, Y., Okamoto, K., & Hirai, S. (2000). Age-related amyloid beta protein accumulation induces cellular death and macrophage activation in transgenic mice. *Journal of Pathology, 191,* 93–101.

Skulachev, V. P. (1996). Why are mitochondria involved in apoptosis? Permeability transition pores and apoptosis as selective mechanisms to eliminate superoxide-producing mitochondria and cell. *FEBS Letters, 397,* 7–10.

Spaulding, C., Guo, W., & Effros, R. B. (1999a). Resistance to apoptosis in human CD8+ T cells that reach replicative senescence after multiple rounds of antigen-specific proliferation. *Experimental Gerontology, 34,* 633–644.

Spaulding, C., Guo, W., & Effros, R. B. (1999b). Resistance to apoptosis in human CD8+ T cells that reach replicative senescence after multiple rounds of antigen-specific proliferation. *Experimental Gerontology, 34,* 633–644.

Sperandio, S., De Belle, I., & Bredesen, D. E. (2000). An alternative, non-apoptotic form of programmed cell death. *Proceedings of the National Academy of Sciences, USA, 97,* 14376–14381.

Tanzi, R. E. (1990). The Alzheimer's disease-associated amyloid beta protein precursor gene and familial Alzheimer disease. *Progress in Clinical Biology Research, 360,* 187–199.

Tata, J. R. (1966). Requirement for RNA and protein synthesis for induced regression of tadpole tail in organ culture. *Developmental Biology, 13,* 77–94.

Telford, W. G., & Miller, R. A. (1999). Aging increases CD8 T cell apoptosis induced by hyperstimulation but decreases apoptosis induced by agonist withdrawal in mice. *Cell Immunology, 191,* 131–138.

Thompson, C. B. (1995). Apoptosis in the pathogenesis and treatment of disease. *Science, 267,* 1456–1462.

Tobin, D. J., Hagen, E., Botchkarev, V. A., & Paus, R. (1998). Do hair bulb melanocytes undergo apoptosis during hair follicle regression (catagen)? *Journal of Investigative Dermatology, 111,* 941–947.

Tortorella, C., Piazzolla, G., Spaccavento, F., Jirillo, E., & Antonaci, S. (1999). Age-related effects of oxidative metabolism and cyclic AMP signaling on neutrophil apoptosis. *Mechanisms of Ageing and Development, 110,* 195–205.

Trump, B. F., & Berezesky, I. K. (1995). Calcium-mediated cell injury and cell death. *FASEB Journal, 9,* 219–228.

Trump, B. F., & Berezesky, I. K. (1998). The reactions of cells to lethal injury: Oncosis and necrosis—the role of calcium. In R. A. Lockshin, Z. Zakeri, & J. L. Tilly (Eds.), *When cells die: A comprehensive evaluation of apoptosis and programmed cell death* (pp. 57–96). New York: Wiley-Liss.

Van Hoesen, G. W., Hyman, B. T., & Damasio, A. R. (1986). Cell-specific pathology in neural systems of the temporal lobe in Alzheimer's disease. *Progress in Brain Research, 70,* 321–335.

Vogelstein, B., & Kinzler, K. W. (1992). p53 function and dysfunction. *Cell, 70,* 523–526.

Wadewitz, A. G., & Lockshin, R. A. (1988). Programmed cell death. Dying cells synthesize a coordinated unique set of proteins in two different episodes of cell death. *FEBS Letters, 241,* 19–23.

Wallace, D. C. (1992). Mitochondrial genetics: A paradigm for aging and degenerative diseases? *Science, 256,* 628–632.

Wang, E. (1995). Senescent human fibroblasts resist programmed cell death, and failure to suppress bcl2 is involved. *Cancer Research, 55,* 2284–2292.

Wang, E. (1997). Regulation of apoptosis resistance and ontogeny of age-dependent diseases. *Experimental Gerontology, 32,* 471–484.

Wang, J., & Watanabe, T. (1999). Expression and function of Fas during differentiation and activation of B cells. *International Review in Immunology, 18,* 367–379.

West, M. J., Kawas, C. H., Martin, L. J., & Troncosco, J. C. (2000). The CA1 region of the human hippocampus is a hot spot in Alzheimer's disease. *Annals of the New York Academy of Sciences, 908,* 255–259.

Wyllie, A. H. (1993). Apoptosis (The 1992 Frank Rose Memorial Lecture). *British Journal of Cancer, 67,* 205–208.

Wyllie, A. H., & Golstein, P. (2001). More than one way to go. *Proceedings of the National Academy of Sciences, USA, 98,* 11–13.

Xue, L., Fletcher, G. C., & Tolkovsky, A. M. (1999). Autophagy is activated by apoptotic signalling in sympathetic neurons: An alternative mechanism of death execution. *Molecular and Cellular Neuroscience, 14,* 180–198.

Yakes, F. M., & Van Houten, B. (1997). Mitochondrial DNA damage is more extensive and persists longer than nuclear DNA damage in human cells following oxidative stress. *Proceedings of the National Academy of Sciences, USA, 94,* 514–519.

Yuan, J., Shaham, S., Ledoux, S., Ellis, H. M., & Horvitz, H. R. (1993). The *C. elegans* cell death gene *ced-3* encodes a protein similar to mammalian interleukin-1b-converting enzyme. *Cell, 75,* 641–652.

Yuan, J., & Yankner, B. A. (1999). Caspase activity sows the seeds of neuronal death [news]. *Natural Cell Biology, 1,* E44–E45.

Yuan, J., & Yankner, B. A. (2000). Apoptosis in the nervous system. *Nature, 407,* 802–809.

Zakeri, Z., Bursch, W., Tenniswood, M., & Lockshin, R. A. (1995). Cell death. Programmed, apoptosis, necrosis, or other? *Cell Death Differentiation, 2,* 87–96.

Zakeri, Z. F., Quaglino, D., Latham, T., & Lockshin, R. A. (1993). Delayed internucleosomal DNA fragmentation in programmed cell death. *FASEB Journal, 7,* 470–478.

Zamzami, N., Susin, S. A., Marchetti, P., Hirsch, T., Gomez-Monterrey, I., Castedo, M., & Kroemer, G. (1996). Mitochondrial control of nuclear apoptosis. *Journal of Experimental Medicine, 183,* 1533–1544.

Zhou, T., Edwards, C. K., III, & Mountz, J. D. (1995). Prevention of age-related T cell apoptosis defect in CD2-fas-transgenic mice. *Journal of Experimental Medicine, 182,* 129–137.

CHAPTER 7

Models in Aging Research: A Critical Assessment

HARRIET GERSHON
DEPARTMENT OF IMMUNOLOGY
RAPPAPORT FACULTY OF MEDICINE

DAVID GERSHON
FACULTY OF BIOLOGY
TECHNION-ISRAEL INSTITUTE OF TECHNOLOGY
HAIFA, ISRAEL

CHOOSING AN APPROPRIATE MODEL FOR GERONTOLOGICAL RESEARCH

Interest in the study of the phenomenon of aging has flourished in the last two decades with the advent of new research methodology in developmental and cellular biology and molecular genetics. The demand for accelerating the pace of research has led to a search for relatively simple experimental models that can provide rapid results. It is important at present to critically review some of the current models used in biological gerontology research and evaluate their contribution to advancing our understanding of senescence.

Aging in Biological Terms

Biological aging is characterized by a gradual decline in the capacity to respond to environmental challenges. When this decline reaches a certain threshold, the survival capacity of the organism is compromised. Gradual changes in the structure and function of the organism that are not due to curable disease or random accidents lead to an increased probability of death as a function of time.

Primary Factors of Aging Versus Secondary Age-associated Phenomena

To avoid confusion between primary causes of aging and secondary age-associated phenomena, Strehler has suggested criteria for identifying underlying mechanisms that lead to age-related changes (Strehler, 1977). We suggest that there are four criteria (the first three adopted from Strehler) for primary age-correlated alterations.

1. *Intraspecies universality:* For a process or phenomenon to be considered fundamental to aging it must be observed in all the older members of the species. The age at which these basic senescence phenomena are expressed can vary, within certain limits, among individuals in any given population. This criterion does not exclude the possibility that the increased propensity to develop diseases in older organisms is due to basic underlying mechanisms of senescence. It does however exclude specific (and quite rare) life-shortening genetic defects or diseases that are caused by special, drastic environmental conditions.
2. *Intrinsicality:* Basic aging mechanisms are innate to the organism and not fully dependent upon modifiable environmental effects.
3. *Progressiveness:* Aging is a gradual process and not the result of sudden events. It commences relatively early in life and progresses as the cumulative effect of small steps. A large number of small interrelated events must take place in order to reach such a complex phenomenon as aging and mortality. This gives the total process a seemingly gradual smoothness.
4. *Interspecies universality and relevance to human aging:* The choice of any paradigm that is not human should take into account a basic premise that some of the most fundamental aging mechanisms are common to all eukaryotes. Care must be taken to avoid making global conclusions from the study of certain peculiar species-specific causes of death, for example, the endocrinologically based programmed death of the Pacific salmon or the rainbow trout (Robertson & Wexler, 1959; Robertson et al., 1961) or the programmed senescence and death of annual plants.

Because it is not possible to extensively review the multitude of theories associated with aging, the reader is referred to the *Handbook of Theories of Aging* (Bengtson & Schaie, 1999) and reviews (Cristofalo, Tresini, Francis, & Volker, 1999; Finch & Seeman, 1999; Solomon, 1999). However, the salient theories of aging can be broadly classified into two main categories.

1. *Programmed aging* implies a built-in program in the genome that when activated at a certain stage of the life cycle leads to death. Such theories

suggest evolutionary selection for genes that specify the onset and progression of senescence leading to morbidity and consequently to mortality. Two major hypotheses can be tested with regard to this group of theories.

(a) A program exists that controls the activation of a cascade of genes whose function is to implement senescence. This implies that interference with the activity of any gene belonging to this chain, particularly via mutation, will modulate the life span of the organism. This gene modification should have a minimal effect on other functions such as the development and fecundity of the organism.
(b) Genes have emerged in the course of evolution that perform an essential early function during either the developmental or reproductive stages of the life cycle and whose continued activity in the postreproductive stage is detrimental (see Cristofalo et al., 1999). Alterations in these genes should then affect the development and/or reproduction of the organism.

2. *Aging as a result of stochastic events* postulates that senescence is a result of random damage that is incurred and accumulates throughout the life span. The damage, caused by environmental factors, affects innate mechanisms that are essential for metabolism, signal transduction, intercellular communication, and response to various forms of stress. Such damage causes gradual reduction in efficiency of overall function and eventually results in death.

The alternative theories can be evaluated by the use of well-chosen experimental paradigms. It is imperative, however, that the limitations and merits of the selected paradigm be taken into account prior to the evaluation of experimental results.

Criteria for Choosing a Model

The purpose of experimental paradigms is to test and evaluate existing theories that attempt to explain the causes and underlying mechanisms of observed phenomena. Because aging is a complex phenotype, it has to be dissected into components. A variety of experimentally suitable models should be used to investigate each component separately.

Biological phenomena are comprised of interrelated pathways that are often controlled by complex mechanisms, so observations must be interpreted in the broad context of the process of senescence. Each system should be examined at all levels of organization, from molecules and genes to tissues, organs, and ultimately the whole organism. In addition, the interaction of the organism with its environment in its natural habitat must be considered in the selection and evaluation of any particular experimental paradigm.

The specific requirements of a model are as follows:

1. The model should be simple and suitable for experimental manipulation. Knowledge of the developmental program of the organism may be an important factor in the selection of the model system.

2. Laboratory conditions under which the organism (or cell culture) is kept should mimic as accurately as possible the prevailing conditions in its natural habitat. Parameters to be considered here include nutrition, temperature, humidity, oxygen tension, photoperiodism and population density. Possible exposure to viruses, bacteria, and other invasive organisms in the natural habitat ought to be taken into account also. All of these conditions are variable and oscillating in the natural habitat, and survival depends upon adaptability of the organism. The artificial laboratory conditions used in order to achieve high fecundity and optimal welfare of laboratory organisms include "unnatural" nutrition, constant temperature and humidity, and for certain models improper oxygen tension, inappropriate photoperiodism, and population density. These present very artificial living conditions for most experimental organisms.

3. Consideration should also be given to the fact that some of our most widely used models *(C. elegans)* have undergone thousands or hundreds (rodent strains) of generations of breeding under ad libitum feeding conditions on diets entirely foreign to those encountered in the natural environment (for example, the feeding of *C. elegans* with *E. coli*, an alien microorganism with the mandatory addition of cholesterol instead of plant sterols).

On the assumption that the ultimate goal of our gerontological research is the understanding of human aging, it behooves us to evaluate, at least theoretically, the relevance of the model system to mammals in general and humans in particular. Caution should be exercised in extrapolating results and their interpretation from lower to higher eukaryotes.

THE BUDDING YEAST AS A MODEL ORGANISM

The unicellular eukaryotic budding yeast *(Saccharomyces cerevisiae)* has a relatively uncomplicated and short life cycle. *S. cerevisiae* has a small, completely sequenced and extensively mapped genome (Goffeau et al., 1996). This organism lends itself to the use of molecular genetic tools that have contributed significantly to the understanding of some of the major processes in cell biology such as signal transduction (Whitmarsh & Davis,

1998); control of cell cycle progression and the basis of the switch from mitosis to meiosis (Nasmyth, 1996); genetic recombination (Stahl, 1996); intracellular trafficking of proteins (Kim, Schilke, Craig, & Horwitz, 1998); response to stress (for example, heat shock genes) (Glover & Lindquist, 1998), and protein degradation (Xie & Varshavsky, 1999).

Yeasts are cheap to grow in large quantities on simple medium. They can be plated as single cells and observed for clonal growth and can be separated from progeny cells by micromanipulation. Yeasts can be manipulated genetically with ease. They have a well-developed system of homologous recombination and lend themselves to relatively simple knockout of individual genes. They can also be maintained and studied in the haploid state. The authors published a detailed review of the yeast model (see Gershon & Gershon, 2000a).

The budding yeast *Saccharomyces cerevisiae* and the fission yeast *Schizosaccharomyces pombe* have been widely studied. The former has also been used extensively in aging research. Both species can proliferate in the haploid and diploid states. As long as nutrients are abundant, proliferation in the diploid state takes place. Upon starvation, they undergo meiosis and spore formation. With improvement of nutritional conditions these haploid progeny germinate and start propagating. Under conditions of deprivation, spores can survive for enormously long periods of time in proportion to the length of the cell cycle (months vs. hours).

The budding yeast, and perhaps the fission yeast (Barker & Walmsley, 1999), divides asymmetrically to form a "mother" cell and a bud. The asymmetric division entails programmed unequal distribution of a transcription repressor that is localized specifically in the bud (O'Shea and Herskowitz, 2000).

Methodology: Observing Time-Dependent Changes in Yeast Cells

Two major approaches have been used to determine "senescence" and "life span" in yeast: budding and the stationary phase.

1. *Budding Life Span:* Mortimer and Johnston first measured the rate of bud production from single cells by observing individual cells and separation of mothers from progeny buds (Mortimer & Johnston, 1959). The number of buds produced by a cell was determined to be finite, with the last two to three rounds of budding of longer duration after which the cell ceases to divide. Nondividing cells eventually die (*vide infra* for a discussion of the validity of this evidence). The number of buds produced by a cell varies considerably depending on genotype, nutritional conditions and perhaps temperature.

Studies by Jazwinski and Guarente (Kennedy, Austriaco, & Guarente, 1994; Kim, Kirchman, Benguria, & Jazwinski) use the method of Mortimer and Johnston (1959) to observe the budding capacity of individual cells as a function of time in culture. In this approach, the finite number of buds produced by a mother cell is determined and is designated the "budding life span." Overcrowding, which may drive the cells into stationary state (Werner-Washburne, Braun, Crawford, & Peck, 1996), must be prevented by separating each "daughter" cell from the mother cell by micromanipulation.

Death verification is not always the endpoint, but rather it is implicitly accepted that postmitotic cells are dead cells. It is quite possible that a fraction of these cells are quiescent rather than dead. A similar problem (and misconception) of equating a postmitotic cell to a dead cell prevails in the studies of in vitro cell cultures of vertebrates.

What does "budding life span" mean in the context of "chronological life span"? Does the finite number of buds a mother cell produces have any relation to its chronological age? It has been reported that daughter cells of both old and young mother cells have the same reproductive capacity (Egilmez & Jazwinski, 1989) and conversely that "maternal" age affects the fecundity of daughter cells (Kennedy et al., 1994). This controversial point is particularly relevant since it has become obvious that mammalian cells in culture do not exhibit a correlation between donor age and number of population doublings (Cristofalo, Allen, Pignolo, Martin, & Peck, 1998).

2. *Stationary Phase:* In this model, whole populations are maintained in liquid medium until cell number reaches a plateau (Longo, 1999). The cells are then maintained for an additional period on either the expired medium or distilled water (Liou et al., 2000). Viability is determined by the ability of individual cells plated from aliquots removed periodically from the cultures to form colonies on agar plates. Viability is also verified by other techniques including estimation of the percentage of cells that are metabolically active (Longo, 1999). Taken together these essential criteria, which are not considered in the budding system, are more relevant to the determination of life span than just the determination of the budding capacity used in the individually plated cells of the budding life span method.

Cells initially grow rapidly in glucose-rich medium and energy production is primarily derived from fermentation. When the glucose in the medium is depleted, growth slows down, mitochondria begin to use stored substrates, there is a switch from fermentation to mitochondrial respiration, and the cells enter a stationary phase. Cells maintained in the expired medium show increased mortality attributed primarily to the production of reactive oxygen species generated by the increasingly active mitochondria (Longo, 1999). In an alternative protocol, after depletion of the glucose in the medium the population is transferred to water in which it can be kept for weeks in a nondividing but viable state presumably due to a 100-fold reduction in the rate of metabolism with no switch to oxidative respiration.

Use of the stationary phase system for the study of chronological, rather than budding, life span involves growing the cells to a stationary phase on minimal glucose medium. In this experimental protocol, the cells maintain high rates of metabolism, as determined by oxygen consumption, virtually throughout the life span (Liou et al., 2000).

In either variation of this approach, the major observation recorded is actually the effect of nutrient deprivation and possibly the accumulation of toxic compounds in the medium. It is highly questionable whether this is relevant to understanding the underlying mechanisms of aging.

There have also been studies on individual yeast genes as life span or longevity modulators.

1. For the purpose of facilitating laboratory research, yeast strains have been adapted—by selection of mutants or by genetic engineering—to efficient growth under the artificial laboratory conditions. These strains contain genes that are not essential for viability under laboratory conditions. It has been pointed out that "it is likely that a large number of apparently redundant yeast genes are required to deal with physiological challenges that are not encountered in the laboratory environment but that yeast commonly encounters in the natural habitat" (Goffeau et al., 1996). Most of the mutations that affect longevity under laboratory growth conditions are part of the process of transition from genotypes that are adapted to natural habitat to those that are better adapted to the artificial laboratory environment. All the strains used as wild type in laboratory models are auxotrophs that survive well in the laboratory. These strains would be feeble, if at all viable, under the much more demanding conditions in nature. It should be noted that the laboratory environment also eliminates many of the conditions of stress that prevail in nature such as extreme temperatures, deprivation of nutrients, and large fluctuations in humidity.

(a) The wild-type strains currently under investigation carry various mutant alleles such as the W303 strain which bears ade2-1, his3-11-15, trp1-1, leu2-3,112, and can1-100 (Austriaco & Guarente, 1997); the EG103 strain, which bears DBY 746; MATα, leu2-3,112, his3$\triangle$1, trp1-289, ura3-52, GAL$^+$ genes (Longo, Ellerby, Bredesen, Valentine, & Gralla, 1997); the YPK4.7 strain, which bears MATα, ura3-52, lys2-801^{amber}, ade 2-101^{ochre}, trp1-$\triangle$63, his3-$\triangle$200, and leu2-$\triangle$1 (Kim, Benguria, Lai, & Jazwinski, 1999b).

(b) Genotypic modifications can have complex phenotypic ramifications. All of these genetic variants are auxotrophs for several nutrients. Under various conditions these mutations may have a significant effect on the expression of other genes (Padilla, Fuge, Crawford, Errett, & Werner-Washburne, 1998).
(c) The basis for the comparative evaluation of life-span studies carried out by the different research groups who use different strains is very difficult at best and is made more difficult when the results obtained with haploid strains are compared to those from diploid strains (e.g., Kim, Benguria, et al., 1999).
(d) Because most mutations in essential genes have a detrimental effect, most, if not all, so-called life-shortening mutations bear very low relevance to the aging process. Mutations in many yeast-regulatory, or even housekeeping genes will exert a range of effects that include lethality, lower fecundity and declining adaptability to the environment. Interference with the delicate and intricate intragenomic balance of an organism is likely to be detrimental. Therefore, claims that certain individual genes have an essential role in the determination of senescence because when mutated they shorten the life span are unwarranted.
(e) Are the mutations (or deletions) of genes that appear to increase life span such as Ras2 really relevant to aging? It has to be demonstrated that yeast with mutations in these "life span assuring genes" are not at a selective disadvantage during exponential growth when mixed in a population of wild type cells. If they are eliminated in a population consisting of various genotypes because of poor competitive capacity (and yeast in nature do not grow under solitary conditions), then the genes in question have highly questionable relevance to the determination of cellular life span.
(f) It is likely that "longevity" mutations carry pleiotropic effects on metabolic functions, cell-cycle progression, and fecundity. In the laboratory under clonal budding conditions where the cells are solitary these mutations can be sustained. It can thus be reasonably assumed (but this assumption should be tested) that in mixed-genotype suspension culture, cells bearing these mutations would be at a selective disadvantage.

2. Is **Ras 2** a longevity modulator?
(a) Ras proteins are GTP-binding switch proteins which function in the response of cells to external signals. In higher eukaryotes, the binding of certain hormones or growth factors to specific cell surface receptors induces the activation of Ras.
(b) In yeast, Ras-1 and Ras-2 are closely related genes with overlapping functions in normal growth (Werner-Washburne, Braus, Johnston,

& Singer, 1993), invasive growth and filamentation (Mosch, Kubler, Krappmann, Fink, & Braus, 1999), spore germination (Herman & Rine, 1997), and stress resistance (Toda et al., 1985).

(c) Conflicting results have been presented for the significance of Ras in the determination of life span.

(i) It has been reported that mutation in Ras-2 increases the life span of stationary phase cells (Liou et al., 2000). Overexpression of Ras-2 causes death in stationary phase cells (Longo, 1999). In contrast to these findings it has been reported that overexpression of Ras-2 increases budding life span (Kale, Childress, Pinswagdi, & Jazwinski, 1994).

(ii) Reconciliation of these results in terms of life-span modifications would require the illogical assumption that there are two types of life span in yeast. Ras activity thus appears to be required under the solitary cell cultures in the budding system and extraneous or even detrimental under the conditions of the cell suspension system. If so, Ras mutations do not appear to be relevant to aging, despite their antistress functions (e.g., Jazwinski, 2000; Liou et al., 2000).

3. Purported roles of Sir2, histone deacetylases, gene silencing, and rDNA circles in determination of yeast life span and aging. Conflicting findings render hard to accept the theory of rDNA circles as a major factor in yeast "aging," and no such phenomenon has been observed in cells of higher organisms (Guarente, 2000).

(a) Silent information regulator (SIR) genes encode a group of proteins involved in transcription silencing. In a recent review, Guarente (2000) offers an overview of the function Sir2 associated with gene silencing and its relationship to yeast aging. There are four SIR genes in yeast that are required for repression of the chromosomal regions encoding for mating type, telomeres, and ribosomal DNA (rDNA). Sir2, Sir3, and Sir4 are involved in chromatin silencing at the mating type loci and telomeres, whereas Sir2 is solely responsible for silencing of ribosomal DNA genes of yeast. Of the four SIR genes, abrogation of Sir2 activity was sufficient to reduce the number of buds produced (Kaeberlein, McVey, & Guarente, 1999). Conversely, an extra copy of Sir2, increased the number of buds produced per cell (Kaeberlein et al., 1999) ("life span," according to the authors).

(b) Guarente has made the point that rDNA circles accumulate in mother cells with age. Accumulation, due to loss of gene silencing in the ribosomal gene chromosomal domain, resulted in increased homologous recombination and thus formation of extra-chromosomal rDNA circles. It has been proposed that this accumulation of circles is a central cause of yeast aging (Sinclair & Guarente, 1997; also see model in Guarente, 2000).

(c) Jazwinski and colleagues explored the function of the RPD3 deacetylase gene in relation to the effect of Sir2 on the number of buds produced per cell (Kim, Benguria, et al., 1999). They found that the life-span shortening in Sir2 mutants is due to increased loss of rDNA silencing *without* increased presence of rDNA circles.

(d) Using the stationary stage protocol it has been found that rDNA circles play no role in aging of cells (Longo, personal communication, 2000).

(e) Unlike in yeast, overexpression of Sir2 in human cells does not affect growth. Moreover, the product of the human Sir2 ortholog is cytoplasmic whereas it is nuclear in yeast (Afshar & Murnane, 1999). This is a good example of orthologs changing function during evolution and serves as a call for caution in interpreting the fact that certain genes are orthologous between lower and higher eukaryotes. The cellular location of their protein products and their functions have got to be strictly compared in yeast and mammalian cells.

(f) Gene silencing involves chromatin acetylation in both yeast and higher eukaryotes. In higher eukaryotes this is associated with DNA methylation. No DNA methylation occurs in yeast. Thus the mechanism of gene silencing differs in important details between the two systems and simple extrapolation from yeast to higher metazoans is, at best, risky.

4. Stress genes (see reviews by Jakubowski, Bilinski, & Bartosz, 2000; Longo, 1999).

(a) The failure to distinguish between aging mechanisms and survival under adverse conditions has led to misconceptions. Survival of yeast cells, as well as cells of multicellular organisms and bacteria, depends among other things on protection against various stressors such as oxidative, thermal, and osmotic adversity. Interference with the genes that control these protective mechanisms will inevitably lead to changes in viability. The effect of mutations in these genes is influenced by genetic background and selection. In the case of the laboratory yeast, many generations of selection under laboratory conditions—which entail minimal environmental stress and "engineering" for certain characteristics that are desirable to the investigator—introduce artificial effects of stress genes whose allelic forms are suitable for a very narrow set of environmental conditions. It is therefore deemed that the effect on cell "longevity" of mutations in stress genes in yeast is of little relevance to the natural aging of multicellular organisms. Moreover, we suggest that these genes may carry different allelic forms and that their functions may even be differently regulated in real wild-type strains of *S. cerevisiae* freshly isolated from their natural habitat.

The question becomes, is the use of yeast as a paradigm a matter of convenience that overlooks basic inadequacies? There are contradictory findings regarding the number of progeny produced by early and late buds removed from the same mother cell. Kennedy et al. claim that maternal age affects the longevity of daughter cells (Kennedy et al., 1994), while Egilez and Jazwinski (1989) report that daughter cells of older mother cells have the same reproductive capacity as those from younger mothers. The former claimed that their data could be interpreted as an accumulation of "senescence substance" in mother cells as a function of time that is transmitted to the progeny buds. This is not supported by Egilez and Jazwinski's observation.

The discrepancies observed in metabolic behavior and longevity between cells in rich medium, minimal medium, and water in stationary-phase and budding-life-span methods raise the fundamental question of how we define life span in yeast. Longo (1999) suggests that the stationary phase system reveals "chronological age" rather than "budding life span. Ashrafi, Sinclair, Gordon, and Guarente (1999) have made an attempt to reconcile the two systems by demonstrating that the mean replicative life span gradually decreases with the length of time the cells are maintained in stationary phase. This is in contrast to Jazwinski's observations that the progeny of any budding cycle have the capacity for full life span (Jazwinski, 2000) regardless of whether they are derived from early or late buds.

Another puzzling difference between the two systems emerges from studies on the Ras2 gene. This gene has been claimed as cardinal in the modulation of the life span of yeast in both culture systems (e.g., Jazwinski, 1999; Liou et al., 2000). Disturbingly, Ras2 has been shown to have opposite effects on survival in cells in the budding-life-span system and in the stationary-phase system. Added to this variability in experimental approach and results is the variety of yeast strains with different genetic make up that are utilized in the various studies. In his chapter on methodology in yeast aging studies, Jazwinski recommends the following:

> The strain chosen as the 'wild type' control may depend upon the experiments you wish to perform; however, several things should be considered. One consideration that is very important in choosing a strain is the ease with which the buds can be removed from the individual cells. . . . *the life span of your control strain is also an important consideration. A strain with a life span that is too short makes it hard to examine variables that shorten the life span,*

while a strain with a life span that is too long may make it difficult to detect extensions and take too long to assay. (Kim, Kirchman, et al., 1999; italics added for emphasis)

In our view this approach is seriously flawed. Extending the life span of a short-lived strain or shortening that of a long-lived strain is meaningless to the study of the fundamental processes of senescence. Mutations in nonredundant genes borne by a strain or inflicted experimentally are normally expected to exert a deleterious effect on survival capacity. Thus the reported findings on the "extension of life span" by mutations have no direct relationship to senescence but rather to adaptation to relatively new laboratory environmental conditions. This is part of a process of forced mini-evolution in the laboratory.

The use of both diploid and haploid strains is also problematic. Some labs use a diploid strain chosen according to the above criteria for the "proper life span," while others use a haploid wild-type strain (Kennedy et al., 1994). Using a haploid strain, it has been claimed that genome instability is a major determinant of the life span (Park, DeFossez, & Guarente, 1999). Genomic instability in a haploid strain cannot effectively represent the situation in diploid yeast or in higher eukaryotes. The use of a haploid strain may lead to problems of interpretation, and its usefulness for studying the complex phenotype of aging is highly questionable.

It has been claimed that yeast mother cells undergo a finite number of mitoses (buddings) and then perish. It has been suggested, therefore, that the budding yeast may serve as a model for replicative cell senescence, particularly for those metazoan cellular systems that divide throughout the life span of a multicellular organism (Kim, Kirchman, et al., 1999; Sinclair, Mills, & Guarente, 1998). Implicit in this assertion is the concept that dividing individual cells in metazoa undergo replicative senescence (Hayflick, 1965). The Hayflick theory in its original form contributed considerably to the serious misconception that a postmitotic cell is a dead cell. Most somatic cell types in higher multicellular organisms are postmitotic yet survive and maintain their functional capacity for many years. The relevance of Hayflick's theory to organismal aging has recently been placed in further doubt. In this regard the reader is referred to the article by Cristofalo and colleagues in which it has been critically shown that there is no correlation between donor age and the number of population doublings attained by fibroblasts in culture (Cristofalo et al., 1998). Thus, the doubtful validity of the contention that individual dividing mammalian cells undergo replicative senescence in vivo opens to *serious* question one of the major incentives for considering yeast as a good model for aging research.

Problems: Using Unicellular Organisms as Models for the Aging of Multicellular Organisms

Although there is a superficial resemblance to aging mechanisms in multicellular organisms, yeast, like bacteria, are basically immortal at the population level. Immediately after the death of the multicellular organism, individual cells maintain viability and can be cultured in vivo, albeit without the ability to re-form the total organism. Barring environmental disasters, populations of unicellular organisms go on multiplying indefinitely even though a proportion of cells die. Moreover, the budding yeast is an exception even among unicellular organisms in that the mother cell produces progeny and ceases to reproduce after a number of buddings. This does not occur among most other unicellular organisms including, for instance, the related fission yeast *Saccharomyces pombe.*

Yeast cells respond to unfavorable environmental conditions by radically reducing their metabolic rate through spore formation. Spores are highly viable cells with a very low metabolic rate (~1% of the normal rate of proliferating cells). The greater longevity of spores is not an extension of the life span. It should be considered as an unusual adaptive mechanism for survival under extreme adversity. Such adaptation is infrequent among higher eukaryotes and cannot be a basic underlying mechanism of aging, as is explained in our previous review (Gershon & Gershon, 2000b). In lower metazoa, similar but not identical adaptation occurs in many but not all species, for example, dauer larvae in *C. elegans;* some mammals hibernate as a regularly programmed phenomenon. However, this is not a general phenomenon and therefore cannot be a decisive underlying mechanism of longevity determination.

One of the major features of aging in multicellular organisms is that the differentiation and specialization of cells to perform specific functions with very high efficiency is lacking in the yeast model. Because of programmed, limited repertoire of cellular functions in multicellular organisms, cellular survival is dependent on communication with and support of other cells over various distances. The failure of this communication is a major contributor to aging of the multicellular organism. As examples of this phenomenon, one can cite skeletal muscle deterioration due to loss of communication via cholinergic synapses (Herscovich & Gershon, 1987) and reduced ability to respond to hormones due to alterations in structure or control of synthesis of appropriate receptors (Supakar & Roy, 1996). This intercellular communication is weak in unicellular organisms. Multicellular organisms are composed of many types of highly specialized cells and have thus established systemic homeostatic environments. Very few cells are directly exposed to external environmental conditions. Stress is dealt with in parallel in the individual cell and at the systemic levels. As a rule, multicellular organisms have diverse functions that are mainly endocrinological and neurological and involve intercellular communication to counteract many forms of stress and afford external protection to individual cells. These essential intercellular communication systems with their fail-safe mechanisms are absent in unicellular organisms like the yeast.

NEMATODES IN GENERAL AND *C. ELEGANS* IN PARTICULAR AS MODEL ORGANISMS IN AGING RESEARCH

The choice of nematodes as a model organism for aging research was first described in 1970 (Gershon, 1970). Free-living nematodes have been deemed suitable for such research due to the following considerations: (a) They have a high degree of cell differentiation and specialization; (b) free-living nematodes of the Rhabditis family are relatively simple multicellular organisms, composed of a small number of cells with very well-defined cell types (c) the developmental lineage of all *C. elegans* cells has been delineated (Horvitz, 1988; Sulston, 1988); (d) these nematodes possess distinct somatic and germinal cell lineage; and (e) the somatic cells are essentially postmitotic like most somatic cell systems in mammals (see detailed discussion in Gershon, 1970; Johnson, 1984; Klass, 1977; Reznick & Gershon, 1999).

These nematodes can be raised and maintained in large populations under relatively simple and cheap laboratory conditions both axenically on defined media (Dougherty, Hansen, Nicholas, Mollett, & Yarwood, 1959; Rothstein & Cook, 1966) and monoxenically on *E. coli* (Sulston & Hodgkin, 1988).

Experimental Nematodes and Their Environment

C. elegans

A ubiquitous, soil-dwelling, free-living nematode, *C elegans* has been used as a model for experimental work and raised under laboratory conditions for more than 40 years (e.g., Dougherty et al., 1959).

In the soil it feeds on microorganisms and decaying organic matter, which supplies plant sterols. In the laboratory, *C. elegans* is generally cultured monoxenically on lawns of *E. coli*. These bacterial cells, which are not encountered in the natural habitat, appear to satisfy the nutritional requirements of the worms except for sterols, which are provided by addition of cholesterol to the medium. The sterol sources for *C. elegans* in the soil are plant sterols (Chitwood & Lusby, 1991). The extent of reactive oxygen-dependent peroxidative damage, which accumulates with age, is dependent on levels and composition of lipids and fatty acids. The fact that laboratory nutritional conditions are quite different from those encountered in the natural habitat must be seriously considered in dealing with life span determination. This is particularly so because the membrane composition of lipids and polyunsaturated fatty acids is greatly influenced by the diet and even temperature of growth used in the laboratory (Tanaka et al., 1996).

During larval development, *C. elegans* has a highly effective stress-resistance mechanism that involves sensing unfavorable environmental conditions, particularly food deprivation, and leads to the formation of dauer larva, a state of diapause at the third larval stage. Riddle and Albert (1997) give an excellent overview of dauer larva formation and characteristics. As a result of gut blockage and shrinking of the intestinal lumen, dauer larvae do not feed. In this form they can survive at least 8 to 10 times longer than the normal worm life span. When environmental conditions improve, dauer larvae revert to normal development through a very well-defined genetic program. The revertants exhibit the same post-larval life span as well-fed unstressed animals. A large number of genes are involved in the dauer developmental program and exit from the dauer stage (Riddle & Albert, 1997). Many of the so-called life extending mutations described for nematodes involve entrance into a unique partial dauer state that has no equivalent in mammals.

Hermaphrodites Versus Dioecious Species

C. elegans is a hermaphrodite that reproduces primarily by self-fertilization. Therefore, under most circumstances, populations of this nematode are composed of clones of essentially homozygous organisms. Males are produced (at about 0.1%–0.3% frequency) by a mechanism of X-chromosome nondisjunction and can mate with the hermaphrodites thus allowing for genetic analysis.

Currently there is little if any work on free-living, dioecious nematodes such as we performed in the 1970s with *Turbatrix aceti*, a dioecious outbred species related to *C. elegans* (Gershon & Gershon, 1970; Reznick & Gershon, 1977, 1979; Zeelon, Gershon & Gershon, 1973). The use of genetically heterogeneous species is closer to the situation in human populations.

The Problem of Using Laboratory Strains for Aging Research

The *C. elegans* strains used in practically all basic biological research, including aging research, are derived from a single isolate from the late 1950s (Dougherty et al., 1959). The N2 strain that is used as wild type was introduced in the late 1960s (Brenner, 1974). Thus, almost all research is being carried out with a strain of *C. elegans* raised under laboratory conditions for thousands of generations (considering a generation time of 3 days).

After growth for thousands of generations in the laboratory, it can be speculated that certain genotypes that have adapted to such conditions of limited stress have been preferentially selected. Strains that are used as laboratory wild type have thus probably undergone considerable loss of fitness with regard to stress in the wild.

In order to facilitate the observation of worms for the duration of their life span under laboratory conditions, they are raised individually rather than in populations, which is the usual situation in nature. In liquid population cultures, reproduction is inhibited by a DNA replication inhibitor such as fluorodeoxyuridine (FUDR) as initially used by Erlanger and Gershon (1970). FUDR does not affect the life span of *C. elegans* (Vanfleteren & Braeckman, 1999).

Fitness in Nature Versus Fitness Under Laboratory Conditions

In the soil this organism encounters considerable environmental fluctuations in the availability of food, temperature, humidity, light exposure, and most likely oxygen tension. It is also subjected to attack by fungi and other organisms. In culture it is subjected to minimal environmental stress.

The Nematode and Relevant Findings in Aging Research

Inactive enzyme molecules accumulate with age. Using the dioecious nematode *Turbatrix aceti,* it was shown that with age there is an accumulation of inactive enzyme molecules (Gershon & Gershon, 1970; Reznick & Gershon, 1977; Zeelon et al., 1973). This was later corroborated in mammalian systems (Gershon & Gershon, 1973a, 1973b).

There is a decline in protein degradation rate with age. Accumulation of inactive enzyme molecules could be at least partially attributed to a decline in protein degradation (Reznick & Gershon, 1979; Zeelon et al., 1973). This mechanism was also demonstrated later in mammals (Lavie, Reznick, Gershon, 1982; Reznick, Lavie, Gershon, & Gershon, 1981; Reznick, Rosenfelder, Shpund, & Gerhson, 1985). These and other observations led to the refutation of Orgel's "error catastrophe" theory of aging since they demonstrated no consequences of misincorporation of amino acids (Gershon, 1979).

Oxidative stress is a major factor in the determination of the life span. Using the nematode *C. briggsae* (which was probably *C. elegans;* see Friedman, Platzer, & Eby, 1977) it was shown that oxidative damage accumulates as a function of age. This damage could be reduced by the use of α-tocopherol with a concomitant extension of the life span (Epstein, Himmelhoch, & Gerhshon, 1972; Epstein & Gershon, 1972).

Are "Gerontogenes" a Laboratory-specific Phenomenon?

A search for mutations that affect life span was initiated by Klass and Hirsh (1976) and by Klass (1977). A large number of genes have been identified that when mutated shorten the life span. Purportedly much more interesting are those that upon mutation extend the life span. For a comprehensive discussion of these genes the reader is directed to the review of Braeckman, Houthoffd, and Vanfleteren (2000). These "gerontogenes" fall into three main categories: genes affecting diapause, dauer formation, and consequently longevity; clock (Clk) genes; and genes involved in reduced food consumption and presumed dietary restriction.

Genes Involved in Dauer Larva Formation (daf)

All the studies on the diapause-related genes indicate that the wild type alleles *decrease* the life span. This observation has created a concept, first proposed by Johnson (Johnson & Lithgow, 1992), of gerontogenes. Thus, there are genes that have alleles that shorten life span, and when these life-shortening alleles are mutated the life span increases. Implicit in this concept is the suggestion that aging is genetically programmed and that one can disrupt the program and thus extend the life span.

A number of the genes involved in dauer larva formation (daf) affect longevity when mutated. This group includes daf-2, age-1 (Friedman & Johnson, 1988a, 1988b), daf 12, daf 16, and daf 18. (We do not intend to comprehensibly review the large number of publications on this group of genes. They are described in Braeckman et al., 2000). Both daf-2 and age-1 alleles that reduce functional capacity increase the life span (Friedman & Johnson, 1988a, 1988b; Kenyon, Chang, Gensch, Rudner, & Tabtiang, 1993).

Clk Genes

Clk genes regulate physiological, developmental, and behavioral clocks during the progression of the life cycle of the nematode. When mutated, the genes involved (for example, clk-1, clk-2, clk-3, and gro-1) cause increases in the length of the life cycle and lengthening of the developmental stages of the larvae and the adults, and decreases in pharyngeal pumping (which is involved in food intake and initial digestion), egg laying, and worm movement (Lakowski & Hekimi, 1996).

All clock genes show maternal inheritance, and there is evidence that these clk mutations cause a reduction in metabolic rate and by implication result in a lower production of reactive oxygen species. However, the direct role in the increase of life span of these mutations is not completely clear.

While all the clk mutants show but a moderate increase in life span, when combined with daf-2 as double mutants they may cause a two-to-three fold increase in the life span (Lakowski & Hekimi, 1996). This is presumably due to the fact that on their own the clk mutations increase the length of the developmental stages and the daf mutants exert, at least partially, dauer larva formation. The combined effect results in a considerable delay in reaching adulthood in the double mutants.

Eat Genes and the Genetics of Dietary Restriction in C. elegans

The life span of N2 is at least twice as long on axenic medium as on *E. coli* monoxenic cultures (Vanfleteren & Braeckman, 1999). This has been widely considered proof that dietary restriction (DR) increases the life span in *C. elegans*. However, there is no direct evidence that the axenic conditions actually involve DR.

There is a direct negative correlation between life span and the concentration of bacteria in the culture (Klass, 1977) suggesting that there are some low levels of toxicity and infectivity exerted by the *E. coli*, which is not normally encountered in the natural habitat. Some "long lived" strains show higher resistance to *E. coli* infection (Fabian & Johnson, 1995). This negative effect of *E. coli* on the nematodes may increase with old age (Croll, Smith, & Zuckerman, 1977; Fabian & Johnson, 1995).

Eat mutants have limited food intake due to reduced pharyngeal activity (Lakowski & Hekimi, 1998). Although eat mutants have a permanent defect in the function of the pharynx, which is of course an essential factor in the feeding process of the nematode, many have problems in parts of the nervous system in addition to the neurons that innervate the pharynx muscle. There is a severe compromise in the physiological functions of the eat mutants that must be related to a serious loss of fitness under natural growth conditions. The reader is referred to a very brief and disconcerting description of the serious defects expressed in these mutants (Hodgkin, 1997).

We suggest that even partial loss of control of feeding would be detrimental under natural conditions that entail varied availability of food, particularly if the mutants have to compete with wild type in a mixed population. A related and indicative experiment, as suggested for nematodes (Reznick & Gershon, 1999) and yeast (Gershon and Gershon, 2000a), has recently been performed (Walker, McColl, Jenkins, Harris, & Lithgow, 2000). Age-1 mutants, shown to have an "extended" life span, were mixed with N2 worms at various ratios. The mixed population retained original strain proportions for several generations under normal laboratory conditions of ad libitum feeding with *E. coli*. However, under starvation conditions made to emulate natural conditions where food is often scarce, the age-1 mutant strain was almost completely eliminated from the mixed populations within six generations. Thus, the bearers of this "life-extending" mutation have reduced fitness under conditions of stress. It should be borne in mind that starvation is but one stress condition in nature. The worms are also exposed in the soil to large fluctuations of temperatures and periods of hypoxia among other things, the effects of which are compounded with the stress of food deprivation. This complex deprivation of types of stress was not addressed in the experiments of Walker and colleagues (2000). We suggest that the age-1 mutant would have been rapidly eliminated under the multiple stress forms that exist in the natural habitats of a soil nematode.

The Role of Individual Genes in the Context of the Whole Genome in Determining Life Span

We suggest that this phenomenon of life extension of N2, the laboratory wild type strain of *C. elegans,* by loss of function alleles results from an evolutionary process, occurring in the laboratory, that involves an adaptive switch from natural habitat conditions to an artificial laboratory ecosystem. In this process, alleles of many genes, including those already described for daf and clk and probably of genes that are yet to be discovered, are in the process of being selected to replace redundant alleles.

The requisite characteristics of such new alleles of gerontogenes are as follows: Such genes are expected to increase the fitness of the organism in order to affect life span. All the mutations in the age-1, daf, and clk genes that increase the levels of SOD and catalase activities may contribute to improved adaptation to culture conditions, which involve growth under atmospheric oxygen (21% oxygen) rather that 1% to 2% oxygen in their natural habitat. Thus, bolstered protective antioxidative mechanisms indirectly bring the life span closer to its potential in nature. This is not new, as we showed in 1972 that tocopherol in the medium decreases oxidative damage in the nematode and concomitantly increases life span (Epstein & Gershon, 1972).

As for the fitness of gerontogene mutants under conditions close to those encountered in nature:

- Almost any gene that has been fixed in the genome is the product of an evolutionary process that made the organism optimally fit to conditions in its natural habitat. Therefore, a mutation in a considerable number of genes will result in diminished fitness under the natural conditions in which the organism evolved. Such a mutation in what has been termed a gerontogene—even when it shows life-span extension under the artifactual laboratory setting—is meaningless in the gerontological sense, although perhaps interesting academically. This is because it will have very little impact on the life span in a mixed-genotype population, as its bearers will be eliminated within a short time due to diminished fitness such as low fecundity, delayed development, and reduced capacity to cope with altered environmental conditions or any combination of these factors.

- Age-1 mutants have been shown to have low competitive ability under stress conditions (Walker et al., 2000).
- It has recently been claimed that mutations that result in loss of sense organ function promote increased life span (Apfeld & Kenyon, 1999). The loss of sense-organ function may be dispensable under the minimally demanding conditions of the laboratory that include adequate nutrition and the culture of individuals rather than growth in populations (as is the prevalent situation in nature). In nature these organs are absolutely indispensable for finding food, escaping from predation, evading adverse environmental conditions, and finding mates. When grown in a mixture with wild-type organisms these mutants would be eliminated almost immediately under even mild stress conditions.

We suggest that all the gerontogene mutations have occurred many times during the evolution of *C. elegans* in the wild and were efficiently selected against because of their biological disadvantage under adverse environmental conditions. We also suggest, as succinctly discussed by Strohman (2001), that aging is a very complex phenotype that requires the interaction of hundreds if not thousands of genes. Therefore the genomics of aging as currently envisaged will at present yield little valuable information because complex and intricate multigenic interactions are involved and tools for the analysis of such complexity are not yet available. Thus, the current search for individual genes that affect this complex phenotype yields negligible contribution to the elaboration of the biological basis of aging.

Problems in the Direct Application of Experimental Findings in *C. elegans* to Mammalian Systems

Wild type *C. elegans* as currently used in the laboratory setting has been selected for adaptation to narrow, minimal-stress laboratory conditions. Therefore, it carries many genes that are essential in its natural habitat yet are either dispensable or have a nonessential function for development and survival in the laboratory. It might be argued that humans who have considerable control over their environment also have a reduced need for the function of many (stress) genes. There are, however, no human populations even in the most developed countries that are not intermittently subjected to temperature stress (climate), pathogens, fluctuations in diurnal-nocturnal timing, and even nutritional stress. Also, competition among individuals in genetically variable populations, as experienced by humans, is not a factor in the experimental nematode system that is genetically homogeneous or, even worse, that is composed of isolated individuals.

Perspectives for Nematodes in Aging Research

1. Culture conditions should more closely mimic those encountered by *C. elegans* in its natural habitats and should include limited nutrition on microorganisms (other than *E. coli*) and organic matter (including plant sterols), temperature fluctuations, oxygen partial tension, and minimal light exposure that approximate those in the habitat of the nematode.
2. Wild type N2 should be compared to new isolates from nature, a consequence of which perhaps might be the introduction of new wild-type strains.
3. More studies should be performed on nematode life span in populations rather than on isolated individual animals.
4. Research on aging should also be performed on dioecious species with populations composed of a variety of genotypes and heterozygous individuals, which would be more relevant to human aging.

CELL CULTURES AS A MODEL FOR WHOLE ORGANISM AGING

The Concept of "Cellular Senescence" In Vitro

Hayflick first described the finite replicative capacity of fetal fibroblasts in culture (Hayflick, 1965; Hayflick & Moorhead, 1961) and interpreted these findings as demonstrative of cellular aging in vitro (Harley, West, Campisi, & Hayflick, 1995). This research erroneously considered postmitotic cells to be dead cells. Another misconception derived from these studies is that the number of cell divisions is a limiting factor that serves as a clock that determines the life span of a multicellular organism. Another misconception is the recent suggestion that the gradual shortening of average telomere length as a function of time and number of population doublings in culture functions as a clock (Harley et al., 1990).

Basic Observations on Cell Culture Methodology

The paradigm of mammalian cells in culture as used for the study of aging is fraught with serious faults. Culture conditions are potentially very damaging to primary cultured cells with most cells not surviving the early period of cultivation.

The accepted protocol of repeated trypsinization of cells in order to transfer cells in culture is very damaging as trypsin degrades receptors, ion channels, extracellular matrix (ECM)-binding proteins, and other surface proteins. In addition, the intracellular environment changes in an unexpected way. For example, Yamanaka and Deamer (1974) described a substantial and sustained reduction of mitochondrial SOD activity following cell trypsinization. All of these effects of trypsin bear harmful consequences on cell responsiveness to environmental cues and cell survival.

Culture under atmospheric oxygen (21%) rather than the low oxygen tension that cells encounter in vivo (1% to 5%) introduces substantial oxidative stress, which cells that are freshly removed from tissues are not equipped to respond to adequately. The result is severe damage to cell functions and viability (Colombatto, Giribaldi, Vargin, & Grillo, 1994; Eppig & Wigglesworth, 1995; Khaliq et al., 1995; Krieger, Landsiedel, & Lawrence, 1996; LaIuppa, Papoutsakis, & Miller, 1998; Ono & Alter, 1995; Reykdal, Abboud, & Liesueld, 1999; Saito, Hammond, & Moses, 1995). Indeed when tested, growth at low oxygen tension has been shown to allow better proliferation of primary keratinocytes and melanocytes in culture (Horikoshi, Balin, & Carter, 1991).

Despite the buffers included in media, fluctuation of pH in culture is much greater than in vivo with damaging consequences (Eagle, 1973).

It must be emphasized that the conditions that are provided in cell cultures are far from optimal due to incomplete understanding of all the factors required by cells (cytokines, hormones, and extracellular matrix components) to normally fulfill functions such as proliferation, differentiation, and programmed cell death. Indeed it is quite surprising that some normal diploid cell types can survive at all under these conditions. It is well known that it is difficult to culture and maintain many cell types as successfully as fibroblasts in culture. Hepatocytes can serve as an example for this and the same is the case for many epithelial cell types.

There is evidence that under culture conditions, connective tissue cells cease dividing as a result of entering a differentiation program. Such a program culminates in a G_0 state that is a normal consequence of terminal differentiation of most cell types in vivo (Bayreuther, Franez, Gogol, & Kontermann, 1992).

Extensive work on various cell types in vivo has not revealed any serious attenuation in the proliferative capacity as a function of age (Daniel, 1977; Harrison, Astle, & DeLaittre, 1988; Krohn, 1966).

Studies Do Not Support the Concept of Depletion of Cell Production with Age

There is no evidence for a "Hayflick limit" in the proliferative capacity of cells in vivo, in fact, there is substantial evidence that points to a lack of proliferative limits in vivo.

- *Serial skin transplants:* Prior to Hayflick's studies Krohn performed serial skin transplants between two mouse strains and their F_1 hybrids, as well as transplantations of grafts from young and old donors into young and old hosts (Krohn, 1966). Proliferation far exceeded that necessary for one mouse life span. The capacity for proliferation in skin transplants did not change significantly between young and old grafts.

- *Serial murine mammary tissue transplants* demonstrate that mammary epithelium cells exhibit a proliferative capacity that far exceeds that required for a single life span (Daniel, 1977).
- *Serially transplanted bone marrow cells* and rescued lethally irradiated mice (Harrison, 1985). Here again proliferative capacity exceeded that required for the life span of a mouse. Moreover, in most experiments the cells of old individuals proliferated as well as young individuals when transplanted into young recipients.
- *Maintenance of stable hematocrit* throughout the life span of healthy rats and humans has been demonstrated (Glass, Gershon, & Gershon, 1983, 1985). We demonstrated that in rats the rate of turnover of erythrocytes doubles with age. Thus the rate of supply of erythrocytes doubles and yet the system remains stable. Thus there is no proliferative limit in this system in vivo.
- *The lack of correlation between donor age and the number of population doublings of skin fibroblasts grown* in vitro was unequivocally demonstrated by Cristofalo and colleagues (1998) who showed that fibroblasts from healthy individuals (not from cadavers) have the same proliferative capacity regardless of donor age. More convincingly, they showed that cells of the same individual at different ages showed the same proliferative capacity.

Lessons from the Cell Culture Model

1. Is the study of cells in culture a measure of cellular resistance to abuse or a model for the study of senescence? We propose that the "Hayflick phenomenon" is a result of abuse in vitro. Without such abuse, in vivo systems have a proliferative capacity that far exceeds the needs for the maintenance of cellular proliferation throughout the life span of the organism.

2. Has the study of cells in culture provided an understanding of whole organism aging? Despite a vast volume of work on senescence in vitro there is scant information provided by tissue culture systems that has advanced our understanding of in vivo aging. The in vitro system lacks the major factors involved in the determination of functions and survival of organisms: intercellular communication (between cell types) and the overall homeostatic environment in which cells exist in vivo. Homeostasis provides both protection against abrupt environmental changes, and intercellular communication influences the stages that cells

undergo from proliferation to differentiation and even programmed cell death. Cells in culture are essentially deprived of these factors and therefore make a very poor model for aging. There is some limited value to the approach taken to compare cells derived from donors of various ages in vitro. Even this approach is questionable, as it is more logical to directly study the tissues removed from individuals of various ages without subjecting them to the artificial conditions of tissue culture.

RODENTS AS MODELS FOR AGING RESEARCH

Inbred Strains and Causes of Concern

Many of the ideas and concerns expressed here have also been comprehensively and lucidly discussed by Austad and by Miller (Austad, 1997; Miller et al., 1999, 2000; Phelan & Austad, 1994).

The use of inbred mouse strains specifically adapted to laboratory conditions has been one of the cornerstones of modern experimental biology. The use of these strains has yielded important insights in the fields of developmental biology, molecular genetics, immunology, virology, and oncology. The main advantage of these laboratory-selected strains is the introduction of domesticated animals that are relatively easy to raise under defined husbandry with significant fecundity (large litters) and relatively short generation time.

A major aim in creating these strains was to create genetically homogeneous populations that would serve to circumvent complications in the analysis of experiments that inevitably arise with populations of animals comprising a spectrum of varied genotypes. For this purpose, animals (particularly mice and to a lesser extent rats) were subjected to extensive inbreeding via intersibling crosses. The strains were developed by selection for specific characteristics that interested investigators from the 1930s through the 1970s. It is important to note that none of the existing strains have been selected with longevity in mind. The main emphasis in their development was centered on characteristics that involved developmental, prepuberty, and fertility factors. Longevity was not a considered criterion in the development of laboratory rodent strains.

The inbred strains of mice primarily used in current research are indeed composed of virtually identical homozygous individuals. Due to their homozygosity, which also entails an increased expression of detrimental alleles, inbred strains have specific inborn, idiosyncratic pathological traits. These in many cases are rare in heterozygous, genetically diverse wild mice.

During the domestication of laboratory animals, which involves selection for genotypes that are better adapted to laboratory conditions, some serious alterations are created in the genetic makeup of the organism, particularly involving genes that are essential for survival and longevity in nature. Biological aging is characterized by a decline in the capacity of an organism to respond to adverse environmental conditions. Survival in the natural habitat of any species involves a combination of stress-response genes that must be expressed under the variable and sometimes extreme environmental conditions present in the habitat. Such adverse conditions are excluded from the laboratory environment. Rather, the animals are raised under conditions of ad libitum feeding, fixed temperature (daily and seasonal), humidity, and light-dark periods, and pathogen-free conditions. After exposure to these conditions over 100 generations one can expect that many stress-response genes have become redundant and that at least part of their allelic makeup has undergone a significant transition. It is deemed therefore that caution be exercised in the interpretation of results obtained from experimental rodents. For instance, it would be very important to compare the effect of dietary restriction on the life span of wild mice whose nutrition is vastly different from that of laboratory animals. Of course, like the wild mouse human populations are genetically diverse, comprising an extensive spectrum of genotypes.

Outbred Strains and F_1 Hybrids

The use of outbred animals may resolve some of the problems of homozygosity and the expression of detrimental alleles of a variety of genes. Some of these genes are particular to certain inbred strains and others may be common to a few strains. This means that the choice of combinations of parental strains to be used for obtaining F1 progeny must be carefully planned. The F1 hybrids will be genetically homogeneous, albeit heterozygous for many alleles, and so experiments using them will eliminate diversity. However, in order to get more genetic diversity (yet homogeneous experimental populations) using "exotic" strains that are the result of four-way crosses of mice has been suggested (Miller et al., 1999). Undoubtedly the maintenance of hybrid populations of experimental animals is somewhat more burdensome than that of inbred strains: however, the relevance of the model, and not convenience, should be the criterion for adopting an experimental system.

Using Wild Rodents for Aging Research

Despite the difficulty, effort must be devoted to using a heterogeneous population of animals that are adapted to the harsh and stressful (relative to the laboratory conditions) environmental conditions of the natural habitat (Harper & Austad, 2000; Miller et al., 2000). The longevity of these animals will be varied due to the genetic variability of a crossbred population, however, one will be able to derive novel information of the underlying mechanisms of senescence.

For instance, one can study the capacity of such wild animals to respond to stress as a function of age. Recent work in our laboratory (E. Ron and D. Gershon, in preparation) indicates that wild mice isolated from arid areas respond to elevated temperatures differently than do laboratory rodents. In laboratory animals, body temperature increases almost immediately in response to elevated temperatures and thus their heat-shock response at the cellular level is activated early (when body temperature reaches 39°–40° C). Wild animals by contrast maintain normal body temperature for much longer periods under high ambient temperatures by endocrinological and behavioral means. As a result their heat-shock response at the cellular level is much delayed, yet they are more resistant to hyperthermia. Whereas, laboratory animals increase their body temperature more slowly with age and thus do not respond as well to heat shock (Blake, Fargnoli, Gershon, & Holbrook, 1991), wild mice aged (3.5–5 years old) in the laboratory cannot maintain body temperature as well as young animals and thus die earlier before their cellular response is fully activated (albeit at higher temperatures) than the laboratory strains (Ron and Gershon, in preparation). This is a completely different situation whereby wild animals maintain protective homeostatic mechanisms much better than laboratory animals that have lost this capacity during long periods of lack of exposure to environmental stress. Thus the capacity to counteract heat stress is dealt with at different, though slightly overlapping, levels in the laboratory and in wild mice.

In the wild mouse, the response level is very strong, first at the organismal level and then at the cellular level, whereas in the laboratory animal the significance of the homeostatic level is reduced and the cellular level gains more significance. These experiments should caution the experimental gerontologists—who put great emphasis in their research on the cellular and molecular levels—against neglecting the very crucial systemic physiological systems. We contend that the weakened capacity to maintain homeostatic systems in the organism is a crucial cause of senescence. Of course, homeostasis is eventually determined by the activities of cellular systems, but intercellular and intersystem communication play a major role in determining homeostasis. This must be considered more carefully in modern experimental gerontology.

The wide range of variation in the response to stress in the wild mice necessitates using a large number of individuals per experimental group and thus a more complex experimental design. Yet the new information derived from experimenting with the wild animals is bound to be very rewarding as it reveals aspects of organismal response that can be overlooked when one works with engineered laboratory strains.

Proper Environmental Conditions for the Study of Aging

As mentioned earlier, the choice of environmental conditions for the study of aging cannot be separated from the choice of model experimental organisms for meaningful aging research. Misleading results and conclusions can come from the study of laboratory strains (and wild animals) that are subjected for many generations to artificial conditions such as nutrition, temperatures, diurnal cycles, and in some cases, such as *C. elegans*, exposure to oxygen levels not encountered by the organism in its natural habitat. Because it is impractical to study the longevity of populations of organisms in their natural ecological niche, the experimenter must be innovative in devising laboratory conditions that best approximate those encountered in nature. It must be stressed that the organism is exposed to a combination of all these experimental factors, and thus studies in the laboratory must deal with the complex and multiple effects of these simultaneously as well as the contributions of the individual factors to the fitness and survival of the organism.

A few examples will illustrate what types of improvements can be considered in this regard:

1. *Nutrition: C. elegans* can be fed with soil bacteria and plant sterols rather than *E. coli* and cholesterol (which certainly affect membrane composition and properties). Additionally the worms should not be fed ad libitum, that is, on full lawns of bacteria, but much more sparingly as is the situation in nature. With rodents ad libitum feeding should be abolished for most purposes. In the case of mammals, animals must also be allowed a greater opportunity to exercise rather than continue their generally sedentary lifestyle in a cage. If rodents are provided with these conditions, the effect of caloric restriction, which is a natural occurrence, is predicted to be of minor importance. This will be more noticeable when one uses animals that are freshly isolated from nature for the reasons discussed above.
2. *Ambient temperatures:* All organisms (including humans to a certain extent) are exposed to considerable temperature fluctuations under natural conditions and are therefore endowed with homeostatic coping mechanisms. Studies of the response of *C. elegans* and rodents of various ages to these fluctuating conditions at the systemic and cellular levels may yield novel insights into the underlying mechanisms of aging.
3. *Diurnal fluctuations:* Most organisms are exposed to seasonal diurnal fluctuations and are profoundly affected by them physiologically. Circadian rhythms are a very well-studied phenomenon that are certainly photoperiodically affected. Laboratory animals are deprived of these crucial environmental cues, and it is suspected that their physiological

well-being is seriously compromised. The effects of providing seasonal light-dark cycles to the animals will probably afford more insight into the biology of aging.

4. Provision of proper lighting to *C. elegans* is even more serious. This soil organism is minimally exposed to light in its natural environment, yet in the laboratory it is exposed to much more intense light than in nature. This may affect its circadian rhythms and cause photooxidative damage. It is important to minimize drastically the exposure of cultured animals to light. In this case also one may observe some surprising effects with significant insight into age-associated phenomena.

5. There are other environmental factors that should be taken into account such as population versus individual rearing of individuals (interorganismal interactions are important); and exposure to high oxygen levels in the case of *C. elegans* is probably crucial.

ACKNOWLEDGMENTS

The support of the Weisz Foundation for Aging Research, Redox Pharmaceutical Corporation, and the Skillman Foundation enabled the writing of this chapter.

REFERENCES

Afshar, G., & Murnane, J. P. (1999). Characterization of a human gene with sequence homology to Saccharomyces cerevisiae SIR2. *Gene, 234,* 161–168.

Apfeld, J., & Kenyon, C. (1999). Regulation of lifespan by sensory perception in Caenorhabditis elegans [comments]. *Nature, 402,* 804–809.

Ashrafi, K., Sinclair, D., Gordon, J. I., & Guarente, L. (1999). Passage through stationary phase advances replicative aging in Saccharomyces cerevisiae. *Proceedings of the National Academy of Science, USA, 96,* 9100–9105.

Austad, S. N. (1997). Issues in the choice of genetic configuration for animal aging models. *Experimental Gerontology, 32,* 55–63.

Austriaco, N. R., Jr., & Guarente, L. P., (1997). Changes of telomere length cause reciprocal changes in the lifespan of mother cells in Saccharomyces cerevisiae. *Proceedings of the National Academy of Sciences, USA, 94,* 9768–9772.

Barker, M. G., & Walmsley, R. M. (1999). Replicative ageing in the fission yeast Schizosaccharomyces pombe. *Yeast, 15,* 1511–1518.

Bayreuther, K., Francz, P. I., Gogol, J., & Kontermann, K. (1992). Terminal differentiation, aging, apoptosis, and spontaneous transformation in fibroblast stem cell systems in vivo and in vitro. *Annals of the New York Academy of Science, 663,* 167–179.

Bengtson, V. L., & Schaie, K. W. (Eds.). (1999). *Handbook of theories of aging.* New York: Springer.

Blake, M. J., Fargnoli, J., Gershon, D., & Holbrook, N. J. (1991). Concomitant decline in heat-induced hyperthermia and HSP70 mRNA expression in aged rats. *American Journal of Physiology, 260,* R663–R667.

Braeckman, B. P., Houthoofd, K., & Vanfleteren, J. R. (2000). Patterns of metabolic activity during aging of the wild type and longevity mutants of *Caenorhabditis elegans. Age, 23,* 51–69.

Brenner, S. (1974). The genetics of *Caenorhabditis elegans. Genetics, 77,* 71–94.

Chitwood, D. J., & Lusby, W. R. (1991). Metabolism of plant sterols by nematodes. *Lipids, 26,* 619–627.

Colombatto, S., Giribaldi, G., Vargiu, C., & Grillo, M. A. (1994). Modulation of ornithine aminotransferase activity by oxygen in rat hepatocyte cultures. *Biochimica Biophysica Acta, 1224,* 329–332.

Cristofalo, V. J., Allen, R. G., Pignolo, R. J., Martin, B. G., & Beck, J. C. (1998). Relationship between donor age and the replicative lifespan of human cells in culture: A reevaluation. *Proceedings of the National Academy of Sciences, USA, 95,* 10614–10619.

Cristofalo, V. J., Tresini, M., Francis, M. K., & Volker, C. (1999). Biological theories of senescence. In V. L. Bengston & K. W. Schaie (Eds.), *Handbook of theories of aging* (pp. 98–112). New York: Springer Publishing Company.

Croll, N. A., Smith, J. M., & Zuckerman, B. M. (1977). The aging process of the nematode Caenorhabditis elegans in bacterial and axenic culture. *Experiental Aging Research, 3,* 175–189.

Daniel, C. W. (1977). Cell Longevity: In Vivo. In C. E. Finch & L. Hayflick (Eds.), *Handbook of the biology of aging* (pp. 122–158). New York: Van Nostrand Reinhold.

Dougherty, E. C., Hansen, E. L., Nicholas, W. L., Mollett, J. A., & Yarwood, E. A. (1959). Axenic cultivation of Caenorhabditis briggsae with unsupplemented and supplemented chemically defined media. *Annals of the New York Academy of Sciences, 77,* 176.

Eagle, H. (1973). The effect of environmental pH on the growth of normal and malignant cells. *Journal of Cell Physiology, 82,* 1–8.

Egilmez, N. K., & Jazwinski, S. M. (1989). Evidence for the involvement of a cytoplasmic factor in the aging of the yeast Saccharomyces cerevisiae. *Journal of Bacteriology, 171,* 37–42.

Eppig, J. J., & Wigglesworth, K. (1995). Factors affecting the developmental competence of mouse oocytes grown in vitro: Oxygen concentration. *Molecular and Reproductive Development, 42,* 447–456.

Epstein, J., & Gershon, D. (1972). Studies on aging in nematodes. IV. The effect of antioxidants on cellular damage and life span. *Mechanisms of Ageing and Development*, 257–264.

Epstein, J., Himmelhoch, S., & Gershon, D. (1972). Studies on aging in nematodes. III. Electromicroscopical studies on age associated cellular damage. *Mechanisms of Ageing and Development, 1,* 245–255.

Erlanger, M., & Gershon, D. (1970). Studies on aging in nematodes. II. Studies of the activities of several enzymes as a function of age. *Experimental Gerontology, 5,* 13–19.

Fabian, T. J., & Johnson, T. E. (1995). Identification genes that are differentially expressed during aging in Caenorhabditis elegans. *Journal of Gerontology, Biological Science and Medical Science, 50,* B245–B253.

Finch, C. E., & Seeman, T. E. (1999). Stress theories of aging. In V. L. Bengston & K. W. Schaie (Eds.), *Handbook of theories of aging* (pp. 81–97). New York: Springer Publishing Company.

Friedman, D. B., & Johnson, T. E. (1988a). Three mutants that extend both mean and maximum life span of the nematode, Caenorhabditis elegans, define th*e age-1 gene. Journal of Gerontology, 43,* B102–B109.

Friedman, D. B., & Johnson, T. E. (1988b). A mutation in the age-1 gene in Caenorhabditis elegans lengthens life and reduces hermaphrodite fertility. *Genetics, 118,* 75–86.

Friedman, P. A., Platzer, E. G., & Eby, J. E. (1977). Species differentiation in *C. briggsae* and *C. elegans. Journal of Nematology, 9,* 197–203.

Gershon, D. (1970). Studies on aging in nematodes. I. The nematode as a model organism for aging research. *Experimental Gerontology, 5,* 7–12.

Gershon, H., & Gershon, D. (1970). Detection of inactive enzyme molecules in ageing organisms. *Nature, 227,* 1214–1217.

Gershon, H., & Gershon, D. (1973a). Altered enzyme molecules in senescent organisms: Mouse muscle aldolase. *Mechanisms of Ageing and Development, 2,* 33–41.

Gershon, H., & Gershon, D. (1973b). Inactive enzyme molecules in aging mice: Liver aldolase. *Proceedings of the National Academy of Sciences, 70,* 909–913.

Gershon, H., & Gershon, D. (2000a). The budding yeast, *Saccharomyces cerevisiae,* as a model for aging research. *Mechanisms of Ageing and Development, 120,* 1–22.

Gershon, H., & Gershon, D. (2000b). Paradigms in aging research: A critical review and assessment. *Mechanisms of Ageing and Development, 117,* 21–28.

Glass, G. A., Gershon, H., & Gershon, D. (1983). The effect of donor and cell age on several characteristics of rat erythrocytes. *Experimental Hematology, 11,* 987–995.

Glass, G. A., Gershon, D., & Gershon, H. (1985). Some characteristics of the human erythrocyte as a function of donor and cell age. *Experimental Hematology, 13,* 1122–1126.

Glover, J. R., & Lindquist, S. (1998). Hsp104, Hsp70, and Hsp40: A novel chaperone system that rescues previously aggregated proteins. *Cell, 94,* 73–82.

Goffeau, A., Barrell, B. G., Bussey, H., Davis, R. W., Dujon, B., Feldmann, H., Galibert, F., Hoheisel, J. D., Jacq, C., Johnston, M., Louis, E. J., Mewes, H. W., Murakami, Y., Philippsen, P., Tettelin, H., Oliver, S. G. (1996). Life with 6000 genes [comments]. *Science, 274,* 563–567.

Guarente, L. (2000). Sir2 links chromatin silencing, metabolism, and aging. *Genes and Development, 14,* 1021–1026.

Harley, C. B., Futcher, A. B., Greider, C. W. (1990). Telomeres shorten during ageing of human fibroblasts. *Nature, 345,* 458–460.

Harper, J. M., & Austad, S. N. (2000). Fecal glucocorticoids: A noninvasive method of measuring adrenal activity in wild and captive rodents. *Physiological and Biochemical Zoology, 73,* 12–22.

Harrison, D. E. (1985). Cell and tissue transplantation: A means of studying the aging process. In C. E. Finch & E. L. Schneider (Eds.), *Handbook of the biology of aging* (pp. 322–356). New York: Van Nostrand Reinhold.

Harrison, D. E., Astle, C. M., & DeLaittre, J. (1988). Effects of transplantation and age on immunohemopoietic cell growthX in the splenic microenvironment. *Experimental Hematology, 16,* 213–226.

Hayflick, L. (1965). The limited in vitro lifetime of human diploid cell strains. *Experimental Cell Research, 37,* 614–620.

Hayflick, L., & Moorhead, P. S. (1961). The serial cultivation of human diploid cell strains. *Experimental Cell Research, 25,* 585–621.

Herman, P. K., & Rine, J. (1997). Yeast spore germination: A requirement for Ras protein activity during re-entry into the cell cycle. *EMBO Journal, 16,* 6171–6181.

Herscovich, S. & Gershon, D. (1987). Effects of aging and physical training on the neuromuscular junction of the mouse. *Gerontology, 33,* 7–13.

Hodgkin, J. (1997). Appendix 1: Genetics, 1, D. L. Riddle, T. Blumenthal, B. J. Meyer, & J. R. Priess (Eds.), *C. elegans II.* Cold Spring Harbor, NY: Cold Spring Harbor Laboratory Press.

Horikoshi, T., Balin, A. K., & Carter, D. M. (1991). Effects of oxygen tension on the growth and pigmentation of normal human melanocytes. *Journal of Investigative Dermatology, 96,* 841–844.

Horvitz, H. R. (1988). Genetics of cell lineage. In W. B. Wood (Ed.), *The nematode* Caenorhabditis elegans (p. 157). Cold Spring Harbor, New York: Cold Spring Harbor Laboratory Press.

Jakubowski, W., Bilinski, T., & Bartosz, G. (2000). Oxidative stress during aging of stationary cultures of the yeast Saccharomyces cerevisiae [in process citation]. *Free Radical Biology and Medicine, 28,* 659–664.

Jazwinski, S. M. (1999). The RAS genes: A homeostatic device in Saccharomyces cerevisiae longevity. *Neurobiological Aging, 20,* 471–478.

Jazwinski, S. M. (2000). Coordination of metabolic activity and stress resistance in yeast longevity. In S. Hekimi (Ed.), *The molecular genetics of aging* (pp. 21–44). Berlin, Germany: Springer-Verlag.

Johnson, T. E. (1984). Analysis of the biological basis of aging in the nematode, with special emphasis on *Caenorhabditis elegans.* In D. H. Mitchel & T. E. Johnson (Eds.), *Invertebrate models in aging research* (p. 59). Boca Raton, FL: CRC Press.

Johnson, T. E., & Lithgow, G. J. (1992). The search for the genetic basis of aging: The identification of gerontogenes in the nematode Caenorhabditis elegans. *Journal of the American Geriatrics Society, 40,* 936–945.

Kaeberlein, M., McVey, M., & Guarente, L. (1999). The SIR2/3/4 complex and SIR2 alone promote longevity in Saccharomyces cerevisiae by two different mechanisms. *Genes and Development, 13,* 2570–2580.

Kennedy, B. K., Austriaco, N. R., Jr., & Guarente, L., (1994.) Daughter cells of Saccharomyces cerevisiae from old mothers display a reduced life span. *Journal of Cell Biology, 127,* 1985–1993.

Kenyon, C., Chang, J., Gensch, E., Rudner, A., & Tabtiang, R. (1993). A C. elegans mutant that lives twice as long as wild type [comments]. *Nature, 366,* 461–464.

Khaliq, A., Patel, B., Jarvis-Evans, J., Moriarty, P., McLeod, D., & Boulton, M. (1995). Oxygen modulates production of bFGF and TGF-beta by retinal cells in vitro. *Experimental Eye Research, 60,* 415–423.

Kim, S., Kirchman, P. A., Benguria, A., & Jazwinski, S. M. (1999). Experimentation with the yeast model. In B. P. Yu (Ed.), *Methods in aging research* (pp. 191–213). Boca Raton, FL: CRC Press.

Kim, S., Benguria, A., Lai, C. Y., & Jazwinski, S. M. (1999). Modulation of life-span by histone deacetylase genes in Saccharomyces cerevisiae. *Molecular Biology of the Cell, 10,* 3125–3136.

Kim, S., Schilke, B., Craig, E. A., & Horwich, A. L. (1998). Folding in vivo of a newly translated yeast cytosolic enzyme is mediated by the SSA class of cytosolic yeast Hsp70 proteins. *Proceedings of the National Academy of Sciences, USA, 95,* 12860–12865.

Klass, M., & Hirsh, D. (1976). Non-ageing developmental variant of Caenorhabditis elegans. *Nature, 260,* 523–525.

Klass, M. R. (1977). Aging in the nematode Caenorhabditis elegans: Major biological and environmental factors influencing life span. *Mechanisms of Ageing and Development, 6,* 413–429.

Krieger, J. A., Landsiedel, J. C., & Lawrence, D. A. (1996). Differential in vitro effects of physiological and atmospheric oxygen tension on normal human peripheral blood mononuclear cell proliferation, cytokine and immunoglobulin production. *International Journal of Immunopharmacology, 18,* 545–552.

Krohn, P. L. (1966). Transplantation and aging. In P. L. Krohn (Ed.), *Topics of the biology of aging* (pp. 125–138). New York: John Wiley.

LaIuppa, J. A., Papoutsakis, E. T., & Miller, W. M. (1998). Oxygen tension alters the effects of cytokines on the megakaryocyte, erythrocyte, and granulocyte lineages. *Experimental Hematology, 26,* 835–843.

Lakowski, B., & Hekimi, S. (1996). Determination of life-span in Caenorhabditis elegans by four clock genes. *Science, 272,* 1010–1013.

Lakowski, B., & Hekimi, S. (1998). The genetics of caloric restriction in Caenorhabditis elegans. *Proceedings of the National Academy of Sciences, USA, 95,* 13091–13096.

Lavie, L., Reznick, A. Z., & Gershon, D. (1982). Decreased protein and puromycinyl-peptide degradation in livers of senescent mice. *Biochemical Journal, 202,* 47–51.

Linskens, M. H., Harley, C. B., West, M. D., Campisi, J., & Hayflick, L. (1995). Replicative senescence and cell death [letter; comment]. *Science, 267,* 17.

Liou, L-L., Fabrizio, P, Moy, V. N., Vaupel, J. W., Valentine, J. S. Gralla, E. B., & Longo, V. D. (2000). *Ras2 and superoxide regulate survival in yeast* (manuscript submitted for publication).

Longo, V. D. (1999). Mutations in signal transduction proteins increase stress resistance and longevity in yeast, nematodes, fruit flies, and mammalian neuronal cells. *Neurobiological Aging, 20,* 479–486.

Longo, V. D., Ellerby, L. M., Bredesen, D. E., Valentine, J. S., & Gralla, E. B. (1997). Human Bcl-2 reverses survival defects in yeast lacking superoxide dismutase and delays death of wild-type yeast. *Journal of Cell Biology, 137,* 1581–1588.

Miller, R. A., Austad, S., Burke, D., Chrisp, C., Dysko, R., Galecki, A., Jackson, A., & Monnier, V. (1999). Exotic mice as models for aging research: Polemic and prospectus [comments]. *Neurobiological Aging, 20,* 217–231.

Miller, R. A., Dysko, R., Chrisp, C., Seguin, R., Linsalata, L., Buchner, G., Harper, J. M., & Austad, S. (2000). Mouse *(Mus musculus)* stocks derived from tropical islands: New models for genetic analysis of life-history traits. *Journal of Zoology [Lond], 250,* 95–104.

Mortimer, R. K., & Johnston, J. R. (1959). Life span of individual yeast cells. *Nature, 183,* 1751–1752.

Mosch, H. U., Kubler, E., Krappmann, S., Fink, G. R., Braus, G. H. (1999). Crosstalk between the Ras2p-controlled mitogen-activated protein kinase and cAMP pathways during invasive growth of Saccharomyces cerevisiae. *Molocular Biology of the Cell, 10,* 1325–1335.

Nasmyth, K. (1996). At the heart of the budding yeast cell cycle. *Trends Genet, 12,* 405–412.

Ono, K., & Alter, B. P. (1995). Effects of low oxygen tension and antioxidants on human erythropoiesis in vitro. *Experimental Hematology, 23,* 1372–1377.

O'Shea, E. K., & Herskowitz, I. (2000). The ins and outs of cell-polarity decisions [news]. *Nature Cell Biology, 2,* E39–E41.

Padilla, P. A., Fuge, E. K., Crawford, M. E., Errett, A., & Werner-Washburne, M. (1998). The highly conserved, coregulated SNO and SNZ gene families in Saccharomyces cerevisiae respond to nutrient limitation [published erratum appears in *Journal of Bacteriology* 1998, December, *180(24)* 6794]. *Journal of Bacteriology, 180,* 5718–5726.

Park, P. U., Defossez, P. A., & Guarente, L. (1999). Effects of mutations in DNA repair genes on formation of ribosomal DNA circles and life span in Saccharomyces cerevisiae. *Molecular Cell Biology, 19,* 3848–3856.

Phelan, J. P., & Austad, S. N. (1994). Selecting animal models of human aging: Inbred strains often exhibit less biological uniformity than F1 hybrids. *Journal of Gerontology, 49,* B1–11.

Reykdal, S., Abboud, C., & Liesveld, J. (1999). Effect of nitric oxide production and oxygen tension on progenitor preservation in ex vivo culture. *Experimental Hematology, 27,* 441–450.

Reznick, A., & Gershon, D. (1999). Experimentation with nematodes. In B. P. Yu (Ed.), *Methods in aging research* (pp. 167–190). Boca Raton, FL CRC Press.

Reznick, A. Z., & Gershon, D. (1977). Age-related alterations in purified fructose-1,6-diphosphate aldolase from the nematode Turbatrix aceti. *Mechanisms of Ageing and Development, 6,* 345–353.

Reznick, A. Z., & Gershon, D. (1979). The effect of age on the protein degradation system in the nematode Turbatrix aceti. *Mechanisms of Ageing Development, 11,* 403–415.

Reznick, A. Z., Lavie, L., Gershon, H. E., & Gershon, D. (1981). Age-associated accumulation of altered FDP aldolase B in mice. Conditions of detection and determination of aldolase half life in young and old animals. *FEBS Letters, 128,* 221–224.

Reznick, A. Z., Rosenfelder, L., Shpund, S., & Gershon, D. (1985). Identification of intracellular degradation intermediates of aldolase B by antiserum to the denatured enzyme. *Proceedings of the National Academy of Sciences, USA, 82,* 6114–6118.

Riddle, D. L., & Albert, P. S. (1997). Genetic and environmental regulation of Dauer larva development. In D. L. Riddle, T. Blumenthal, B. J. Meyer, & J. R. Priess (Eds.), C. Elegans II (pp. 739–768). Cold Spring Harbor, NY: Cold Spring Harbor Laboratory Press.

Robertson, O. H., Drupp, M. A., Thomas, S. F., Favom, C. B., Hane, S., & Wexler, B. C. (1961). Hyperadrenocorticism in spawning migratory and non-migratory rainbow trout *(Salmo gairdnerii):* Comparison with Pacific salmon *(genus Oncorhynchus). Endocrinology, 1,* 473–484.

Robertson, O. H., & Wexler, B. C. (1959). Hyperplasia of the adrenal cortical tissue in Pacific salmon and rainbow trout accompanying sexual maturation and spawning. *Endocrinology, 65,* 225–238.

Rothstein, M., Cook, E. (1966). Nematode biochemistry. VI. Conditions for axenic culture of Turbatrix aceti, Panagrellus redivivus, Rhabditis anomala and Caenorhabditis briggsae. *Comparative Biochemistry and Physiology, 17,* 683–692.

Saito, H., Hammond, A. T., & Moses, R. E. (1995). The effect of low oxygen tension on the in vitro-replicative life span of human diploid fibroblast cells and their transformed derivatives. *Experimental Cell Research, 217,* 272–279.

Sinclair, D. A., & Guarente, L. (1997). Extrachromosomal rDNA circles—A cause of aging in yeast. *Cell, 91,* 1033–1042.

Sinclair, D. A., Mills, K., & Guarente, L. (1998). Molecular mechanisms of yeast aging. *Trends in Biochemical Science, 23,* 131–134.

Solomon, D. (1999). The role of aging processes in aging-dependent diseases. In V. L. Bengtson & K. W. Schaie (Eds.), *Handbook of theories of aging* (pp. 133–152). New York: Springer Publishing Co.

Stahl, F. (1996). Meiotic recombination in yeast: coronation of the double-strand-break repair model. *Cell, 87,* 965–968.

Strehler, B. L. (1977). *Time, cells, and aging* (1st ed.). New York: Academic Press.

Strohman, R. C. (2001). Genomics and human life span—what's left to extend? *Nature Biotechnology, 19,* 195.

Sulston, J. (1988). Cell Lineage. In W. B. Wood (Ed.), *The nematode* Caenorhabditis elegans (p. 123). Cold Spring Harbor, NY: Cold Spring Harbor Laboratory Press.

Sulston, J. & Hodgkin, J. (1988). Methods. In W. B. Wood (Ed.), *The nematode* Caenorhabditis elegans (p. 587). Cold Spring Harbor, NY: Cold Spring Harbor Laboratory Press.

Sun, J., Kale, S. P., Childress, A. M., Pinswasdi, C., & Jazwinski, S. M. (1994). Divergent roles of RAS1 and RAS2 in yeast longevity. *Journal of Biological Chemistry, 269,* 18638–18645.

Supakar, P. C., & Roy, A. K. (1996). Role of transcription factors in the age-dependent regulation of the androgen receptor gene in rat liver. *Biological Signals, 5,* 170–179.

Tanaka, T., Ikita, K., Ashida, T., Motoyama, Y., Yamaguchi, Y., & Satouchi, K. (1996). Effects of growth temperature on the fatty acid composition of the free-living nematode Caenorhabditis elegans. *Lipids, 31,* 1173–1178.

Toda, T., Uno, I., Ishikawa, T., Powers, S., Kataoka, T., Broek, D., Cameron, S., Broach, J., Matsumoto, K., & Wigler, M. (1985). In yeast, RAS proteins are controlling elements of adenylate cyclase. *Cell, 40,* 27–36.

Vanfleteren, J. R., & Braeckman, B. P. (1999). Mechanisms of life span determination in Caenorhabditis elegans. *Neurobiology of Aging, 20,* 487–502.

Walker, D. W., McColl, G., Jenkins, N. L., Harris, J., & Lithgow, G. J. (2000). Evolution of lifespan in C. elegans. *Nature, 405,* 296–297.

Werner-Washburne, M., Braun, E., Johnston, G. C., & Singer, R. A. (1993). Stationary phase in the yeast Saccharomyces cerevisiae. *Microbiological Reviews, 57,* 383–401.

Werner-Washburne, M., Braun, E. L., Crawford, M. E., & Peck, V. M. (1996). Stationary phase in Saccharomyces cerevisiae. *Molecular Microbiology, 19,* 1159–1166.

Whitmarsh, A. J., & Davis, R. J. (1998). Structural organization of MAP-kinase signaling modules by scaffold proteins in yeast and mammals. *Trends in Biochemical Science, 23,* 481–485.

Xie, Y., & Varshavsky, A. (1999). The N-end rule pathway is required for import of histidine in yeast lacking the kinesin-like protein Cin8p. *Current Genetics, 36,* 113–123.

Yamanaka, N., & Deamer, D. (1974). Superoxide dismutase activity in WI-38 cell cultures: Effects of age, trypsinization and SV-40 transformation. *Physiological and Chemical Physiology, 6,* 95–106.

Zeelon, P., Gershon, H., & Gershon, D. (1973). Inactive enzyme molecules in aging organisms. Nematode fructose-1,6- diphosphate aldolase. *Biochemistry, 12,* 1743–1750.

CHAPTER 8

Modern Approaches to the Mechanisms of Aging: Molecular Genetics and Genomics

S. MICHAL JAZWINSKI
DEPARTMENT OF BIOCHEMISTRY AND MOLECULAR BIOLOGY
LOUISIANA STATE UNIVERSITY HEALTH SCIENCES CENTER

A BRIEF HISTORY OF GENETIC APPROACHES TO AGING

Although thought previously had been given to the number and nature of the genes that are important in aging, the beginning of genetic research on aging began in the early 1980s. Modern genetics uses a variety of molecular tools, such as the polymerase chain reaction (PCR) in genotyping. However, the use of such technology in the study of aging should not be equated with genetics, at least as it is considered here. Genetics establishes a cause and effect relationship between a genotype and a phenotype. This relationship is not always as direct as we would like, but it strives to go beyond the realm of a correlation. Thus, for example, the finding that the expression of a certain gene changes with age is not sufficient to brand that gene as one that affects the aging process. The reverse is certainly interesting; namely, the determination that the expression of the gene, and whatever it affects, is influenced by aging.

Genes that are instrumental in the aging process have, as a group, been given a variety of names. The most frequently encountered include "gerontogenes" and "longevity genes," which are often called longevity-determining or longevity-assurance genes. The designation "aging genes" has not met with favor, because it seems to indicate that the wild type functions in a program promoting aging and death. This in turn suggests the existence of natural selection for aging, something that is not likely to occur (Rose, 1991). We will use the term "longevity gene" in this chapter, predicated on the fact that most of the genes in this category were implicated in aging through their effect on the life span of the organism. It is difficult to put forth biomarkers that define physiological age better than nominal age itself, making life span the best available predictor of longevity.

The designation "longevity genes," or "gerontogenes," skirts a difficult issue in aging research: the distinction between disease and aging. There are two schools of thought in this area, the first of which considers aging the accumulation of disease processes. The second postulates an aging process that results in an increase in the risk of disease. It will be of obvious interest to find out whether longevity genes fall into the category of disease genes or whether they encode proteins that are involved in various fundamental biological processes, which they affect in ways that take a life span to become evident as aging.

This chapter would end right here if our subject was purely human aging and it were being studied in the intact human. It is instructive to note that pharmaceuticals are always tested first on animals rather than on humans. There must be some degree of correspondence between the physiology of humans and nonhuman animals. Furthermore, the carcinogenicity of chemicals is screened most readily in the Ames test in bacteria and in yeast, suggesting the utility of these "lowly" organisms in human biology. Arguably, much of what we know in fundamental molecular and cell biology has been derived from the study of lower eukaryotes. If aging has no cellular basis, we are out of luck examining simple organisms. Although the jury is still out, most of what has to be said of the genetics of aging is based on studies in invertebrates. Apart from any relevance to the human condition, their aging, however defined, has intrinsic biological interest.

With these preliminary considerations out of the way, we can examine the broad approaches to the genetic analysis of the biological aging process. They are selection, mutagenesis, associative genetics, and quantitative genetics. These four distinct methodologies have been variously applied to different aging organisms (Table 8.1).

The beginning of genetics of aging in the proper sense dates back to the selection of *Drosophila* lines that exhibited extended longevity. This experiment was carried out initially by Rose and Charlesworth (1981), and then perfected by Rose (1984) and Luckinbill, Arking, Clare, Cirocco, and Buck, (1984). Fruit flies were essentially selected for delayed reproduction by collecting eggs laid by older and older flies in each generation. This procedure facilitated the accretion of alleles, extant in the starting population, which were conducive to long life. This approach has been duplicated since then by others (Partridge & Fowler, 1992; Hillesheim & Stearns, 1992; Zwaan, Bijlsma, & Hoekstra, 1995). Most analyses subsequently concentrated on the physiological correlates of extended longevity, with the goal

TABLE 8.1 Genetic Approaches to Aging

Organism	Methodology
Saccharomyces cerevisiae	Mutagenesis • forward genetics • reverse genetics
Caenorhabditis elegans	Mutagenesis • forward genetics • reverse genetics Selection Quantitative genetics
Drosophila melanogaster	Mutagenesis • forward genetics • reverse genetics Selection Quantitative genetics
Mouse	Mutagenesis • forward genetics • reverse genetics Selection Quantitative genetics Associative genetics
Human	Associative genetics

of identifying potential candidate longevity genes. The flies that display extended longevity have been subjected to quantitative genetic analysis, with the same goal in mind. The selection approach, in a different guise, has also been applied to the nematode worm *Caenorhabditis elegans* with success (Ebert et al., 1993). The worms that were obtained have been subjected to quantitative genetic analysis. Selection has also been applied to mice (Covelli et al., 1989; Nagai, Lin, & Sabour, 1995), although there is some criticism of the studies.

The mutagenesis approach has proven spectacularly successful in the identification of longevity genes as "single gene" traits. It is the subject of two of the following sections, that deal with forward and reverse genetics. Associative genetics has been applied to the study of aging in mice and humans. This approach simply examines whether there is any difference in the frequency of alleles at a candidate gene locus between long- and short-lived individuals. In the mouse, it has served to implicate certain alleles at the major histocompatibility complex with longevity

(Yunis & Salazar, 1993). Quantitative genetics designates the genetics of continuous phenotypes. Certainly, aging possesses the features of just such a trait. The advent of methods for identification of quantitative trait loci (QTL) has provided a modus operandi for identification of chromosomal regions that possess genes that play a role in the aging process. QTL analysis is now being applied to the study of aging in *C. elegans* (Shook & Johnson, 1999), the fruit fly (Resler et al., 1998), and in mice (Miller, Chrisp, & Atchley, 2000). It is being used both in conjunction with selection, as well as directly without any selection. This methodology has facilitated the identification of a putative locus that affects the variation in the life span of individuals among lines of mice with otherwise identical mean life spans (de Haan, Gelman, Watson, Yunis, & Van Zant, 1998).

MOLECULAR GENETICS

Classical genetics involves the treatment of genes as abstract entities, subject to the laws of assortment. In molecular genetics, these entities have become physical elements that can be further dissected and analyzed. Although in forward genetics they can be considered these abstract moieties, the goal, often achieved in aging research, has been to provide them with a physical garb.

The distinction between forward and reverse genetics is sometimes confused. Here, we consider forward genetics to designate methods that start with a phenotype of interest, having as their goal the identification of the responsible genes. Reverse genetics begins with a known gene and has as its goal the identification of the phenotype that the gene controls. Thus, it is distinguished from forward genetics by its targeted nature. In this chapter, we will only discuss genes that have actually been cloned and sequenced, and not simply genes identified as mutants.

Forward Genetics

Yeast and Other Fungi

The budding yeast *Saccharomyces cerevisiae* has a finite life span, measured by the number of times individual cells divide (Mortimer & Johnston, 1959; Müller, Zimmerman, Becker, & Flömer, 1980). (The replicative life span of the fission yeast *Schizosaccharomyces pombe* has been similarly defined [(Barker & Walmsley, 1999).] The survival of *S. cerevisiae* cells in stationary phase, after most growth has ceased in batch culture, has been termed the chronological life span (Longo, 1999). There may be some relationship between replicative and chronological life span (Ashrafi, Sinclair, Gordon, & Guarente, 1999; Jazwinski, 1999a). Another ascomycete, the filamentous fungus *Podospora anserina*, has long been a model in aging studies (Osiewacz & Borghouts, 2000), in which chronological age and growth are correlated measures of longevity. These fungi are discussed because the genetics of aging has progressed in these organisms to the level of identification and further analysis of individual genes and the processes in which they participate.

Some 30 genes that determine the *S. cerevisiae* replicative life span have been identified and cloned (Table 8.2). In addition, *SOD1* and *SOD2* have been shown to be important for maintaining chronological life span. In *Podospora*, the *grisea* and copper-transporter genes have been demonstrated to play a role in aging (Osiewacz & Borghouts, 2000). The various longevity genes described in these systems are involved in a broad array of biochemical functions, suggesting the participation of several pathways or processes in life-span determination. Nevertheless, it is possible from these analyses to discern the role of four broad physiological principles in aging: metabolic control, resistance to stress, gene dysregulation, and genetic stability.

Forward genetics has identified two of the genes alluded to, *SIR4* and *UTH4* in *S. cerevisiae*. These were among four gene mutants isolated for survival in stationary phase at low temperature. These mutants not only had a longer life span, but they were resistant to a variety of stresses (Kennedy, Austriaco, Zhang, & Guarente, 1995). *SIR4* was already known as a crucial component of the silencing apparatus, which prevents the transcription of genes located at the heterochromatic silent-mating-type and subtelomeric loci. The role of *UTH4* is less clear, but it appears to function in the transport and intracellular localization of the silencing complexes (Kennedy et al., 1997).

Caenorhabditis elegans

The bulk of worm longevity genes has been identified through forward genetics (Table 8.3). The first of these genes was *age-1*, which was also identified later as *daf-23* (Friedman & Johnson, 1988; Klass, 1983). This gene encodes a subunit of phosphatidylinositol-3-OH kinase (Morris, Tissenbaum, & Ruvkun, 1996), which is part of a signal transduction pathway (Figure 8.1) with the insulin/IGF-1-like receptor, DAF-2, at its head (Kenyon, Chang, Gensch, Rudner, & Tabtiang, 1993; Larsen, Albert, & Riddle, 1995; Kimura, Tissenbaum, Liu, & Ruvkun, 1997). Downstream of *age-1* are the *akt-1* and *akt-2* genes, which code for protein kinase B homologs (Paradis & Ruvkun, 1998). The target of this signaling pathway is the forkhead transcription factor encoded by *daf-16* (Ogg et al., 1997; Lin, Dorman, Rodan, & Kenyon, 1997), whose activity is required for extended longevity (Larsen et al., 1995; Dorman, Albinder, Shroyer, & Kenyon, 1995). DAF-16 is functionally most similar to the forkhead transcription factor FKHR,

TABLE 8.2 Yeast Longevity Genes

Gene	Function	References
LAG1	Endoplasmic reticulum (ER) protein; GPI-anchored protein transport, sphingolipid metabolism	D'mello et al. (1994)
LAC1	Homolog of *LAG1;* ER protein; GPI-anchored protein transport, sphingolipid metabolism	Jiang et al. (1998)
RAS1	GTP-binding (G-) protein; signal transduction	Sun et al. (1994)
RAS2	G-protein; signal transduction	Sun et al. (1994)
CDC35	Adenylate cyclase	Sun et al. (1994); Lin et al. (2000)
BCY1	Regulatory subunit of protein kinase A	Sun et al. (1994)
PHB1	Mitochondrial protein; membrane-bound mitochondrial protein chaperone	Jazwinski (1996); Coates et al. (1997); Berger & Yaffe (1998)
PHB2	Mitochondrial protein; homolog of *PHB1;* membrane-bound mitochondrial protein chaperone	Coates et al. (1997); Berger & Yaffe (1998)
CDC7	Protein kinase; cell cycle control	Jazwinski et al. (1989)
BUD1	G-protein; cell polarity	Jazwinski et al. (1998)
RTG2	Unknown; retrograde response	Kirchman et al. (1999)
RTG3	Basic helix-loop-helix/leucine zipper transcription factor; retrograde response	Kirchman et al. (1999); Jiang et al. (2000)
RPD3	Histone deacetylase; chromatin-dependent gene regulation	Kim et al. (1999)
HDA1	Histone deacetylase; chromatin-dependent gene regulation	Kim et al. (1999)
SIR2	Histone deacetylase; chromatin-dependent transcriptional silencing	Kim et al. (1999); Imai et al. (2000)
SIR4	Transcriptional silencing	Kennedy et al. (1995)
UTH4	Unknown	Kennedy et al. (1997)
YGL023	Unknown; homolog of *UTH4*	Kennedy et al. (1997)

TABLE 8.2 ***(Continued)***

Gene	Function	References
SGS1	DNA helicase; DNA recombination	Sinclair et al. (1997); Heo et al. (1999)
RAD52	DNA repair	Park et al. (1999)
FOB1	Replication block	Defossez et al. (1999)
CDC25	GDP-GTP exchange factor for *RAS*	Lin et al. (2000)
TPK2	Protein kinase A catalytic subunit	Lin et al. (2000)
GPR1	Glucose-binding protein	Lin et al. (2000)
GPA2	G-protein	Lin et al. (2000)
ZDS1	Transcriptional silencing	Roy & Runge (2000)
ZDS2	Transcriptional silencing	Roy & Runge (2000)
NMT1	N-myristoyltransferase	Ashrafi et al. (2000)
SIP2	Unknown; N-myristoylprotein	Ashrafi et al. (2000)
SNF1	AMP-activated protein kinase homolog	Ashrafi et al. (2000)
SNF4	Regulatory subunit of Snf1 complex	Ashrafi et al. (2000)
SOD1	Cu, Zn-superoxide dismutase	Wawryn et al. (1999); Barker et al. (1999)
SOD2	Mn-superoxide dismutase	Wawryn et al. (1999)

which is involved in insulin and glucocorticoid signaling (Nasrin et al., 2000). The *pdk-1* gene is also part of the *daf-2* pathway; it encodes a homolog of the phosphatidylinositol-dependent kinase, which activates protein kinase B (Paradis, Ailion, Toker, Thomas, & Ruvkun, 1999). The *daf-18* gene modulates this pathway. This gene is a homolog of the human tumor suppressor gene PTEN, which encodes a phosphatidylinositol 3,4,5-triphosphate 3-phosphatase activity (Ogg & Ruvkun, 1998). All of the genes just described (and *daf-12*, which follows) were identified on the basis of the secondary phenotype of dauer larva formation, an altered developmental stage that functions as a dispersal form.

It has been shown that *daf-2* acts nonautonomously in cells to regulate life span (Apfeld & Kenyon, 1998). The study suggested interactions between multiple cell types. Indeed, signals from both the germ line and the somatic gonad play a role (Hsin & Kenyon, 1999). The *daf-12* gene plays a role in these interactions. This gene had already been implicated

TABLE 8.3 ***C. elegans*** **Longevity Genes**

Gene	Function	References
age-1	Phosphatidylinositol-3-OH kinase	Klass, 1983; Friedman & Johnson (1988)
daf-2	Insulin/IGF-1-like receptor	Kenyon et al. (1993); Larsen et al. (1995)
akt-1	Protein kinase B	Paradis & Ruvkun (1998)
akt-2	Protein kinase B	Paradis & Ruvkun (1998)
daf-16	Forkhead transcription factor	Larsen et al. (1995); Dorman et al. (1995)
pdk-1	Phosphatidylinositol-dependent protein kinase	Paradis et al. (1999)
daf-18	Phosphatidylinositol 3,4,5-triphosphate 3-phosphatase	Ogg & Ruvkun (1998)
daf-12	Steroid-thyroid hormone-vitamin D receptor/retinoic acid receptor superfamily member	Larsen et al. (1995)
osm-6	Intraflagellar transport particle homolog	Apfeld & Kenyon (1999)
osm-3	Kinesin-like protein	Apfeld & Kenyon (1999)
tax-4	Cyclic nucleotide-gated channel component	Apfeld & Kenyon (1999)
unc-64	Syntaxin homolog	Ailion et al. (1999)
unc-31	CAPS homolog	Ailion et al. (1999)
spe-26	Kelch and scruin homolog	Varkey et al. (1995)
mev-1	Succinate dehydrogenase cytochrome b	Ishii et al. (1998)
clk-1	Ubiquinone biosynthesis	Ewbank et al. (1997)
old-1	Tyrosine kinase receptor	Murakami & Johnson (1998)
ctl-1	Cytoplasmic catalase	Taub et al. (1999)

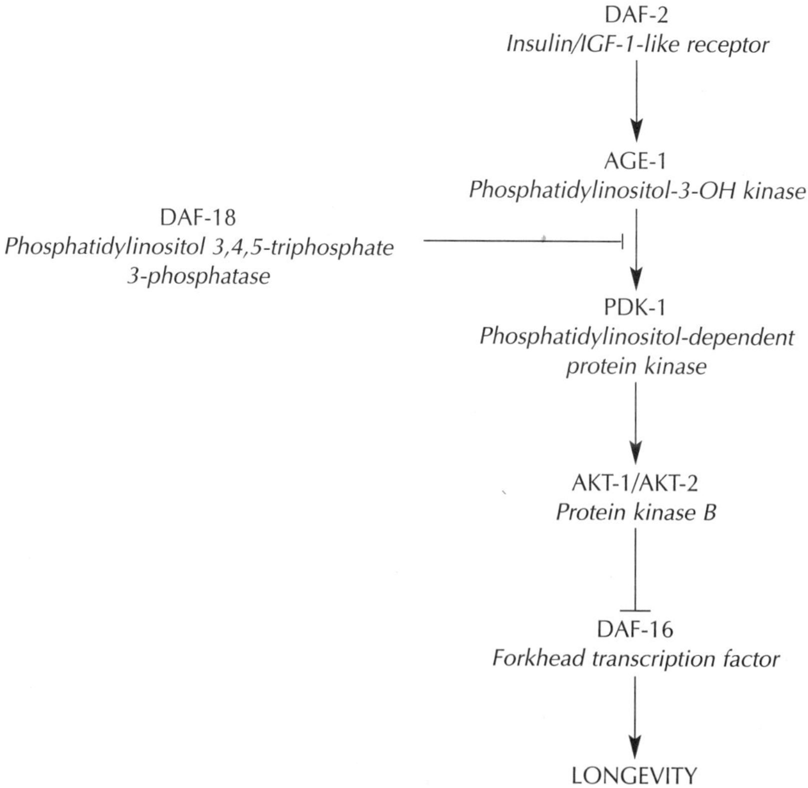

FIGURE 8.1 The *C. elegans* DAF pathway for life-span determination.

in life-span determination (Larsen et al., 1995). DAF-12 belongs to the glucocorticoid-thyroid hormone-vitamin D receptor/retinoic acid receptor superfamilly (Antebi, Yeh, Tait, Hedgecock, & Riddle, 2000; Snow & Larsen, 2000). However, it appears that the nervous system may be a pacesetter for longevity (Wolkow, Kimura, Lee, & Ruvkun, 2000). Sensory neurons play a particularly important role. It has been shown that mutants affecting sensory neuron development, structure, and function affect worm life span (Apfeld & Kenyon, 1999). Thirteen genes were identified in this way, and three have been cloned. They include *osm-6*, a homolog of an intraflagellar transport particle required for assembly of a cilium-like structure that is analogous to one found in worm sensory neurons; *osm-3*, encoding a kinesin-like protein; and *tax-4*, a component of a cyclic nucleotide-gated channel. The studies suggest that the pathway these sensory mutants define acts only partly through *daf-16* or that the *daf-16* pathway functions in parallel. Some evidence is available that indicates the former possibility. Additional evidence for the role of sensory neuron function has been presented. The *unc-64* and *unc-31* genes, which encode homologs of syntaxin and CAPS (proteins that mediate calcium-regulated secretion) also determine worm life span (Ailion, Inoue, Weaver, Holdcraft, & Thomas, 1999). These two genes act through *daf-16.*

Essentially all of the longevity genes that have been identified in the worm are involved in stress resistance (Johnson et al., 2000). The stresses that were tested included heat, ultraviolet radiation, and oxidants. The *spe-26* gene also belongs to this category. This gene codes for a protein that is similar to the actin-associated proteins kelch and scruin (Varkey, Muhlrad, Minniti, Do, & Ward, 1995). As is the case with the *daf* mutants, all of the other longevity gene mutants were identified first through a secondary phenotype. Mutations in the *mev-1* gene, which encodes succinate dehydrogenase cytochrome b, results in oxidative stress and accelerated aging in the worm (Ishii et al., 1998).

Another pathway to extended longevity is described by the *clk* mutants (Lakowski & Hekimi, 1996). The prototype is the gene *clk-1,* which encodes a homolog of the yeast *COQ7* gene that is required for ubiquinone biosynthesis (Ewbank et al., 1997). The *clk* mutants all display a slowing of an array of diverse developmental and behavioral processes, and they also cause an irregular periodicity. The *clk-1* mutant displays maternal effects. The slowing of the worm's physiological processes includes respiration (Felkai et al., 1999); however, the effect on mitochondrial function is slight. This has prompted the conclusion that *clk-1* performs a regulatory function by participating in a signaling pathway from the mitochondrion to the nucleus (Branicky, Benard, & Hekimi, 2000). This conclusion has been disputed in a recent study that shows there is a primary defect in ubiquinone biosynthesis that is rescued by the ubiquinone provided in the bacterial diet of the worm (Jonassen, Larsen, & Clarke, 2001). Another point of contention is the place of *clk-1* and the other *clk* genes in worm pathways for extended longevity. Originally, it was shown that the *clk-1* mutant was not suppressed by *daf-16* mutants. However, such suppression was demonstrated in another study, in which it was also shown that *clk-1* affects stress resistance in the worm and that this is suppressed by *daf-16* mutants (Murakami & Johnson, 1996).

Drosophila melanogaster

The number of fly longevity genes is much less impressive than that for yeast or worms. There are only two genes that have been discovered using forward genetics. They are *methusaleh* (Lin, Seroude, & Benzer, 1998) and *indy* (Rogina, Reenan, Nilsen, & Helfand, 2000). The first of these genes encodes a putative guanosine triphosphate–binding protein-coupled seven-transmembrane domain receptor and enhances resistance to starvation, heat, and free radical generators. The second is similar to a mammalian sodium dicarboxylate cotransporter, a membrane protein found in the kidney that transports Krebs cycle intermediates. Given its expression in the fly in the fat body, midgut, and oenocytes, it has been proposed that the mutant *indy* causes a metabolic state mimicking caloric restriction. This would be an exciting conclusion if validated.

Mouse

The Snell dwarf mouse has been reported to live longer than its normal control under laboratory conditions (Bartke, 2000). This mouse has a mutation in a single gene, *pit-1,* which is involved in the differentiation of somatotrophs, lactotrophs, and thyrotrophs in the pituitary. The pit-1 protein binds to the promoters of the growth hormone, prolactin, and thyroid-stimulating hormone-β genes causing their activation. These dwarf mice are smaller than their wild-type litter mates, have a reduced body temperature and metabolic rate, and are characterized by hypothyroidism and hypogonadism. However, they seem to have an improved capacity for removal of reactive oxygen species. They represent an interesting model for study of the aging process. Unfortunately, the molecular identity of the *prop-1* gene that is mutated in the counterpart to the Snell dwarf, the Ames dwarf mouse, is not known at present, although it appears to regulate *pit-1* activity.

An attempt to generate a transgenic mouse resulted in the insertional mutagenesis in a gene called *klotho* (Kuro-o et al., 1997). The mutant mouse displayed multiple abnormalities, which conjured up a syndrome of premature human aging for the researchers. The phenotype displayed by the mouse suggests a widespread connective tissue disorder, and it resembles more a maturational defect than premature aging. The protein encoded by the gene is similar to microbial β-glucosidases. It appears to exist in both membrane-bound and secreted forms (Matsumura et al., 1998). It has been proposed that it functions in an endocrine mechanism of aging.

Human

Werner's syndrome is a segmental progeroid syndrome, which presents many of the phenotypic characteristics of normal aging and some features that distinguish it from normal aging. In a sense, it is a caricature of the aging process. The gene that is defective in this disorder has been cloned. The *WRN* gene encodes a DNA helicase in the recQ family (Yu et al., 1996). This gene has been the subject of intensive study. It appears to affect several DNA transactions, including replication, recombination, repair, and transcription. This would easily explain its pleiotropic effects, which manifest themselves as premature aging. Because aging is a process that is characterized by multiple, seemingly random deficits that accumulate with time, it is perhaps not surprising that a gene having pleiotropic effects might mimic aging. This does not necessarily indicate that *WRN* is involved in normal aging. However, study of *WRN* may reveal something about processes that contribute to normal aging.

Reverse Genetics

Saccharomyces cerevisiae

In contrast to the situation in *C. elegans,* the majority of yeast longevity genes (Table 8.2) have been identified using the reverse genetics approach. The first yeast longevity gene cloned as such is *LAG1* (D'mello et al., 1994), which was originally identified among several genes that are differentially expressed during the yeast life span (Egilmez, Chen, & Jazwinski, 1989). In fact, this was the first longevity gene cloned from any species. The Lag1p affects the kinetics of transport of glycosylphosphatidylinositol-anchored proteins from the endoplasmic reticulum to the Golgi (Barz & Walter, 1999). However, this appears to be a secondary effect. Lag1p has been shown to play a role in sphingolipid metabolism (Brandwagt et al., 2000). The human and *C. elegans* homologs of yeast *LAG1* have been cloned (Jiang, Kirchman, Zagulski, Hunt, & Jazwinski, 1998). These homologs functionally complement the yeast gene. Indeed, the human Lag1p supports a full life span in the yeast cell. *LAG1* possesses a homolog in yeast called *LAC1,* whose function is redundant (Jiang et al., 1998).

The yeast *RAS* genes, which are homologs of the protooncogene *HRAS1,* encode GTP-binding proteins that are important in signal transduction. They are longevity genes that have divergent effects on yeast life span (Sun, Kale, Childress, Pinswasdi, & Jazwinski, 1994). *RAS2* activity extends life span, whereas the opposite holds for *RAS1.* The involvement of these genes in yeast aging was already evident from the life span–extending effect of v-*H-ras* in yeast (Chen, Sun, & Jazwinski, 1990). The *RAS* genes function as a homeostatic device in yeast longevity by modulating several pathways and processes that play a role in yeast aging (Jazwinski, 1999a). These pathways function in metabolic control (Kirchman, Kim, Lai, & Jazwinski, 1999), heat (Shama, Kirchman, Jiang, & Jazwinski, 1998; Shama, Lai, Antoniazzi, Jiang, & Jazwinski, 1998) and ultraviolet radiation (Kale & Jazwinski, 1996) resistance, and cell polarity and transcriptional silencing, (Jazwinski, Kim, Lai, & Benquria, 1998). The role that *RAS2* plays depends on whether the cell is subject to stress (Jazwinski, 1999b). This is important, because it demonstrates that one cannot separate the genotype from the environment. The *CDC25, CDC35, BCY1* and *TPK2* genes, which lie in one of the *RAS* signaling pathways, function as longevity genes in yeast (Sun et al., 1994; Lin, Defossez, & Guarente, 2000). Cdc25p is the Ras protein GTP-GDP exchange factor. Cdc35p is adenyate cyclase, and Bcy1p and Tpk2p are regulatory and catalytic subunits, respectively, of protein kinase A.

The prohibitin genes are highly conserved throughout phylogeny, just as the *RAS* genes. The yeast homologs *PHB1* and *PHB2* affect life span (Jazwinski, 1996; Coates, Jamieson, Smart, Prescott, & Hall, 1997; Berger & Yaffe, 1998). They encode proteins that are embedded within the inner mitochondrial membrane (Berger & Yaffe, 1998). Prohibitins regulate membrane protein degradation by the AAA protease in mitochondria (Steglich, Neupert, & Langer, 1999), but this may be a consequence of their primary function as a membrane-bound chaperone of mitochondrial proteins (Nijtmans et al., 2000).

There are two metabolic mechanisms of aging that have been identified in yeast. The first was the retrograde response, which is an intracellular signaling pathway from the mitochondrion to the nucleus that communicates loss of mitochondrial function (Parikh, Morgan, Scott, Clements, & Butow, 1987). Mitochondrial damage and loss of function are a feature of the aging process in many organisms (Shigenaga, Hagen, & Ames, 1994). The retrograde response results in a reprogramming of nuclear gene expression, involving potentially hundreds of genes (Traven, Wong, Xu, Sopta, & Ingles, 2000). The result is an adjustment of metabolism and the enhancement of stress responses (Liu & Butow, 1999; Traven et al., 2000). Induction of the retrograde response results in an extension of life span (Kirchman et al., 1999). This pathway is modulated by *RAS2*, as indicated earlier. The retrograde response acts like a rheostat, making adjustments commensurate with the amount of mitochondrial dysfunction.

The *RTG* genes mediate the retrograde response. The Rtg1 and Rtg3 proteins are the subunits of a basic helix-loop-helix/leucine zipper transcription factor that acts at the retrograde response element in the promoters of retrograde response genes (Liao & Butow, 1993; Jia, Rothermel, Thornton, & Butow, 1997). Rtg2p binds to this transcription factor, activates it, and is involved in its translocation from the cytoplasm to the nucleus (Rothermel, Thornton, & Butow, 1997; Sekito, Thornton, & Butow, 2000). The Rtg1p-Rtg3p complex and Hap complex (heme-dependent transcriptional activator) regulate the expression of many of the same metabolic enzyme genes. There is a switch from the Hap to the Rtg complex under conditions of metabolic duress caused by mitochondrial dysfunction. The *RTG2* gene functions as a longevity gene in the retrograde response (Kirchman et al., 1999).

Limitation of glucose or amino acids results in an extension of life span in yeast that resembles caloric restriction in mammals (Jiang, Jaruga, Repnevskaya, & Jazwinski, 2000). This metabolic mechanism is distinct from the retrograde response, because there is no requirement for *RTG2*.

Indeed, *RTG3* prevents the realization of the full benefits of the caloric restriction pathway to extended longevity in yeast (Jiang et al., 2000). This is reminiscent of the mutually exclusive roles in part of the Rtg and Hap complexes noted earlier. There is likely to be more than one pathway involved in caloric restriction in yeast. One of these may be defined by *GPR1* and *GPA2* (Lin et al., 2000) and another by *SNF1* (Ashrafi, Lin, Manchester, & Gordon, 2000), which are longevity genes in yeast. Gpr1p is a glucose-signaling membrane-protein, while Gpa2p is an associated G-protein. Snf1p encodes the yeast homolog of the AMP-dependent protein kinase, which in mammals acts as a fuel gauge.

The yeast histone deacetylase genes *RPD3* and *HDA1*, which are homologs of the human *HDAC* genes, play a role in determining yeast life span (Kim, Benguria, Lai, & Jazwinski, 1999). They maintain equilibrium between silenced and transcriptionally active chromatin. Similarly, *SIR2*, which has homologs in other organisms, is a histone deacetylase that contributes to this balance (Kim et al., 1999; Imai, Armstrong, Kaeberlein, & Guarente, 2000). Sir2p is NAD-dependent, providing a potential link between metabolism and aging (Imai et al., 2000; Lin et al., 2000). There are three known heterochromatic regions in the yeast genome, which are known to be affected by these enzymes. They are the silent mating-type loci, the telomeric regions, and the rDNA cluster. There is a loss of silencing at the former two during aging (Smeal, Claus, Kennedy, Cole, & Guarente, 1996; Kim, Villeponteau, & Jazwinski, 1996). The silencing status of the rDNA locus is particularly important for longevity (Kim et al., 1999). It has been proposed that events at this locus contribute to longevity through their role in the maintenance of the protein synthetic capacity of the cell (Jazwinski, 2000). There are other silencing proteins that play a role in determining life span. Recently, two new ones have been added. They are the products of the genes *ZDS1* and *ZDS2* (Roy & Runge, 2000).

The yeast recQ DNA helicase family member *SGS1* affects yeast life span (Sinclair, Mills, & Guarente, 1997). It has been touted as the *WRN* homolog in yeast. However, it is now clear that it is more closely related to the Bloom's syndrome gene, *BLM* (Heo et al., 1999). Defects in *SGS1* shorten life span and result in nucleolar fragmentation (Sinclair et al., 1997). This has been ascribed to recombination events at the rDNA tandem repeats in the rDNA cluster, which lead to the formation of extrachromosomal rDNA circles (Sinclair, Mills, & Guarente, 1998), although this has been disputed more recently (Heo et al., 1999). It is clear that the rDNA circles can kill yeast cells. However, the induction of the retrograde response causes circles to accumulate (Conrad-Webb & Butow, 1995), and yet the yeasts live longer (Kirchman et al., 1999). Thus, the circles are not sufficient to cause aging, at least under all conditions.

Caenorhabditis elegans

Two worm longevity genes have been found using reverse genetics, and one additional gene is a probable. The *tkr-1* gene, which has been renamed *old-1*, was identified in a screen of transgenic worms containing cosmids carrying fragments of the worm genome (Murakami & Johnson, 1998). This resulted in transgenics containing many copies of the gene. This longevity gene encodes a putative tyrosine kinase receptor, and it not only confers extended longevity but also resistance to heat and ultraviolet light.

Another longevity gene was identified by screening mutant worms for ones that underexpress the catalase activity (Taub et al., 1999). The mutation in *ctl-1* causes a shortened life span. It also suppresses the life extension seen in *daf-2, age-1,* and *clk-1*. The *ctl-1* gene encodes a cytoplasmic form of catalase. The results support the importance of resistance to oxidative stress in determining worm life span. However, there is some criticism of the interpretation. The life span shortening that was observed in the wild-type worm carrying the *ctl-1* mutation complicates the interpretation of the suppression of the life extension seen in the other mutants.

It has been shown that a mutant in the *tph-1* gene screened using the PCR in strains of chemically mutagenized worms displayed reduced rates of feeding and other metabolic and behavioral changes coupled to reduced food sensation and ingestion (Sze, Victor, Loer, Shi, & Ruvkun, 2000). These worms displayed a longer reproductive life span, which would suggest they would also have a longer total adult life span. Surprisingly this was not examined. The *tph-1* gene encodes tryptophan hydroxylase, which catalyzes the rate-limiting step in serotonin biosynthesis. Serotonin is involved in the control of mammalian feeding and metabolism. The serotonin signaling in the worm seems to operate through transforming growth factor-β and insulin-like signals.

Drosophila

The reverse genetic approach in the fruit fly has been directed at the implication of genes involved in protection against oxidative stress. These attempts have focused on both Cu-, Zn- *(SOD1)* and Mn-superoxide dismutases *(SOD2)*, in which there is a long history. They have included catalase and glutathione peroxidase as well. The first clear evidence for a life-extending effect of transgenes carrying *SOD1* and catalase genes also demonstrated a reduction in oxidative damage with no diminution of oxygen consumption during the lifetime (Orr & Sohal, 1994). It was found that a rather precise proportion of both enzymes was required to observe the positive effect on life span. This made sense, because the product of the dismutase reaction generates the substrate for the catalase reaction. A similar study which directed human rather than fly *SOD1* expression only to motorneurons achieved similar results (Parkes et al., 1998). Both these studies have been criticized because there is no good control in the experiment. This is because each transgenic line differs by the random targeting of the transgene, with no control for possible effects on life span of insertion. As we have seen, *indy* was discovered by the effects of just such a random insertion.

These criticisms have been allayed with a different approach toward obtaining the transgenic line (Sun & Tower, 1999). *SOD1* overexpression was obtained in a transgenic line in which the promoter-enhancer is brought in juxtaposition with the coding region of the transgene by a site-specific recombination event promoted by the yeast FLP recombinase. This occurs when the recombinase is provided by mating with another strain which carries that transgene, which can later be crossed out. The *SOD1* transgenic line is its own control, when recombination has not been induced to allow expression. In sum, these studies provide good evidence that resistance to oxidative stress is an important factor determining fly longevity.

Mouse

A gene whose activity has been altered by accident is the urokinase-type plasminogen activator (Miskin & Masos, 1997). A transgenic mouse was deliberately generated, but expression did not occur as expected. Ectopic expression in the brain resulted in the spontaneous reduction of food consumption, retardation of growth and body weight, and an increase in longevity. It has been proposed that these mice are spontaneously calorie restricted due to overproduction of the protein in brain sites that control feeding behavior.

The targeted mutation of the $p66^{shc}$ gene in the mouse resulted in an extension of life span (Migliaccio et al., 1999). It also caused an increase in resistance to paraquat, a free-radical generator. Cells from these mice showed enhanced resistance to oxidative stress and apoptosis induced by either hydrogen peroxide or ultraviolet radiation. The Shc protein is a cytoplasmic signal transducer operating between tyrosine kinase growth factor receptors and Ras. However, this p66 variant of Shc may not be involved in Ras activation. It is not clear at present how this p66 affects Ras signaling. This study raises some interesting questions. For example, how is it that a mouse defective in apoptosis can survive longer, suggesting that cancer development is delayed.

GENOMICS

Genomics is often defined as the study of genes and their function. I do not like this definition, because genetics, biochemistry, and molecular biology already are dedicated to this task, so why invent a new terminology? On the other hand, I can accept this definition if it is enlarged to state that this study is in the context of the whole genome. By this definition, genomics would become an integrative approach. It seems to me that this modified definition is already being applied, albeit tersely. *Functional genomics* has already been coined to describe genome-wide scans of gene activity using microarray technology.

Microarray Analysis

Microarrays for the analysis of gene expression profiles are of two kinds in terms of the medium that is utilized. They can be prepared on hybridization membranes, usually nylon, or they can be prepared on glass slides or similar media. The latter allows an impressive miniaturization, providing for the deposit of more than 100,000 probes rather than just a few thousand. Categorization of microarrays is also based on the nature of the probes. They can be oligonucleotides specific for various genes, or they can be cDNAs derived from the respective mRNAs. The two categories each has its strengths and weaknesses. The method of detection can be based on radioisotopes or fluorescent dyes. Fluorescent dye techniques allow the direct comparison of expression under two, or theoretically more, conditions, when the dye-labeled nucleotides are chosen judiciously. This provides estimates of the ratios of mRNA levels under the two or more conditions that are analyzed. When standardized properly, radioisotopic methods allow the data obtained to be combined with other data at will. The use of gene arrays in the study of aging has been discussed previously (Vijg, 1999).

Caloric Restriction

Changes in the expression of specific genes during aging and caloric restriction have been analyzed extensively during the past decade. However, it is only with the advent of microarray technology that genome-wide profiles of gene expression during aging and caloric restriction have been assessed. To date there are three relevant studies.

The gene expression profile of aging mouse skeletal muscle (Lee, Klopp, Weindruch, & Prolla, 1999) and brain (Lee, Weindruch, & Prolla, 2000) have been analyzed and the effects of caloric restriction assessed. Each study was carried out with only three mice for each condition: young and old, calorie-restricted, and ad libitum–fed. More than 6,000 selected mouse genes, representing 5% to 10% of the genome, were scanned using the Affymetrix system. As little as 1.5-fold differences in expression level were deemed significant. In both tissues, the number of detectable gene expression changes during aging numbered approximately 2% to 3%

of the total genes scanned, distributed more or less equally among increases and decreases. Caloric restriction attenuated both increases and decreases in gene expression. In skeletal muscle, this attenuation affected approximately 30% of the genes partially and another 30% completely. In brain, the effects were similar in the neocortex but more extensive (75%) in the cerebellum, lumping together partial and complete attenuation. Caloric restriction also affected in similar numbers the expression of many genes whose activity does not change with age.

There were common features in the gene-expression profiles of aging skeletal muscle and brain. Aging resulted in an increase in stress responses, which was reversed by caloric restriction. In muscle, there was a decline in energy metabolism, which was also reversed. In brain, there was an increase in inflammatory responses, which was reversed. Caloric restriction stimulated protein turnover and biosynthesis in muscle, while in brain it stimulated growth and trophic factors. The authors of these studies in brain and muscle are correct in noting that these changes in gene expression may not translate to changes in protein levels. Indeed, a study in yeast demonstrated that there is no clear correlation for less abundantly expressed genes (Gygi, Rochon, Franza, & Aebersole, 1999). However, there are other difficulties in interpreting the specific profiles of gene expression.

It is not clear how reproducible individual gene changes actually are in each case or the statistical significance. Given the multiple comparisons involved in these determinations, it is likely that a substantial number of false positives were detected. This type of analysis is valuable as an exploratory method leading to hypotheses that can be subjected to further testing. Indeed, 6 of the approximately 500 gene-expression changes in the brain were verified by a quantitative PCR method.

A study using cDNA expression arrays on membranes containing 588 genes was used to examine aging and caloric restriction in mouse liver (Han, Hilsenbeck, Richardson, & Nelson, 2000). This study detected six gene-expression changes with age, only one of which was attenuated by caloric restriction. In addition, four other genes were differentially expressed between old ad libitum–fed and old calorie-restricted mice. The relative abundance of gene expression changes was similar to that seen in brain and skeletal muscle. Clearly, there is no wholesale reprogramming in gene expression associated with aging or caloric restriction, although this conclusion must be tempered by the fact that the genes on the microarrays were not chosen at random. It is important to note that four of the six genes subjected to further validation by Northern and PCR methods showed patterns of change corresponding to those seen on the microarrays. The statistical methodology used for quantitation of expression differences differed substantially from the other two studies that were discussed.

Human Fibroblast Aging

The Affymetrix system has also been applied to the profiling of gene expression changes in skin fibroblasts from human donors of various ages and to progeria patients (Hutchinson-Gilford syndrome) (Ly, Lockhart, Lerner, & Schultz, 2000). This study is subject to the same criticisms as the work on caloric restriction in skeletal muscle and brain, and more so because no verification of changes in gene expression was attempted. However, this is somewhat tempered by the additional comparisons that were made. Of the 6,000 genes screened, the authors observed changes in expression in about 1% between young and middle-aged individuals, using a 2-fold change as the cutoff. More than one half of these genes are involved in cell cycle progression and maintenance and remodeling of the extracellular matrix. Additional changes were found when old individuals were compared. These included changes in stress response and metabolic enzyme genes similar to those found in skeletal muscle in the study described earlier. The changes seen in progeria fibroblasts mimicked those found in fibroblasts from old donors. Finally, many of the changes observed conjure up the presence of age-related pathologies. The authors suggest that the changes in cell cycle progression genes lead to errors in the mitotic machinery in later life and that this dysfunction leads to genetic instability and misregulation of genes.

Centenarian Studies

Associative Genetics

We have behind us a decade of studies attempting to identify human longevity genes. All these studies have depended on testing the frequency of alleles of various candidate genes in nonagenarians and centenarians, as compared to younger controls. This procedure is known as associative genetics. It requires facile procedures for typing polymorphisms at selected loci, and thus it is based on molecular techniques. The advantage of this approach for aging studies is that it does not require families with a history of longevity. Indeed, it does not depend on the availability of siblings or parents. It is particularly useful for mapping complex traits such as longevity, because it allows the assignment of an allele to a trait even if that allele is responsible for only a fraction of the variance for that trait (Lander & Schork, 1994). There is a severe problem associated with this technique, however. It is population admixture, in which the association of an allele with a trait is due to the prevalence of the allele in a subgroup of the population that happens to be enriched in the trait for other reasons. The association can also be discovered because the actual causal factor is in linkage disequilibrium with the allele that is being studied. The first of these difficulties can be circumvented by studying relatively homogeneous populations, which has largely been the case. Replication of a finding in an unrelated population provides additional reassurance.

Early studies focused on HLA antigen frequencies (Proust et al., 1982; Takata, Suzuki, Ishii, Sekiguchi, & Iri, 1987). The populations were very different (French and Japanese), and the results were not replicated in the case of the antigen common to both studies (DR). HLA phenotypes were revisited recently in a study of a Chinese population (Yong-Xing et al., 1997). The results obtained with the C_w7 antigen flatly contradicted the French findings. Similarly, the association found for A9 was not seen in the French study. Apolipoprotein E phenotypes were examined in a Finnish population (Kervinen et al., 1994). The frequency of the E4 isoform was reduced in nonagenarians. The same study associated an *APOB* polymorphism (*Eco*RI) with longevity, while finding no association for another allele (*Xba*I polymorphism). Another Finnish study (Louhija et al., 1994) confirmed the *APOE* results at the genetic level, and it found in addition that the ε2 allele has a higher frequency in centenarians. Furthermore, this study replicated the lack of association of the *Xba*I polymorphism in *APOB* with longevity, but identified an increased frequency of an *APOC* allele in centenarians. The *APOE* results of this study have been replicated in a French population (Schachter et al., 1994). This French study also associated the D allele of *ACE* with longevity, a surprising finding given the increased incidence of myocardial infarction associated with this allele. Loci in the Huntington's disease region and *BCL-2* were also examined in this study with no associations with longevity reported. An Italian study has confirmed the association of *APOB* with longevity found in the Finnish population (De Benedictis et al., 1997). However, it was not the *Eco*RI polymorphism that was implicated. It was a multiallelic marker (VNTR) that facilitated the association. In the same study, no association of a *TPO* gene VNTR with longevity was detected. The *THO* gene, but not *REN, PARP,* and *SOD2,* has also been associated with longevity in Italian centenarians (De Benedictis et al., 1998), as has *PAI-1* (Mannucci et al., 1997). The allelic association is counterintuitive, as seen with *ACE.* Similarly, the presence in healthy centenarians of *p53* variants predisposing to cancer (Bonafe et al., 1999) provides food for thought. The development of methodologies that utilize both genetic and demographic information (Yashin et al., 1999) may add a new dimension to association studies and enrich the interpretation of the apparent paradoxes presented by *ACE, PAI-1,* and *p53.* It is comforting that not all genes tested associate with longevity, at least for certain polymorphisms in certain populations (Muiras, Verasdonck, Cottet, & Schachter, 1998).

Mitochondrial genotypes have also been examined for their association with longevity (Tanaka, Gong, Zhang, Yoneda, & Yagi, 1998). A rare mitochondrial haplogroup was associated with longevity in this Japanese centenarian study. This polymorphism is located in the gene encoding NADH dehydrogenase subunit 2. The value of examination of allele frequencies in several age groups was demonstrated. The results are consistent with the association of the mitochondrial polymorphism with susceptibility to adult-onset diseases. In a French study, a nucleotide substitution in *ATP6*, which encodes a subunit of ATP synthase, was detected more frequently in centenarians (Ivanova, Lepage, Charron, & Schachter, 1998). More recently, the mitochondrial J haplogroup was shown to be notably higher in frequency in Italian centenarians (De Benedictis et al., 1999). A polymorphic variant of the Werner gene *(WRN)* has been associated with increased incidence of myocardial infarction in the general Japanese population (Ye et al., 1997). This is an interesting finding, because *WRN* is responsible for a segmental progeroid syndrome, one of whose trademarks is death from myocardial infarction (Yu et al., 1996). This polymorphism is not associated with longevity in the Finnish population (Castro et al., 1999). In all of the human studies, the candidate genes were chosen because they constitute a risk factor, however well documented, for a disease whose incidence increases with age.

One might ask whether the confirmation that a particular allele is associated with long life indicates the beneficial effect of the allele in question or the lack of a detrimental effect. This question is usually difficult to answer for lack of knowledge of the functional consequences. In some cases, the association is counterintuitive, as indicated previously. The rationale is sound only in the case of the *APOE* gene. The E4 isoform of this lipoprotein is associated with increased risk for myocardial infarction and Alzheimer's disease.

Linkage Disequilibrium

The proper choice of a candidate gene in associative genetic studies is essential. The identity of the gene must somehow conjure an association with aging. With an association in hand, however, it is necessary to demonstrate a reasonable functional ramification for the particular allelic variant detected. There is still another difficulty to address: the possibility that the variant detected is simply a recurring mutation in the population, a mutation that is not really causative.

The latter difficulty can be addressed by examining haplotypes and not simply isolated polymorphisms. The notion behind this is that a stable hereditary factor responsible for longevity should be passed intact from generation to generation. It should be identical by descent. One would therefore expect in such a case to see an entire genomic region, with its various polymorphisms, associated with longevity because of linkage disequilibrium. This test has not been typically employed in aging studies. It requires analysis of genetic markers in and around the candidate gene and more sophisticated statistical analyses.

Single-nucleotide polymorphisms (snp) are coming to the fore in the genetic analysis of complex traits (Nelson, 2001). Their density can provide fine mapping. However, the expense of doing whole-genome scans makes the candidate-gene approach especially attractive when employing snp's. With snp's, it is less likely to find a gratuitous recurring mutation. Thus, the identity by descent is virtually assured, especially when embedded within a haplotype.

SUMMARY AND PERSPECTIVES

The genetics of aging is further along in lower organisms as compared to humans. Studies in lower organisms have implicated a large number of genes that function in a number of different pathways. The range of different biochemical functions supported by these genes is quite large, yet the broad physiological mechanisms that are involved is surprisingly small. It appears that metabolism and stress resistance are especially important, and gene dysregulation and genetic instability may also play a role. This is encouraging because it coincides nicely with studies of caloric restriction in mammals. The correspondence between the physiological mechanisms that underlie aging in the various organisms studied suggests a more general applicability.

The availability of homologs of the various longevity genes identified in lower organisms allows the testing of their relevance to mouse and human aging. Studies in the mouse will require transgenic and knockout approaches, and such studies are already in progress. Studies in humans will take the associative genetic approach. More than the genes themselves, however, it is the physiological processes and pathways they support that are important. The genetics of aging in lower organisms allows the formulation of hypotheses that can be tested on the substrate of the mouse or human, targeting the genes relevant to each pathway or process and each organism.

The specific aspects of aging can be classified as major or minor in each species (Jazwinski, 1993). The utility of comparative aging research lies in the fact that aging processes differ in their intensity from species to species. Thus, a major aspect in one may be a minor one in another. It is much easier to study a major process in one species and to apply the knowledge gained to another.

ACKNOWLEDGMENTS

Research in the author's laboratory was supported by grants from the National Institute on Aging of the National Institutes of Health (USPHS).

REFERENCES

Ailion, M., Inoue, T., Weaver, C. I., Holdcraft, R. W., & Thomas, J. H. (1999). Neurosecretory control of aging in *Caenorhabditis elegans. Proceedings of the National Academy of Sciences, USA, 96,* 7394–7397.

Antebi, A., Yeh, W. H., Tait, D., Hedgecook, E. M., & Riddle, D. L. (2000). daf-12 encodes a nuclear receptor that regulates the dauer diapause and developmental age in *C. elegans. Genes and Development, 14,* 1512–1527.

Apfeld, J., & Kenyon, C. (1998). Cell nonautonomy of *C. elegans daf-2* function in the regulation of diapause and life span. *Cell, 95,* 199–210.

Apfeld, J., & Kenyon, C. (1999). Regulation of lifespan by sensory perception in Caenorhabditis elegans. *Nature, 402,* 804–809.

Ashrafi, K., Lin, S. S., Manchester, J. K., & Gordon, J. I. (2000). Sip2p and its partner Snf1p kinase affect aging in *S. cerevisiae. Genes and Development, 14,* 1872–1885.

Ashrafi, K., Sinclair, D., Gordon, J. I., & Guarente, L. (1999). Passage through stationary phase advances replicative aging in *Saccharomyces cerevisiae. Proceedings of the National Academy of Sciences, USA, 96,* 9100-9105.

Barker, M. G, Brimage, L. J., & Smart, K. A. (1999). Effect of Cu,Zn superoxide dismutase disruption mutation on replicative senescence in *Saccharomyces cerevisiae. FEMS Microbiology Letters, 177,* 199–204.

Barker, M. G., & Walmsley, R. M. (1999). Replicative ageing in the fission yeast *Schizosaccharomyces pombe. Yeast, 15,* 1511–1518.

Bartke, A. (2000). Delayed aging in Ames dwarf mice. Relationships to endocrine function and body size. *Results and Problems in Cell Differentiation, 29,* 181–202.

Barz, W. P., & Walter, P. (1999). Two endoplasmic reticulum (ER) membrane proteins that facilitate ER-to-Golgi transport of glycosylphosphatidylinositol-anchored proteins. *Molecular Biology of the Cell, 10,* 1043–1059.

Berger, K. H., & Yaffe, M. P. (1998) Prohibitin family members interact genetically with mitochondrial inheritance components in *Saccharomyces cerevisiae. Molecular and Cellular Biology, 18,* 4043–4052.

Bonafé, M., Olivieri, F., Mari, D., Baggio, G., Mattace, R., Sansoni, P., De Benedictis, G., De Luca, M., Bertolini, S., Barbi, C., Monti, D., &

Franceschi, C. (1999). p53 variants predisposing to cancer are present in healthy centenarians. *American Journal of Human Genetics, 64,* 292–295.

Brandwagt, B. F., Mesbah, L. A., Takken, F. L., Laurent, P. L., Kneppers, T. J., Hille, J., & Nijkamp, H. J. (2000). A longevity assurance gene homolog of tomato mediates resistance to Alternaria alternata f. sp. lycopersici toxins and fumonisin B1. *Proceedings of the National Academy of Sciences, USA, 97,* 4961–4966.

Branicky, R., Benard, C., & Hekimi, S. (2000). *clk-1,* mitochondria, and physiological rates. *Bioessays, 22,* 48–56.

Castro, E., Ogburn, C. E., Hunt, K. E., Tilvis, R., Louhija, J., Penttinen, R., Erkkola, R., Panduro, A., Riestra, R., Piussan, C., Deeb, S. S., Wang, L., Edland, S. D., Martin, G. M., & Oshima, J. (1999). Polymorphisms at the Werner locus: I. Newly identified polymorphisms, ethnic variability of 1367Cys/Arg, and its stability in a population of Finnish centenarians. *American Journal of Medical Genetics, 82,* 399–403.

Chen, J. B., Sun, J., & Jazwinski, S. M. (1990). Prolongation of the yeast life span by the v-*Ha-RAS* oncogene. *Molecular Microbiology, 4,* 2081-2086.

Coates, P. J., Jamieson, D. J., Smart, K., Prescott, A. R., & Hall, P. A. (1997). The prohibitin family of mitochondrial proteins regulate replicative lifespan. *Current Biology, 7,* 607-610.

Conrad-Webb, H., & Butow, R. A. (1995). A polymerase switch in the synthesis of rRNA in *Saccharomyces cerevisiae. Molecular and Cellular Biology, 15,* 2420–2428.

Covelli, V., Mouton, D., Di Majo, V., Bouthillier, Y., Bangrazi, C., Mevel, J. C., Rebessi, S., Doria, G., & Biozzi, G. (1989). Inheritance of immune responsiveness, life span, and disease incidence in interline crosses of mice selected for high or low multispecific antibody production. *Journal of Immunology, 142,* 1224–1234.

De Benedictis, G., Carotenuto, L., Carrieri, G., De Luca, M., Falcone, E., Rose, G., Cavalcanti, S., Corsonello, F., Feraco, E., Baggio, G., Bertolini, S., Mari, D., Mattace, R., Yashin, A. I., Bonafé, M., & Franceschi, C. (1998). Gene/longevity association studies at four autosomal loci *(REN, THO, PARP, SOD2). European Journal of Human Genetics, 6,* 534–541.

De Benedictis, G., Falcone, E., Rose, G., Ruffolo, R., Spadafora, P., Baggio, G., Bertolini, S., Mari, D., Mattace, R., Monti, D., Morellini, M., Sansoni, P., & Franceschi, C. (1997). DNA multiallelic systems reveal gene/longevity associations not detected by diallelic systems. The APOB locus. *Human Genetics, 99,* 312-318.

De Benedictis, G., Rose, G., Carrieri, G., De Luca, M., Falcone, E., Passarino, G., Bonafé, M., Monti, D., Baggio, G., Bertolini, S., Mari, D., Mattace, R., & Franceschi, C. (1999). Mitochondrial DNA inherited variants are associated with successful aging and longevity in humans. *FASEB Journal, 13,* 1352–1536.

de Haan, G., Gelman, R., Watson, A., Yunis, E., & Van Zant, G. (1998). A putative gene causes variability in lifespan among genotypically identical mice. *Nature Genetics, 19,* 114–116.

Defossez, P. A., Prusty, R., Kaeberlein, M., Lin, S. J., Ferrigno, P., Silver, P. A., Keil, R. L., & Guarente, L. (1999). Elimination of replication block protein Fob1 extends the life span of yeast mother cells. *Molecular Cell, 3,* 447–455.

D'mello N. P., Childress, A. M., Franklin, D. S., Kale, S. P., Pinswasdi, C., & Jazwinski, S. M. (1994). Cloning and characterization of *LAG1,* a longevity-assurance gene in yeast. *Journal of Biological Chemistry, 269,* 15451–15459.

Dorman, J. B., Albinder, B., Shroyer, T., & Kenyon, C. (1995). The *age-1* and *daf-2* genes function in a common pathway to control the lifespan of *Caenorhabditis elegans. Genetics, 141,* 1399–1406.

Ebert, R. H., Cherkasova, V. A., Dennis, R. A., Wu, J. H., Ruggles, S., Perrin, T. E., & Shmookler Reis, R. J. (1993). Longevity-determining genes in *Caenorhabditis elegans:* Chromosomal mapping of multiple noninteractive loci. *Genetics, 135,* 1003–1010.

Egilmez, N. K., Chen, J. B., & Jazwinski, S. M. (1989). Specific alterations in transcript prevalence during the yeast life span. *Journal of Biological Chemistry, 264,* 14312–14317.

Ewbank, J. J., Barnes, T. M., Lakowski, B., Lussier, M., Bussey, H., & Hekimi, S. (1997). Structural and functional conservation of the *Caenorhabditis elegans* timing gene *clk-1. Science, 275,* 980–983.

Felkai, S., Ewbank, J. J., Lemieux, J., Labbe, J. C., Brown, G. G., & Hekimi, S. (1999). CLK-1 controls respiration, behavior and aging in the nematode *Caenorhabditis elegans. EMBO Journal, 18,* 1783–1792.

Friedman, D. B., & Johnson, T. E. (1988). A mutation in the *age-1* gene in *Caenorhabditis elegans* lengthens life and reduces hermaphrodite fertility. *Genetics, 118,* 75–86.

Gygi, S. P., Rochon, Y., Franza, B. R., & Aebersold, R. (1999). Correlation between protein and mRNA abundance in yeast. *Molecular and Cellular Biology, 19,* 1720–1730.

Han, E., Hilsenbeck, S. G., Richardson, A., & Nelson, J. F. (2000). cDNA expression arrays reveal incomplete reversal of age-related changes in gene expression by calorie restriction. *Mechanisms of Ageing and Development, 115,* 157–174.

Heo, S. J., Tatebayashi, K., Ohsugi, I., Shimamoto, A., Furuichi, Y., & Ikeda, H. (1999). Bloom's syndrome gene suppresses premature ageing caused by Sgs1 deficiency in yeast. *Genes to Cells, 4,* 619–625.

Hillesheim, E., & Stearns, S. C. (1992). Correlated responses in life-history traits to artificial selection for body weight in *Drosophila melanogaster. Evolution, 46,* 745–752.

Hsin, H., & Kenyon, C. (1999). Signals from the reproductive system regulate the lifespan of *C. elegans*. *Nature, 399*, 362–366.

Imai, S., Armstrong, C. M., Kaeberlein, M., & Guarente, L. (2000). Transcriptional silencing and longevity protein Sir2 is an NAD-dependent histone deacetylase. *Nature, 403*, 795–800.

Ishii, N., Fujii, M., Hartman, P. S., Tsuda, M., Yasuda, K., Senoo-Matsuda, N., Yanase, S., Ayusawa, D., & Suzuki, K. (1998). A mutation in succinate dyhydrogenase cytochrome b causes oxidative stress and ageing in nematodes. *Nature, 394*, 694–697.

Ivanova, R., Lepage, V., Charron, D., & Schachter, F. (1998). Mitochondrial genotype associated with French Caucasian centenarians. *Gerontology, 44*, 349.

Jazwinski, S. M. (1993). The genetics of aging in the yeast *Saccharomyces cerevisiae*. *Genetica, 91*, 35–51.

Jazwinski, S. M. (1996). Longevity, genes, and aging. *Science, 273*, 54–59.

Jazwinski, S. M. (1999a). The RAS genes: A homeostatic device in *Saccharomyces cerevisiae* longevity. *Neurobiology of Aging, 20*, 471–478.

Jazwinski, S. M. (1999b). Molecular mechanisms of yeast longevity. *Trends in Microbiology, 7*, 247–252.

Jazwinski, S. M. (2000). Metabolic control and ageing. *Trends in Genetics, 16*, 506–511.

Jazwinski, S. M., Kim, S., Lai, C. Y., & Benguria, A. (1998). Epigenetic stratification: The role of individual change in the biological aging process. *Experimental Gerontology, 33*, 571–580.

Jia, Y., Rothermel, B., Thornton, J., & Butow, R. A. (1997). A basic helix-loop-helix-leucine zipper transcription complex in yeast functions in a signaling pathway from mitochondria to the nucleus. *Molecular and Cellular Biology, 17*, 1110–1117.

Jiang, J. C., Jaruga, E., Repnevskaya, M. V., & Jazwinski, S. M. (2000). An intervention resembling caloric restriction prolongs life span and retards aging in yeast. *FASEB Journal, 14*, 2135–2137.

Jiang, J. C., Kirchman, P. A., Zagulski, M., Hunt, J., & Jazwinski, S. M. (1998). Homologs of the yeast longevity gene LAG1 in *Caenorhabditis elegans* and human. *Genome Research, 8*, 1259–1272.

Johnson, T. E., Cypser, J., de Castro, E., de Castro, S., Henderson, S., Murakami, S., Rikke, B., Tedesco, P., & Link, C. (2000). Gerontogenes mediate health and longevity in nematodes through increasing resistance to environmental toxins and stressors. *Experimental Gerontology, 35*, 687–694.

Jonassen, T., Larsen, P. L., & Clarke, C. F. (2001). A dietary source of coenzyme Q is essential for growth of long-lived *Caenorhabditis elegans clk-1* mutants. *Proceedings of the National Academy of Sciences, USA, 98*, 421–426.

Kale, S. P., & Jazwinski, S. M. (1996). Differential response to UV stress and DNA damage during the yeast replicative life span. *Developmental Genetics, 18,* 154–160.

Kennedy, B. K., Austriaco, N. R., Zhang, J., & Guarente, L. (1995). Mutation in the silencing gene *SIR4* can delay aging in *S. cerevisiae. Cell, 80,* 485–496.

Kennedy, B. K., Gotta, M., Sinclair, D. A., Mills, K., McNabb, D. S., Murthy, M., Pak, S. M., Laroche, T., Gasser, S. M., & Guarente, L. (1997). Redistribution of silencing proteins from telomeres to the nucleolus is associated with extension of life span in *S. cerevisiae. Cell, 89,* 381–391.

Kenyon, C., Chang, J., Gensch, E., Rudner, A., & Tabtiang, R. (1993). A *C. elegans* mutant that lives twice as long as wild type. *Nature, 366,* 461–464.

Kervinen, K., Savolainen, M. J., Salokannel, J., Hynninen, A., Heikkinen, J., Ehnholm, C., Koistinen, M. J., & Kesaniemi, Y. A. (1994). Apolipoprotein E and B polymorphisms—longevity factors assessed in nonagenarians. *Atherosclerosis, 105,* 89–95.

Kim, S., Benguria, A., Lai, C.-Y., & Jazwinski, S. M. (1999). Modulation of life-span by histone deacetylase genes in *Saccharomyces cerevisiae. Molecular Biology of the Cell, 10,* 3125–3136.

Kim, S., Villeponteau, B., & Jazwinski, S. M. (1996). Effect of replicative age on transcriptional silencing near telomeres in *Saccharomyces cerevisiae. Biochemical and Biophysical Research Communications, 219,* 370–376.

Kimura, K. D., Tissenbaum, H. A., Liu, Y., & Ruvkun, G. (1997). *daf-2,* an insulin receptor-like gene that regulates longevity and diapause in *Caenorhabditis elegans. Science, 277,* 942–946.

Kirchman, P. A., Kim, S., Lai, C.-Y., & Jazwinski, S. M. (1999). Interorganelle signaling is a determinant of longevity in *Saccharomyces cerevisiae. Genetics, 152,* 179–190.

Klass, M. R. (1983). A method for the isolation of longevity mutants in the nematode *Caenorhabditis elegans* and initial results. *Mechanisms of Ageing and Development, 22,* 279–286.

Kuro-o, M., Matsumura, Y., Aizawa, H., Kawaguchi, H., Suga, T., Utsugi, T., Ohyama, Y., Kurabayashi, M., Kaname, T., Kume, E., Iwasaki, H., Iida, A., Shiraki-lida, T., Nishikawa, S., Nagai, R., & Nabeshima, Y. I. (1997). Mutation of the mouse *klotho* gene leads to a syndrome resembling ageing. *Nature, 390,* 45–51.

Lakowski, B., & Hekimi, S. (1996). Determination of life-span in *Caenorhabditis elegans* by four clock genes. *Science, 272,* 1010-1013.

Lander, E. S., & Schork, N. J. (1994). Genetic dissection of complex traits. *Science, 265,* 2037–2048.

Larsen, P. L., Albert, P. S., & Riddle, D. L. (1995). Genes that regulate both development and longevity in *Caenorhabditis elegans. Genetics, 139,* 1567–1583.

Lee, C. K., Klopp, R. G., Weindruch, R., & Prolla, T. A. (1999). Gene expression profile of aging and its retardation by caloric restriction. *Science, 285,* 1390–1393.

Lee, C. K., Weindruch, R., & Prolla, T. A. (2000). Gene-expression profile of the ageing brain in mice. *Nature Genetics, 25,* 294–297.

Liao, X., & Butow, R. A. (1993). *RTG1* and *RTG2:* Two yeast genes required for a novel path of communication from mitochondria to the nucleus. *Cell, 72,* 61–71.

Lin, K., Dorman, J. B., Rodan, A., & Kenyon, C. (1997). *daf-16:* An HNF-3/forkhead family member that can function to double the life-span of *Caenorhabditis elegans. Science, 278,* 1319–1322.

Lin, S. J., Defossez, P. A., & Guarente, L. (2000). Requirement of NAD and SIR2 for life-span extension by calorie restriction in *Saccharomyces cerevisiae. Science, 289,* 2126–2128.

Lin, Y. J., Seroude, L., & Benzer, S. (1998). Extended life-span and stress resistance in the *Drosophila* mutant *methuselah. Science, 282,* 943–946.

Liu, Z., & Butow, R. A. (1999). A transcriptional switch in the expression of yeast tricarboxylic acid cycle genes in response to a reduction or loss of respiratory function. *Molecular and Cellular Biology, 19,* 6720–6728.

Longo, V. D. (1999). Mutations in signal transduction proteins increase stress resistance and longevity in yeast, nematodes, fruit flies, and mammalian neuronal cells. *Neurobiology of Aging, 20,* 479–486.

Louhija, J., Miettinen, H. E., Kontula, K., Tikkanen, M. J., Miettinen, T. A., & Tilvis, R. S. (1994). Aging and genetic variation of plasma apolipoproteins. Relative loss of the apolipoprotein E4 phenotype in centenarians. *Arteriosclerosis and Thrombosis, 14,* 1084–1089.

Luckinbill, L. S., Arking, R., Clare, M. J., Cirocco, W. C., & Buck, S. A. (1984). Selection for delayed senescence in *Drosophila melanogaster. Evolution, 38,* 996–1003.

Ly, D. H., Lockhart, D. J., Lerner, R. A., & Schultz, P. G. (2000). Mitotic misregulation and human aging. *Science, 287,* 2486–2492.

Mannucci, P. M., Mari, D., Merati, G., Peyvandi, F., Tagliabue, L., Sacchi, E., Taioli, E., Sansoni, P., Bertolini, S., & Franceschi, C. (1997). Gene polymorphisms predicting high plasma levels of coagulation and fibrinolysis proteins. A study in centenarians. *Arteriosclerosis, Thrombosis and Vascular Biology, 17,* 755–759.

Matsumura, Y., Aizawa, H., Shiraki-Iida, T., Nagai, R., Kuro-o, M., & Nabeshima, Y. (1998). Identification of the human *klotho* gene and its two transcripts encoding membrane and secreted klotho protein. *Biochemical and Biophysical Research Communications, 242,* 626–630.

Migliaccio, E., Giorgio, M., Mele, S., Pelicci, G., Reboldi, P., Pandolfi, P. P., Lanfrancone, L., & Pelicci, P. G. (1999). The p66shc adaptor protein controls oxidative stress response and life span in mammals. *Nature, 402,* 309–313.

Miller, R. A., Chrisp, C., & Atchley, W. (2000). Differential longevity in mouse stocks selected for early life growth trajectory. *Journal of Gerontology Series A: Biological Sciences and Medical Sciences, 55,* B455–B461.

Miskin, R., & Masos, T. (1997). Transgenic mice overexpressing urokinase-type plasminogen activator in the brain exhibit reduced food consumption, body weight and size, and increased longevity. *Journal of Gerontology Series A: Biological Sciences and Medical Sciences, 52,* B118–B124.

Morris, J. Z., Tissenbaum, H. A., & Ruvkun, G. (1996). A phosphatidylinositol-3-OH kinase family member regulating longevity and diapause in *Caenorhabditis elegans. Nature, 382,* 536–539.

Mortimer, R. K., & Johnston, J. R. (1959). Life span of individual yeast cells. *Nature, 183,* 1751–1752.

Muiras, M. L., Verasdonck, P., Cottet, F., & Schachter, F. (1998). Lack of association between human longevity and genetic polymorphisms in drug-metabolizing enzymes at the *NAT2, GSTM1* and *CYP2D6* loci. *Human Genetics, 102,* 526–532.

Müller, I., Zimmermann, M., Becker, D., & Flömer, M. (1980). Calendar life span versus budding life span of *Saccharomyces cerevisiae. Mechanisms of Ageing and Development, 12,* 47–52.

Murakami, S., & Johnson, T. E. (1996). A genetic pathway conferring life extension and resistance to UV stress in *Caenorhabditis elegans. Genetics, 143,* 1207–1218.

Murakami, S., & Johnson, T. E. (1998). Life extension and stress resistance in *Caenorhabditis elegans* modulated by the *tkr-1* gene. *Current Biology, 8,* 1091–1094.

Nagai, J., Lin, C. Y., & Sabour, M. P. (1995). Lines of mice selected for reproductive longevity. *Growth, Development and Aging, 59,* 79–81.

Nasrin, N., Ogg, S., Cahill, C. M., Biggs, W., Nui, S., Dore, J., Calvo, D., Shi, Y., Ruvkun, G., & Alexander-Bridges, M. C. (2000). DAF-16 recruits the CREB-binding protein coactivator complex to the insulin-like growth factor binding protein 1 promoter in HepG2 cells. *Proceedings of the National Academy of Sciences, USA, 97,* 10412–10417.

Nelson, D. L. (2001). SNP's, linkage disequilibrium, human genetic variation and Native American culture. *Trends in Genetics, 17,* 15–16.

Nijtmans, L. G., de Jong, L., Artal Sanz, M., Coates, P. J., Berden, J. A., Back, J. W., Muijsers, A. O., van der Spek, H., & Grivell, L. A. (2000). Prohibitins act as a membrane-bound chaperone for the stabilization of mitochondrial proteins. *EMBO Journal, 19,* 2444–2451.

Ogg, S., Paradis, S., Gottlieb, S., Patterson, G. I., Lee, L., Tissenbuam, H. A., & Ruvkun, G. (1997). The Fork head transcription factor DAF-16 transduces insulin-like metabolic and longevity signals in *C. elegans. Nature, 389,* 994–999.

Ogg, S., & Ruvkin, G. (1998). The *C. elegans* PTEN homolog, DAF-18, acts in the insulin receptor-like metabolic signaling pathway. *Molecular Cell, 2,* 887–993.

Orr, W. C., & Sohal, R. S. (1994). Extension of life-span by overexpression of superoxide dismutase and catalase in *Drosophila melanogaster. Science, 263,* 1128–1130.

Osiewacz, H. D., & Borghouts, C. (2000). Cellular copper homeostasis, mitochondrial DNA instabilities, and lifespan control in the filamentous fungus podospora anserina. *Experimental Gerontology, 35,* 677–686.

Paradis, S., Ailion, M., Toker, A., Thomas, J. H., & Ruvkun, G. (1999). A PDK1 homolog is necessary and sufficient to transduce AGE-1 PI3 kinase signals that regulate diapause in *Caenorhabditis elegans. Genes and Development, 13,* 1438–1452.

Paradis, S., & Ruvkun, G. (1998). *Caenorhabditis elegans* Akt/PKB transduces insulin receptor-like signals from AGE-1 PI3 kinase to the DAF-16 transcription factor. *Genes and Development, 12,* 2488–2498.

Parikh, V. S., Morgan, M. M., Scott, R., Clements, L. S., & Butow, R. A. (1987). The mitochondrial genotype can influence nuclear gene expression in yeast. *Science, 235,* 576–580.

Park, P. U., Defossez, P. A., & Guarente, L. (1999). Effects of mutations in DNA repair genes on formation of ribosomal DNA circles and life span in *Saccharomyces cerevisiae. Molecular and Cellular Biology, 19,* 3848–3856.

Parkes, T. L., Elia, A. J., Dickinson, D., Hilliker, A. J., Phillips, J. P., & Boulianne, G. L. (1998). Extension of *Drosophila* lifespan by overexpression of human *SOD1* in motorneurons. *Nature Genetics, 19,* 171–174.

Partridge, L., & Fowler, K. (1992). Direct and correlated responses to selection on age at reproduction in *Drosophila melanogaser. Evolution, 46,* 76–91.

Proust, J., Moulias, R., Fumeron, F., Bekkhoucha, F., Busson, M., Schmid, M., & Hors, J. (1982). HLA and longevity. *Tissue Antigens, 19,* 168–173.

Resler, A. S., Kelly, K., Kantor, G., Khazaeli, A. A., Tatar, M., & Curtsinger, J. W. (1998). Genetic analysis of extended life span in *Drosophila melanogaster.* II. Replication of the backcross test and molecular characterization of the N14 locus. *Genetica, 104,* 33–39.

Rogina, B., Reenan, R. A., Nilsen, S. P., & Helfand, S. L. (2000). Extended life-span conferred by cotransporter gene mutations in *Drosophila. Science, 290,* 2137–2140.

Rose, M. R. (1984). Laboratory evolution of postponed senescence in *Drosophila melanogaster. Evolution, 38,* 1004–1010.

Rose, M. R. (1991). *Evolutionary biology of aging.* New York: Oxford University Press.

Rose, M. R., & Charlesworth, B. (1981). Genetics of life history in *Drosophila melanogaster.* II. Exploratory selection experiments. *Genetics, 97,* 187–196.

Rothermel, B. A., Thornton, J. L., & Butow, R. A. (1997). Rtg3p, a basic helix-loop-helix/leucine zipper protein that functions in mitochondrial-induced changes in gene expression, contains independent activation domains. *Journal of Biological Chemistry, 272,* 19801–19807.

Roy, N., & Runge, K. W. (2000). Two paralogs involved in transcriptional silencing that antagonistically control yeast life span. *Current Biology, 10,* 111–114.

Schachter, F., Faure-Delanef, L., Guenot, F., Rouger, H., Froguel, P., Lesueur-Ginot, L., & Cohen, D. (1994). Genetic associations with human longevity at the APOE and ACE loci. *Nature Genetics, 6,* 29–32.

Sekito, T., Thornton, J., & Butow, R. A. (2000). Mitochondria-to-nuclear signaling is regulated by the subcellular localization of the transcription factors Rtg1p and Rtg3p. *Molecular Biology of the Cell, 11,* 2103–2115.

Shama, S., Kirchman, P. A., Jiang, J. C., & Jazwinski, S. M. (1998). Role of RAS2 in recovery from chronic stress: Effect on yeast life span. *Experimental Cell Research, 245,* 368–378.

Shama, S., Lai, C.-Y., Antoniazzi, J. M., Jiang, J. C., & Jazwinski, S. M. (1998). Heat stress-induced life span extension in yeast. *Experimental Cell Research, 245,* 379–388.

Shigenaga, M. K., Hagen, T. M., & Ames, B. N. (1994). Oxidative damage and mitochondrial decay in aging. *Proceedings of the National Academy of Sciences, USA, 91,* 10771–10778.

Shook, D. R., & Johnson, T. E. (1999). Quantitative trait loci affecting survival and fertility-related traits in *Caenorhabditis elegans* show genotype-environment interactions, pleiotropy and epistasis. *Genetics, 153,* 1233–1243.

Sinclair, D. A., Mills, K., & Guarente, L. (1997). Accelerated aging and nucleolar fragmentation in yeast *sgs1* mutants. *Science, 277,* 1313–1316.

Sinclair, D. A., Mills, K., & Guarente, L. (1998). Molecular mechanisms of yeast aging. *Trends in Biochemical Sciences, 23,* 131–134.

Smeal, T., Claus, J., Kennedy, B., Cole, F., & Guarente, L. (1996). Loss of transcriptional silencing causes sterility in old mother cells of *S. cerevisiae. Cell, 84,* 633–642.

Snow, M. I., & Larsen, P. L. (2000). Structure and expression of *daf-12:* A nuclear hormone receptor with three isoforms that are involved in development and aging in *Caenorhabditis elegans. Biochimica et Biophysica Acta, 1494,* 104–116.

Steglich, G., Neupert, W., & Langer, T. (1999). Prohibitins regulate membrane protein degradation by the m-AAA protease in mitochondria. *Molecular and Cellular Biology, 19,* 3435–3442.

Sun, J., Kale, S. P., Childress, A. M., Pinswasdi, C., & Jazwinski, S. M. (1994). Divergent roles of *RAS1* and *RAS2* in yeast longevity. *Journal of Biological Chemistry, 269,* 18638–18645.

Sun, J., & Tower, J. (1999). FLP recombinase-mediated induction of Cu/Zn-superoxide dismutase transgene expression can extend the life span of adult *Drosophila melanogaster* flies. *Molecular and Cellular Biology, 19,* 216–228.

Sze, J. Y., Victor, M., Loer, C., Shi, Y., & Ruvkun, G. (2000). Food and metabolic signalling defects in a *Caenorhabditis elegans* serotonin-synthesis mutant. *Nature, 403,* 560–564.

Takata, H., Suzuki, M., Ishii, T., Sekiguchi, S., & Iri, H. (1987). Influence of major histocompatibility complex region genes on human longevity among Okinawan-Japanese centenarians and nonagenarians. *Lancet, 2,* 824–826.

Tanaka, M., Gong, J. S., Zhang, J., Yoneda, M., & Yagi, K. (1998). Mitochondrial genotype associated with longevity. *Lancet, 351,* 185–186.

Taub, J., Lau, J. F., Ma, C., Hahn, J. H., Hoque, R., Rothblatt, J., & Chalfie, M. (1999). A cytosolic catalase is needed to extend adult lifespan in *C. elegans* daf-C and *clk-1* mutants. *Nature, 399,* 162–166.

Traven, A., Wong, J. M., Xu, D., Sopta, M., & Ingles, C. J. (2000). Interorganellar communication: Altered nuclear gene expression profiles in a yeast mitochondrial DNA mutant. *Journal of Biological Chemistry, 276,* 4020–4027.

Varkey, J. P., Muhlrad, P. J., Minniti, A. N., Do, B., & Ward, S. (1995). The *Caenorhabditis elegans spe-26* gene is necessary to form spermatids and encodes a protein similar to the actin-associated proteins kelch and scruin. *Genes and Development, 9,* 1074–1086.

Vijg, J. (1999). Profiling aging by gene arrays. *Mechanisms of Ageing and Development, 112,* 1–4.

Wawryn, J., Krzepilko, A., Myszka, A., & Bilinski, T. (1999). Deficiency in superoxide dismutases shortens life span of yeast cells. *Acta Biochimica Polonica, 46,* 249–253.

Wolkow, C. A., Kimura, K. D., Lee, M. S., & Ruvkun, G. (2000). Regulation of *C. elegans* life-span by insulin like signaling in the nervous system. *Science, 290,* 147–150.

Yashin, A. I., De Benedictis, G., Vaupel, J. W., Tan, Q., Andreev, K. F., Iachine, I. A., Bonafe, M., DeLuca, M., Valensin, S., Carotenuto, L., & Franceschi, C. (1999). Genes, demography, and life span: The contribution of demographic data in genetic studies on aging and longevity. *American Journal of Human Genetics, 65,* 1178–1193.

Ye, L., Miki, T., Nakura, J., Oshima, J., Kamino, K., Rakugi, H., Ikegami, H., Higaki, J., Edland, S. D., Martin, G. M., & Ogihara, T. (1997). Association of a polymorphic variant of the Werner helicase gene with myocardial infarction in a Japanese population. *American Journal of Medical Genetics, 68,* 494–498.

Yong-Xing, M., Yue, Z., Zan-Shun, W., Chuan-Fu, W., Su-Ying, C., Mao-tong, Z., Gong-Liang, Z., Su-Qin, Z., Jian-Gang, Z., Qi, G., & Lin, H. (1997). HLA and longevity or aging among Shanghai Chinese. *Mechanisms of Ageing and Development, 94,* 191–198.

Yu, C. E., Oshima, J., Fu, Y. H., Wijsman, E. M., Hisama, F., Alisch, R., Matthews, S., Nakura, J., Miki, T., Ouais, S., Martin, G. M., Mulligan, J., & Schellenberg, G. D. (1996). Positional cloning of the Werner's syndrome gene. *Science, 272,* 258–262.

Yunis, E. J., & Salazar, M. (1993). Genetics of life span in mice. *Genetica, 91,* 211–223.

Zwaan, B., Bijlsma, R., & Hoekstra, R. F. (1995). Direct selection on life span in *Drosophila melanogaster. Evolution, 49,* 649–659.

CHAPTER 9

Neuronal Environment and Age-Related Neurodegenerative Disease: Nutritional Modification

JAMES A. JOSEPH, N. A. DENISOVA, K. A. YOUDIM,
D. BIELINSKI, D. FISHER, AND B. SHUKITT-HALE
USDA HUMAN NUTRITION RESEARCH CENTER ON AGING
TUFTS UNIVERSITY

A great deal of research indicates that there are numerous neuronal and behavioral deficits that occur during aging that are independent of, but may contribute to, neurodegenerative disease. These changes may include decrements in calcium homeostasis (see, for example, Landfield & Eldridge, 1994), as well as reductions in the sensitivity of several receptor systems including: (a) muscarinic (Egashira, Takayama, & Yamanaka, 1996; Joseph, Kowatch, Maki, & Roth, 1990; Yufu, Egashira, & Yamanaka, 1994), (b) dopaminergic (Joseph, Berger, Engel, & Roth, 1978; Levine & Cepeda, 1998), (c) adrenergic (Gould & Bickford, 1997), and (d) opioid (Kornhuber, Schoppmeyer, Bendig, & Riederer, 1996; Nagahara, Gill, Nicolle, & Gallagher, 1996).

In the case of muscarinic receptors (MAChR) we (Cutler, Joseph, Yamagami, Villalobos-Molina, & Roth, 1994) and others (Fowler, Cowburn, & Joseph, 1997; Roth, Joseph, & Mason, 1996) have shown that there are significant reductions in receptor-G protein coupling/uncoupling as a function of age and Alzheimer's disease (AD). In the latter, Jope, Song, and Powers (1997) reported a decline of 40% in carbachol-stimulated GTP(S) in the prefrontal cortical membranes of AD versus controls, while Cutler and colleagues (1994) reported significant differences in carbachol stimulated GTPase in striata among AD, aged matched controls, and young controls. This could significantly reduce the subsequent signaling cascade and receptor sensitivity. Interestingly, there was a decline in the basal ganglia in this parameter even in normal aging. Moreover, similar decrements have also been reported in senescent rats (Yamagami, Joseph, & Roth,

1992). This loss in sensitivity is important, since there are data that indicate that MAChRs are intimately involved in various aspects of both neuronal amyloid precursor protein, APP processing, (Rossner, Ueberman, Schleib, Perez-Polo, & Bigl, 1998), and vascular functioning (Elhusseiny, Cohen, & Olivier, 1999). Additionally, research has indicated that MAChR of the M1 subtype modulates excitatory hippocampal synaptic transmission (Marino, Rouse, Levey, Potter, & Conn, 1998).

Thus, given the ubiquitous nature of these changes it is possible that they can be expressed, ultimately, as alterations in both motor (Joseph et al., 1983; Kluger et al., 1997) and cognitive behaviors (Bartus, 1990). Evaluations in the rat (Shukitt-Hale, 1999; Wallace, Krauter, & Campbell, 1980), mouse (Dean et al., 1981; Zornetzer & Rogers, 1983) and humans (Welford, 1977) have consistently demonstrated that motor deficits are directly correlated with the degree of task difficulty. Simple behavioral tasks that require only reflexive behavior show the least amount of change with age, while more complicated tasks that require more balance, muscle strength and coordination (Joseph et al., 1983; Kluger et al., 1997; Shukitt-Hale, 1999) show greater declines.

In the case of memory deficits, evidence indicates that these occur primarily in secondary memory systems and are reflected in the retrieval of newly acquired information. The impairments in retrieval have been attributed to deficits in such encoding processes as motivation, attention, processing depth, and organizational skills (Kausler, 1982; Poon, 1985). Indeed, these characterizations have been supported subsequently by a great deal of research both in animals (Bartus, 1990; Ingram, 1990; Ingram, Jucker, & Spangler, 1994; Joseph & Roth, 1993; Shukitt-Hale, 1999; Shukitt-Hale, Mouzakis, & Joseph, 1998) and humans (Muir, 1997; West, 1996).

Age-related deficits in motor performance are thought to be the result of alterations in the striatal dopamine (DA) system (Joseph, Hunt, Rabin, & Dalton, 1992) or in the cerebellum (Baba & Rotaru, 1983; Bickford, 1993) (especially as it relates to decreases in receptor sensitivity; see above). It appears that age-related memory decrements can occur from alterations in either the hippocampus (which mediates allocentric spatial navigation or place learning) or the striatum (which mediates egocentric spatial orientation or response/cue learning) (Devan, Goad, & Petri, 1996; McDonald & White, 1994; Oliveira, Bueno, Pomarico, & Gugliano, 1997).

The mechanisms involved in the losses of sensitivity in the various receptor systems and the related loss in cognitive and motor behaviors are the subjects of continued research. However, it appears that two related factors may be especially relevant in this regard. The first is that there may be increased amounts of inflammatory markers during aging, including increased glial fibrillary acid-protein expression by middle age to inflammation (Rozovsky, Finch, & Morgan, 1998) which, in older adults occurs even in the absence of an inflammatory stimulus (McGeer & McGeer, 1995). Moreover, it has also been reported that TNFα is produced in higher amounts during cytotoxic reactions in senescence (Chang et al., 1996). A second mechanism that may be important here is enhanced vulnerability by the CNS to oxidative stress (OS), which may be the result of such factors as reduced endogenous protection (e.g., glutathione, GSH) (Olanow, 1992). The critical issue is that additional research has shown that this sensitivity may increase further during aging (Joseph et al., 1996; Cantuti-Castelvetri & Joseph, 1999). As an example, Cantuti-Castelvetri and colleagues (unpublished data) have shown that senescent rats exhibited significantly greater motor behavioral deficits and reduced tyrosine hydroxylase immunoreactivity (pars compacta) than young rats following intra-nigral applications of dopamine.

Previous research has indicated that these increases in vulnerability may be the result of increases in the ratio of oxidized to total GSH (Olanow, 1992), significant lipofuscin accumulation with bcl-2 increases, increases in membrane lipid peroxidation (Migheli, Cavalla, Piva, Giordana, & Schiffer, 1994; Yu, 1994), reduced glutamine synthetase (Carney, Smith, Carney, & Butterfield, 1994), alterations in membrane lipids (Denisova, Strain, & Joseph, 1997) and regional variations in the distribution of OS sensitive receptor subtypes (Joseph et al., unpublished data).

In summary, then it appears that there are changes in neuronal function (e.g., signaling) as a function of age that translate into behavioral deficits in motor and cognitive function. The studies mentioned also suggest that these deficits may result from an increase in brain vulnerability to oxidative stress and inflammation that occurs in aging. The purpose of this review is to elaborate on the possible mechanisms involved in these increases in vulnerability and to discuss possible methods to reduce these increases through dietary administration of fruits, vegetables, or natural products that are high in antioxidants and anti-inflammatory activities.

PUTATIVE MECHANISMS CONTRIBUTING TO INCREASED OS AND INFLAMMATORY VULNERABILITY

Membrane Lipid Changes in Aging

Aging is accompanied by substantial alterations in several aspects of membrane molecular structure including (a) the type of linkage to the glycerol moiety; (b) chemical structure of the polar head; and (c) the structure of the aliphatic chains at *sn*-1 and *sn*-2 positions, etc. (Avrova, Chenykaeva, & Obukhova, 1973; Delion, Chalon, Guilloteau, Besnard, &

Durand, 1996; Denisova, Erat, Kelly, & Roth, 1998; Kelly, Joseph, Denisova, Erat, Mason, & Roth, 1995; Lopez, Ilincheta de Boschero, Castagnet, & Giusto, 1995; Sunshine & McNamee, 1994; Tacconi, Lligona, Salmona, Pitsikas, & Algeri, 1991; Wood, Strong, Williamson, & Wise, 1984; Youdim, Martin, & Joseph, 2000; Zhang, Appelkvist, Kristenssom, & Dallner, 1996). These alterations can result in decreases in both membrane asymmetry and fluidity (Choe, Jackson, & Yu, 1995; Choi & Yu, 1995; Igbavboa, Avdulov, Chochina, & Wood, 1997; Schroeder et al., 1996; Wood et al., 1984). The loss of fluidity is primarily in the exofacial plasma membrane leaflet (Igbavboa, Avdulov, Schroeder, & Wood, 1996; Wood, Schroeder, Avdulov, Chochina, & Igbavboa, 1999), which results in membrane asymmetry (Wood et al., 1999). Such decreases in membrane asymmetry might alter the transport of phosphatidylserine (PS) from the outer to the inner leaflet of the plasma membrane, so that it would accumulate in the outer leaflet, possibly resulting in apoptosis (Bratton et al., 1997; Diaz & Schroit, 1996; Schor et al., 1999). This could have important consequences for neuronal cell death and function.

One important lipid that can significantly affect membrane fluidity is cholesterol (CHL), which comprises over 40 mol% of membrane lipids (Wood et al., 1999; Wood, Schroeder, Rao, Igbavboa, & Avdulov, 1996), and is associated with bulk membrane fluidity (Leibel, Firestone, Legler, Braswell, & Miller, 1987). This lipid generally translocates to the exofacial leaflet (Igbavboa et al., 1996), especially during aging. In this regard it has been shown that CHL that is oxidized in the outer leaflet of synaposomes induced significant reductions in the activity of the Ca^{2+} ATPase "pump" (Wood et al., 1996) and subsequent calcium buffering, possibly creating serious consequences for the cell.

Research has also indicated that sphingomyelin (SPH) has been shown to regulate CHL trafficking (Slotte & Bierman, 1988). More importantly, however, SPH and its metabolites also may have more direct interactions with oxidative stressors that could result in increased vulnerability to OS. For example, when SPH and CHL were increased in PC12 cells to levels seen with respect to brain aging (Denisova et al., 1997), followed by exposure to H_2O_2, the cells showed greater decrements in calcium buffering following 30 mM KCl-induced depolarization than that seen in control cells. Such long-lasting increases in cytosolic calcium may lead to cell death by several mechanisms, including (a) xanthine oxidase activation (Reiter, Teng, & Beckman, 2000); (b) excitotoxicity through glutamate activation (Lynch & Dawson, 1994); and (c) nitric oxide synthase and phospholipase up-regulation (Mishra & Delivoria-Papadopoulos, 1999). OS may enhance calcium dysfunction (Zaidi & Michaelis, 1999) in compromised cells, resulting in subsequent pro-oxidant generation and loss of functional capacity of the cell.

The experimental increases in cellular levels (PC-12 cells) of SPH and CHL were also shown to induce significant reductions in GSH (Denisova, Cantuti-Castelvetri, Hassan, Paulson, & Joseph, 2001). A previous study (Denisova, Fisher, Provost, & Joseph, 1999) had indicated that the SPH metabolite, sphingosine-1-phosphate, significantly increased the sensitivity to OS induced by exposure to hydrogen peroxide following depolarization with 30 mM KCl as assessed via loss of calcium buffering. It also appeared that sphingosine-1-phosphate was extremely effective in lowering GSH levels and that this may have induced the increased oxidative stress vulnerability, since GSH repletion with N-acetylcysteine antagonized the deleterious effects of sphingosine-1-phosphate on the cells at the low (5 μM) but not the high (300 μM) hydrogen peroxide concentration.

Though not affecting oxidative stress sensitivity (via calcium), ceramide, another SPH metabolite, significantly potentiated the effect of hydrogen peroxide on the production of reactive oxygen species (dicholorofluorascine, DCF analysis) in the cells (Denisova et al., 1999). Recent studies also indicate that these SPH metabolites (e.g., ceramide) may interact with the mitochondrial electron transport chain and consequently lead to ROS generation, lipid oxidation, and loss of mitochondrial functions (Garcia-Ruiz, Colell, Mari, Morales, & Fernandez-Checa, 1997; Gudz, Tserng, & Hoppel, 1997).

Taken together these findings indicate that there may be several membrane changes in aging that could enhance the vulnerability to OS. These include alterations in CHL transfer or levels, SPH regulation of CHL transfer, or SPH-CHL induced reductions in GSH levels. Additional studies suggest that membrane fatty-acid-binding proteins (e.g., FABP) may also decrease in aging, further inhibiting normal CHL trafficking (Pu et al., 1999).

Receptor Changes in Aging

As important as they seem to be in increasing vulnerability to OS, lipid modifications appear to act in concert with a second factor that is also important in mediating this sensitivity. This involves qualitative/quantitative differences in receptor subtypes in various neuronal populations. As an example, it has been known for many years that some areas of the brain "age" at a faster rate than others, particularly, the striatum. If variations in OS sensitivity are involved in these selective regional variations in function, it may be the result of differences in the preponderance of certain receptor subtypes in the various brain regions.

As a first step in making these determinations, we chose to examine differential sensitivity to OS among the five muscarinic receptor (MAChR) subtypes. As indicated above, research has indicated that they may be critically important in a variety of neuronal functions and they show declines in sensitivity and signaling in aging. Additionally, studies indicate that there are high concentrations of vulnerable MAChRs in memory control areas (Levey, 1996) and in the vasculature (Elhusseiny et al., 1999), predisposing them to increased oxidative stress vulnerability.

To examine the differential sensitivity to oxidative stress among the 5 MAChR subtypes, we exposed COS-7 cells that were transfected with one of five muscarinic receptor subtypes (M1- M5-AChR) to low concentrations of H_2O_2 (0, 300 or 500 μM for 30 min in growth medium) or dopamine (DA, 1 mM for 4 hrs) and examined intracellular Ca^{2+} levels prior to and following 500 μM oxotremorine (oxo, to induce depolarization), as well as cell death following OS exposure. We employed COS-7 cells for these experiments, because they do not express MAChR and have a long history of usefulness in studying various structural-activity relationships among the MAChR subtypes in isolation (Jakubic & Wess, 1999).

The results of this study indicated that COS-7 cells transfected with M1, 2 or M 4AChR showed the greatest decreases (25%–100%) in calcium buffering following H_2O_2 or dopamine (DA) exposure and oxotremorine-induced depolarization. Those cells transfected with M3 and M5 and exposed to DA- or H_2O_2 showed no loss in calcium buffering. The results paralleled those observed with respect to cell viability when examined in M1 and M3-transfected COS-7 cells as representative for a "vulnerable" and "nonvulnerable" receptor, respectively. Thus, it may be that receptor differences in OS sensitivity may determine, in part, regional susceptibility to cell death.

It has been shown, for example, in the striatum that (a) there are high concentrations of DA, which form a variety of OS-based toxic products (Ben-Shachar, Zuk, & Glinka, 1995; Hastings & Zigmond, 1994); (b) M1 receptor protein is expressed in 78% of the neurons; (c) M4 receptors were localized to 44% of striatal cells (Hersch, Gutekunst, Rees, Heilman, & Levey, 1994); and (d) M2 receptors may be the predominant muscarinic receptor. Therefore, the profound age-related changes in the striatum may be reflective of the interactions between DA and specific populations of OS vulnerable receptors.

These results parallel those seen previously in the aged animal with respect to DA receptor subtype (D1 and D2) vulnerability to OS. In that study age differences in D1- or D2-stimulated GTPase activity following SKF38393 or quinelorane (D1 or D2 agonists, respectively) application to striatal slices obtained from young (6 months) and old (24 months) rats were assessed following exposure to 1 mM DA (Joseph, Erat, Denisova, & Villalobos-Molina, 1998). The results indicated that while DA significantly reduced GTPase activity in both age groups and in both D1 and D2 receptors, the effects of DA were significantly greater in the striatal slices obtained from old animals, with respect to the D1 receptors, even though striatal DA uptake was significantly lower as a function of age. These findings suggest that there are age-related increases in OS vulnerability that may be receptor subtype selective.

As mentioned, because the MAChR are intimately involved in APP processing and in other aspects of vascular functioning, and because AD and vascular dementia can occur simultaneously in the aged, we examined the selectivity of amyloidβ 25-35 toxicity on M1- and M3-transfected COS-7 cells (assessed as described above). The results showed that the pattern of Aβ sensitivity was similar to that seen with respect to DA- or H_2O_2-induced OS. That is that the Aβ-exposed, M1-transfected cells showed greater disruptions in calcium buffering than that seen in M3-transfected cells exposed to Aβ. An additional experiment showed that pretreatment of the M1-transfected cells with the nitrone trap, phenyl-n-tert-butylnitrone (PBN), or the calcium channel antagonists, nifedipine or conotoxin, prevented the Aβ-induced decrements in calcium buffering.

Thus, it is clear from these findings and those stated previously that in addition to the alterations in membranes, the possible differences in vulnerability to oxidative stress seen in aging may involve the regional variability in selective vulnerability of muscarinic and DA-receptor subtypes.

AGING: FERTILE GROUND FOR ALZHEIMER'S DISEASE?

Age–Alzheimer's Disease Parallels

1. *Oxidative Stress.* A great deal of research suggests that the etiology of Alzheimer's disease (AD) is multifactorial and may involve such processes as membrane alterations (Blanchard et al., 2000; Pu et al., 1999; Soderberg, Edlund, Alafuzoff, Kristensson, & Dallner, 1992; Wells, Farooqui, Liss, & Horrocks, 1995); and inflammation (Rosenman, Shrikant, Dubb, Benveniste, & Ransohoff, 1995). A third factor, of course, is OS, which interacts with all of the previous factors and subsequently results in increases in neurodegeneration and loss of cognitive behavioral function. As we have discussed above, these additional factors are also implicated in normal brain aging, and they may indeed increase brain vulnerability to neurodegenerative diseases such as AD.

Thus, it may be that these increases in OS vulnerability, especially as it relates to factors such as alterations in membranes or differential receptor subtypes, may determine, in part, regional susceptibility to cell death that may not be correlated with Aβ deposition. Sayre, Zagorski, Surewicz, Krafft, & Perry, (1997) showed that 4-hydroxynonenal (HNE) in brain tissue from AD and age-matched control patients was identified in about 50% of all neurofibrillary tangles (NFT), but weakly in a minority of senile plaques and dystrophic neurites. Aβ deposits were unlabeled. Age-matched controls showed only background HNE-pyrrole immunoreactivity in hippocampal or cortical neurons. This study provided evidence that OS is pervasive in this disease and that lipid peroxidation (as assessed via HNE) may also play a role in the neuronal death and the cognitive deficits that are associated with AD.

In subsequent studies (Sayre et al., 1997; Smith, Richey Harris, Sayre, Beckman, & Perry, 1997), peroxynitrite-related nitrotyrosine formation was found in all vulnerable neurons, not just the ones containing NFT. These findings indicate there was generalized OS that would be important in influencing disease pathogenesis. Additional evidence for increased OS in AD can be seen from experiments showing that there is impaired iron (Smith, Wehr, Harris, Siedlak, Connor, & Perry, 1998) or metal homeostasis (Sayre et al., 1997; Nishida & Nishino, 1999) in AD brain parenchyma.

Therefore, it might be postulated that OS plays a major role in the cascade of effects associated with AD that are not necessarily associated with Aβ deposition. If the "gerofactor" is included in this mix, it is obvious that these perturbations would be acting upon an organism that is already showing similar increases in vulnerability to OS. It may be that treatments that would alter this vulnerable environment in aging might be very effective at reducing or preventing the deleterious effects associated with AD.

2. *Inflammatory Processes and AD: The Role of Cytokines.* In the introduction we presented some evidence to show that inflammatory processes may be an important contributor to the deleterious effects of brain aging. Products of inflammatory reactions such as cytokines, complement proteins, and adhesion molecules are neurotoxic. They may represent extracellular signals that initiate neuronal degeneration through several processes (Rosenman et al., 1995; Schipper, 1996; Steffen, Breier, Butcher, Schultz, & Engelhardt, 1996; Stella et al., 1997; Woodroofe, 1995). For example they can degrade membrane lipids and induce the accumulation of free fatty acids such as arachidonic acid. The release of this fatty acid can enhance the formation of numerous metabolites with proinflammatory properties (Aisen, 1997; Borgeat, Hamberg, & Samuelson, 1976; Fontana, Kristensen, dubs, Gemsa, & Weber, 1982; Murray, Clements, & Lynch, 1999).

Given these properties, it might be surmised that the release of proinflammatory cytokines plays an important role in the etiology and development of neurodegenerative conditions. Over the life span, direct and collateral damage mediated by AD inflammatory processes appear to play a key role in intensifying the pathogenic processes that give rise to AD. In fact, new observations obtained from animal models and human studies strongly suggest that the inflammation process in AD might be a significant contributor to the AD pathology. Inflammatory events, therefore, appear to be an important factor in the etiology of neurologic processes such as AD (Merrill & Murphy, 1997).

3. *Membrane Alterations in AD.* The data regarding the levels of CHL in AD are mixed. There are studies which have reported significant increases in CHL levels in frontal cortex (Sparks, 1997). Conversely, additional studies have reported decreases in PL, CHL, and gangliosides (which is associated with axodendritic arborization) (Svennerholm, Bostrom, Helander, & Jungber, 1991; Svennerholm & Gottfries, 1994), as well as reductions in the concentration of apolipoprotein (ApoE) (Poirier, 1999).

Investigations of membrane CHL/SPH/ApoE interactions are few in number, but Huang and colleagues (1995) showed that ApoE polymorphism may be an important factor in CHL transport with 30% less (3H)cholesterol released into plasmas of ApoE2/2 and ApoE4/4 individuals compared with those obtained from ApoE3/3 subjects. As a result, there was 50% and 65% more cell-derived (3H)cholesterol in alpha-LpA-I2 than that seen in plasmas of ApoE4/4 and ApoE2/2-subjects.

Although SPH interactions with various ApoE polymorphisms have not been examined, it is clear that their specification in AD might be extremely important, especially as it might relate to increases in OS vulnerability or inflammatory processes. Mattson and coauthors (Mattson, Goodman, Luo, Fu, & Furukawa, 1997) have suggested, for example, that TNF alpha signaling in AD involves the p55 receptor which in turn is linked to a SPH-ceramide NFκB pathway. Because SPH or its metabolites may be altered in the aged brain, this might significantly affect the strength or conduction of this signal and the subsequent effects on microglia and neurons.

Amyloid Beta-Membrane Lipid Interactions

In addition to the factors just discussed, the brain membrane molecular structure may also be a determinant of amyloid-beta peptide-lipid interactions in AD, as amyloid beta may interact with both CHL to which it may preferentially bind (Avdulov et al., 1997; Klunk et al., 1997; Mason et al., 1999) or with phospholipids which may stabilize it. In vitro studies showed that the interaction of AD beta-amyloid peptides with membrane lipids may take on two forms: one that penetrates the membrane, or one that is stabilized by surface binding to phospholipid (PL) head groups (McLaurin, Franklin, Fraser, & Chakrabartty, 1998). It appears that in AD there is a potentiation of the age-related decreases in total frontal cortical and hippocampal PL on a DNA basis (Mason et al., 1999). There also appears to be a GM1-ganglioside membrane bound form of beta-amyloid peptide (Yanagisawa, Odaka, Suzuki, & Ihara, 1995), and it appears that GM1 inhibits AD amyloid beta peptide induced cytokine release, consequently preventing inflammatory responses of neuronal cells in AD (Ariga & Yu, 1999).

Thus, in AD the age-related alterations on membrane lipid composition in various brain regions may create preexisting abnormalities in membrane molecular structure significantly affecting AD beta-amyloid peptide interactions in the membrane microenvironment and subsequent OS and inflammatory processes. This could result in impaired performance and decreased neuronal plasticity. Further elaborations of the age-related changes in the brain plasma (and mitochondrial) membranes should also be of considerable importance in AD. This should allow information to be obtained that is concerned with such factors as (a) locus and mechanisms of oxidative damage in neuronal cell death; (b) the putative sites involved in membrane damage and subsequent alterations in neurotransmitter receptor mediated signal transduction; and (c) interactions between membrane lipids such as CHL, SPM, and OS.

Behavior and Amyloid Beta

There have been inconsistences in the determinations directed toward examining whether amyloid beta is toxic in vivo in the many animal models of AD. A good behavioral model of the memory impairment of AD in animals should utilize tasks and measures which are equivalent to the ones on which Alzheimer patients are impaired. In the case of Aβ injections into rats, there are numerous factors that could account for the inconsistencies in toxic observed behavioral effects including conformational state, dose, and sequence of Aβ; method of administration; pathological endpoints measured, regional variations, hemisphere injected; age of animals used, and species or strain utilized (Sigurdsson, Lee, Dong, Henja, & Lorens, 1997; Winkler et al., 1994). A second factor that may be important in light of the previous discussions about parallels between AD and aging is that perhaps the neuronal environment in some of the mice that are transgenic for amyloid beta or the rats that have been injected with amyloid beta are not sensitive to this insult. For example, one study showed that rats who were injected with either Aβ or vehicle at an early age (3 months), and not tested until they were old (18 months), were impaired in swim maze performance (Winkler et al., 1994), suggesting that even small hippocampal lesions in aging rats caused by two injections produce deficits in behavior.

It is also possible that Aβ alone is not sufficient or necessary for producing the behavioral changes, and it may be that it is most effective when OS or inflammatory processes are activated. Thus, behavioral deficits are more detectable when the microinjections are repeated over a prolonged period of time and the effects are measured at an extended latency postinjection (Cleary, Hittner, Semotuk, Mantyh, & O'Hare, 1995; O'Hare et al., 1999). It may be that the delayed behavioral effects observed are the result of secondary damage to neurons following Aβ-induced activation of glia (O'Hare et al., 1999), or perhaps to the long-term effects of the indwelling cannulae (Cleary et al., 1995) inducing inflammatory changes. In one study, aggregated Aβ was present in the brain 90 days postinjection and was accompanied by substantial gliosis. Behavioral deficits developed slowly and were clearly central in nature as opposed to being an artifact of a general retardation of responding. These findings suggested that the putative toxic effects of Aβ may require the induction of inflammatory responses, or toxins associated with glial activation (O'Hare et al., 1999). Also, Aβ has been shown to adversely affect maze learning after bilateral hippocampus injection when combined with ibotenic acid, but not when injected alone (Dornan, Kang, McCampbell, & Kang, 1993).

In the case of the various mouse models that are transgenic for amyloid precursor protein (APP) mutations or presenilin-1 (PS1) mutations, there are similar inconsistencies in the behavioral effects that have been observed. Moreover, it is not clear whether the deficits that are observed are the result of Aβ deposition, the overexpression of APP or the overexpression of other proteins (Neve & Robakis, 1998). Although there is some evidence in transgenic mice for graded neurodegenerative changes (mainly in the vicinity of the plaques) it is unclear if these changes are due mainly to the neurotoxic effects of Aβ or the large accumulation of Aβ deposits (Sirinathsinghji, 1998). In this respect, despite the robust production and deposition of Aβ, there is no evidence for frank neuronal loss or synaptic loss anywhere in the brain or along specific neuronal pathways (Sirinathsinghji, 1998). As seen with the Aβ injections, there may be other factors that involve inflammation and OS that mediate the putative toxicity of the Aβ, not the least of which may be the aging environment. Moreover, in AD it appears that there are other factors that come into play that can also contribute to the putative toxicity of Aβ. These include the ApoE ratio, presenilins, increased tau phosphorylation, altered cholesterol/phospholipid ratios, and subsequent changes in membranes—factors that once again call into question the necessity and sufficiency of Aβ in the devastating behavioral effects seen in this disease.

FOODS FOR THOUGHT

In the previous sections we have tried to show that there are changes in the vulnerability to OS in aging that are the result of possible alterations in endogenous antioxidants, membrane changes, and possibly differential receptor oxidative stress sensitivity. Additionally, we have shown that there are parallels between the changes seen in aging and those seen with respect to neurodegenerative diseases such as AD and that aging is a central factor in this disease. Therefore, it might be advantageous to focus more research on reducing or forestalling the age-related decrements (for example, increased vulnerability to oxidative stress) that are providing a favorable environment for development of AD and other neurodegenerative diseases. One way of accomplishing this may be through nutritional antioxidants and antiinflammatories.

Phytochemicals: The "Anti-Aging" Properties of Fruits and Vegetables

There is a long history of evidence showing a significant association between fruit and vegetable intake and decreased mortality from cardiovascular disease (Armstrong, Mann, Adelstein, & EsKin, 1975; Hughes, 1995; Mayne, 1996; Verlangieri, Kapeghian, el-Dean, & Bush, 1985). Nutritional supplementation of fruits and vegetables also appears to reduce the incidence and mortality rates of cancer in humans (Doll, 1990; Willett, 1994) and animals (Wattenberg & Coccia, 1991). Even extracts of single foods such as tomato (Sharoni, Giron, Rise, & Levy, 1997) and garlic (Pinto et al., 1997) may have antitumor properties.

Although studies examining the effects of fruit and vegetable consumption on cancer and cardiovascular disease are well documented and numerous, there is far less documentation with respect to the central nervous system and aging. However, there is indirect evidence suggesting that nutritional supplementation may be important in neuronal health. For example, there has been some success in AD treatment with the antioxidant vitamin E (Sano et al., 1997). Additional data (as in the following sections) show that it is possible to increase the antioxidant protection in aged animals and humans by the consumption of the flavonoid glycosides of *Ginkgo biloba* and to improve cognitive performance (Rai, Shovlin, & Wesnes, 1991), difficulties in concentration (Kleijnen & Knipschild, 1992), and Ca^{2+}-induced increases in the oxidative metabolism of brain neurons (Oyama, Hayashi, & Ueha, 1993; Oyama, Fuchs, Katayama, & Noda, 1994). More recent evidence suggests that administration of *Ginkgo biloba* EGb 761 slowed the progression of AD (Kanowski, Herrmann, Stephen, Weirich, & Horr, 1996).

One study (Snowdon, Gross, & Butler, 1996) that investigated the relationship of plasma antioxidants to reduced functional capacity in older adults found a strong positive association between plasma lycopene and the ability of older nuns to perform self-care such as dressing and feeding. (Lycopene is a red pigment found in a small number of vegetables such as tomatoes, watermelons, and pink grapefruit.)

Therefore, it may be that increasing the intake of dietary antioxidants may have protective effects on CNS function similar to those seen with respect to cancer and cardiovascular disease. One important question that we wanted to consider is whether this can be accomplished by increasing the dietary amounts of fruits and vegetables. Subsequent research showed that fruit and vegetable extracts containing high levels of anthocyanins and other flavonoids also exhibited increased levels of total antioxidant activity as assessed via the Oxygen Radical Absorbance Capacity Assay (ORAC). This assay utilizes β-phycoerythrin (β-PE) or R-PE as an indicator protein, 2,2'-Azobis(2-amidino-propane) dihydrochloride (AAPH) as a peroxyl radical generator, and Trolox as a standard (Cao, Verdon, Wu, Wang, Prior, 1995). The assay revealed that the foods showing the highest ORAC activity included spinach, strawberries (Cao, Sofie, & Prior, 1996; Wang, Cao, & Prior, 1996), and blueberries (Prior et al., 1998).

In the first study we examined whether long-term feeding (from 6 to 15 months of age; Fischer 344 rats) with a control diet (AIN-93) or supplemented diet (strawberry extract or spinach extract or vitamin E) would prevent age-related decrements in cognitive or neuronal function. Results indicated that the supplemented diets forestalled the onset of age-related deficits as assessed via several parameters (e.g., signal transduction such as oxotremorine-enhanced striatal dopamine release [ox-K^+-ERDA], as well as cognitive behavior (e.g., Morris water maze performance) (Joseph & Shukitt-Hale, 1998). The most efficacious of the fruit and vegetable supplements was spinach. These results suggested that phytochemicals present in antioxidant rich foods might be effective in forestalling functional age-related deficits.

However, it might be noted that at present, the world population of people over 65 years of age represents more than 50% of all those who have ever lived who have attained this age. Therefore, as important as the prevention of these age-related decrements may be, even more critical is the reversal of these decrements once they occur. Thus, in a subsequent experiment (Joseph, Shukitt-Hale, & Denisova, 1999), we examined whether dietary supplementations (for 8 weeks) with spinach, strawberry, or blueberry extracts in an AIN-93 diet would be effective in reversing age-related deficits in neuronal and behavioral (motor and cognitive) function in aged (19 months) F344 rats. The results showed that overall these supplements, particularly blueberry, were effective in reversing age-related deficits in several neuronal and behavioral parameters. These included oxotremorine-enhancement of K^+-evoked release of dopamine from striatal slices, carbachol-stimulated GTPase activity, and striatal Ca^{45} buffering in striatal synaptosomes.

This observation is particularly striking, as maintaining the functional integrity of the striatum—in particular that of the dopaminergic system—

has been reported to have a major impact on several behavioral parameters (Joseph et al., 1990; Joseph et al., 1983; Joseph, Shukitt-Hale, McEwen, & Rabin, 1999). Furthermore, it is known that a major role is played in PD by reduced release of DA from the decline in the number dopaminergic neurons within the substantia nigra that forms projections into the striatum (Youdim & Riederer, 1997). As such, the ability of blueberry extract to enhance DA release upon stimulation may also have important implications in the etiology of this disease. In fact, in Joseph, Shukitt-Hale, and Denisova (1999) and in a more recent experiment (Youdim et al., 2000), we found that the blueberry diet was effective in reversing motor behavioral performance on the rod-walking and accelerod tasks and Morris water-maze performance (Joseph, Shukitt-Hale, Denisova, et al., 1999). Dr. Paula Bickford and colleagues (Bickford, Shukitt-Hale, & Joseph, 1999; Bickford et al., 2000) also showed reversals in motor learning deficits and losses in cerebellar Purkinje-cell noradrenergic-receptor sensitivity following dietary supplementation with blueberry or strawberry extracts. We are currently investigating the signaling parameters that may mediate these reversals. The changes seen with respect to motor behavior are particularly interesting since it is well known that age-related decrements in motor behavior (e.g., deficits in balance and coordination) have been very resistant to reversal.

These findings suggest that in addition to their known beneficial effects on cancer and heart disease, the phytochemicals in antioxidant-rich foods may be beneficial in reversing the course of neuronal and behavioral aging. However, it is also interesting to note that the diets in these studies were supplemented based on equal antioxidant activity, as determined by the ORAC assay (Cao et al., 1996). Thus, it might be expected that they would have been equipotent in their effects on the various parameters examined. This result would indicate that a simple measure of antioxidant activity (e.g., ORAC) should be carefully scrutinized and perhaps combined with functional assessments, in order to ascertain potency of agents supposedly thought to have high antioxidant activity. Moreover, when two indices of antioxidant activity were examined—ROS production and glutathione levels in the striatum and cerebellum—(Joseph, Shukitt-Hale, Denisova et al., 1999), it was found that the supplementations only resulted in modest effects that could not totally account for the efficacy of these treatments. This would suggest that other beneficial effects of the polyphenolic compounds may be important in this regard. These properties may involve their anti-inflammatory (Krischer, Eisenmann, Bock, & Mueller, 1997) and membrane fluidizing effects (Halder & Bhaduri, 1998). We have shown for example that the anthocyanins and hydroxycinnamates, two polyphenolic classes isolated from blueberries, have very potent antioxidant properties (e.g., against AAPH) and anti-inflammatory properties (against tumor necrosis factor, TNFα) in vascular endothelial cells (unpublished data), and blueberry extract is effective against TNFα-induced decrements in calcium buffering in M1AChR-transfected COS7 cells.

One interesting set of parallel experiments that we have been conducting using the blueberry extract involved examining the effects of pretreatment of the M1-transfected COS-7 cells with this extract on preventing Aβ-induced decrements in calcium buffering. As is well known, Aβ deposition is one of the pathological hallmarks of AD (Steele, 2000). Results indicated that the blueberry extract was extremely efficacious in preventing the deleterious effects of the Aβ on this parameter (unpublished data). We are presently attempting to determine the most effective blueberry polyphenolic or combination that may be inducing this protection. However, it should be clear that in age-related neurodegenerative diseases (AD and PD), the additional insults that are are superimposed upon a nervous system that is already showing increased responsiveness to OS. Therefore, it may be possible to reduce this sensitivity through supplementation with the combinations of antioxidants found in fruits and vegetables. In this effort and in collaboration with Dr. David Morgan we have been examining mice with presenilin-1 mutations, and that are transgenic for Aβ, and that had been supplemented with diets containing blueberry extract or their controls. The preliminary results indicate that there were significant increases in carbachol-stimulated GTPase activity in the blueberry-supplemented mice. These increases were associated with enhancements in Y-maze performance.

Overall, the observations made in the studies cited in this section support the hypothesis that dietary polyphenolics from fruits and vegetables improve age-related decrements in neuronal function and behavior. Studies further suggest that they also may be of some value in the treatment of age-related neurodegenerative diseases such as AD.

Aged Garlic Extract and Red Bell Pepper—Senescence Accelerated Mouse Model

Aged garlic extract (AGlE, *Allium sativum*), which contains S-allycisteine, S-allymercaptocysteine, allicin, and diallosulfides, has been reported to exhibit beneficial effects toward cognitive impairments in the senescence accelerated mouse (SAM) (Moriguchi, Saito, & Nishiyama, 1997; Moriguchi, Takashina, Chu, Saito, & Nishiyama, 1994; Nishiyama, Moriguchi, & Saito, 1997; Zhang, Moriguchi, Saito, & Nishiyama, 1998). The SAM model has been shown to exhibit both morphological and neurological impairments that also have been observed in normal aging (Kawaguchi et al., 1995; Potier et al., 1993a; Potier et al., 1993b; van Eitzen et al., 1998; Yagi et al., 1989). Initial studies found that SAM supplemented with AGlE (2% w/w) displayed both increased life span and improved learning as assessed by active and passive avoidance tests (Moriguchi et al., 1994). Further beneficial effects of AGlE administration have been found in the SAM model where no atrophic morphological changes in neocortex, olfactory cortex, and amygdala were observed (Moriguchi et al., 1997; Nishiyama et al., 1997; Shimada, Ohta, Akiguchi, & Takeda, 1992; Shimada et al., 1994).

While a direct protective effect cannot be dismissed, the beneficial effects promoted by AGlE could also be attributed to improved antioxidant activity within brain regions, which potentially could result in a reduction in membrane lipid peroxidation, an observation that has been observed with AGlE in vitro (Horie, Azawu, Itakura, & Fuwa, 1992; Horie et al., 1989). As already mentioned, such protection may lead to improved neuronal signaling and increased receptor sensitivity, although these have not been directly assessed in this model. Extrapolations from our cited work with respect to fruits and vegetables would suggest that there are a multiplicity of actions that may be responsible for these beneficial effects in addition to those seen with respect to their antioxidant activity.

It has been argued that in addition to antioxidant activity, changes in the immune response may contribute to a number of age-related impairments in cognitive performance (Hauss-Wegrzyniak, Vannucchi, & Wenk, 2000; Yamada et al., 1999). In this regard, a recent study by Zhang and colleagues (1998) found that thymectomized mice supplemented with AGlE displayed marked improvement in a number of markers of immune function. AGlE treatment was found to prevent the reduction of thymectomy-induced antibody production and improve thymectomy-induced deterioration of performance in a passive avoidance and spatial memory task. Interestingly, both AGlE and a high molecular protein fraction of AGlE have been reported to increase oxidative burst in murine macrophages and to enhance T-lymphocyte (Lau, Yamasaki, & Gridley, 1991) and human lymphocyte (Morioka, Sze, Morton, & Irie, 1993) proliferation. Together this evidence would suggest that AGlE may exert some protective effects in SAM through immunomodulatory mechanisms, because it has been shown that unfavorable changes in the immune system result in impairment of learning and memory functions (Hauss-Wegrzyniak et al., 2000; Yamada et al., 1999).

In addition to AGlE, red bell pepper (*Capsicum annuum* L.) has also been employed in the SAM model, and beneficial effects were observed in both memory and acquisition performance (Suganuma, Hirano, & Inakuma, 1999). One of the active compounds in red bell peppers may be the lycopenes. Thus, to the extent that the SAM model is effective in aging, both garlic and red bell pepper may have positive benefits on age-related deficits.

Tea

Although the increased consumption of polyphenolics from tea has been found to correlate with reduced incidence of certain cancers (Suganuma et al., 1998; Suganuma, Okabe et al., 1999), it has also been suggested that they elicit potentially beneficial effects toward improving neuronal function. Matsuoka and colleagues (1995) found that intracisternal injection of epicatechin improved the memory impairment induced by intracisternal glucose oxidase, and IV injection of catechin or epicatechin improved deficits induced by the cerebral ischemia, possibly by inhibiting oxidative and inflammatory processes (Hofbauer et al., 1999; Lin & Lin, 1997; Lin, Tsai, Lin-Shiau, Ho, & Lin, 1999). Both of these parameters are characteristic events during and following ischemic insults (Planas, Soriano, Justicia, & Rodriguez-Farre, 1999; Schafer et al., 2000; Stanimirovic & Satoh, 2000; Stephenson et al., 2000) that ultimately affect behavior (Hauss-Wegrzyniak et al., 2000). Although, these polyphenolics were administered IV, there is evidence to suggest that tea polyphenolics can localize within the brain following dietary consumption (Suganuma et al., 1998) and thus are available to promote actions resulting in cognitive improvements (Matsuoka et al., 1995).

Carotenoids, Vitamin E, and Vitamin C

Unfortunately, there is a paucity of research regarding the effects of dietary supplemenation of vitamins E and C or carotenoids on age-related behavioral or neuronal deficits. the majority of studies that have identified their roles on brain functions have done so through dietary deficiency. Nonetheless, numerous epidemiological studies have reported some positive benefits of dietary carotenoids on age-related impairments in memory and learning performance (Youdim & Joseph, 2001). Parallel with these assessments, correlations with flavonoids and vitamins E and C have also been reported with mixed results. There is however, growing evidence to suggest a potential beneficial effect of these compounds, particularly vitamin E, against the damaging effects of neurodegenerative disorders such as AD and PD (Cantuti-Castelvetri, Shukitt-Hale, & Joseph, 2000).

For the most part, it has been difficult to establish from epidemiological studies whether changes in b-carotene (Jama et al., 1996; Perrig, Perrig, & Stahelin, 1997), vitamin E (La Rue et al., 1997; Perkins et al., 1999; Schmidt et al., 1998), or vitamin C (Goodwin, Goodwin, & Garry, 1983; La Rue et al., 1997; Perrig et al., 1997) preceded or were as the result of impaired cognition. Even more difficult to determine are the mechanisms by which they might provide CNS protection. Additionally, as with any epidemiological investigations, there are always problems with the reliability of information and measurement error that could influence the interpretation of the results.

Ginkgo Biloba (EGb 761)

EGb 761 is a standardized extract of dried *Ginkgo biloba* leaves. It has also been shown to be an effective free-radical scavenger and a potent inhibitor of lipid peroxidation (Diamond et al., 2000). It is one of the most extensively studied extracts of cognitive performance in animal and human studies, and some positive results have been observed with respect to AD (Brailowsky & Montiel, 1997; Christen, 2000; Clostre, 1999; Cohen-Salmon et al., 1997; Gajewski & Hensch, 1999; Grassel, 1992; Hoyer, Lannert, Noldner, & Chatterjee, 1999; Ivaniv, 1998; Kanowski et al., 1996; Pardon et al., 2000; Petkov et al., 1993; Porsolt, Martin, Lenegre, Fromage, & Drieu, 1990; Rapin, Lamproglou, Drieu, & DeFeudis, 1994; Stoll, Scheuer, Pohl, & Muller, 1996; Tadano et al., 1998). A number of very good review articles have recently been published that are solely directed to discussing Ginkgo and its various pharmacological actions, and the reader is referred to these for a comprehensive overview of the literature (Clostre, 1999; Diamond et al., 2000; Kidd, 1999).

Ginkgo has numerous properties that could account for the beneficial effects seen in AD and possibly aging. Some of these effects are as follows:

1. Reduced levels of OS (Oyama, Chikahisa, Ueha, Kanemaru, & Noda, 1996; Oyama et al., 1994; Seif-El-Nasr & El-Fattah, 1995); as we have shown above, OS is implicated in decrements in brain function (see also Floyd, 1999).
2. Increased cerebral blood flow, thereby increasing the amount of oxygen and glucose delivered to the brain.
3. Modulation of membrane fluidity, possibly through protection of membrane fatty acids (al-Zuhair, el-Fattah, & el-Sayed, 1998; Klein, Chatterjee, & Loffelholz, 1997; Rabin et al., 1998; Rodriguez de Turco, Droy-Lafaiz, & Bazan, 1993; Stoll et al., 1996). Changes in membrane fatty acids have been shown to correlate with cognitive performances (Kessler & Yehuda, 1985; Scheuer, Rostock, Bartsch, & Muller, 1999; Suzuki, Park, Tamura, & Ando, 1998).
4. Interaction with the muscarinic cholinergic system (Chopin & Briley, 1992; Deberdt, 1994). In addition to the parameters cited earlier, the muscarinic cholinergic system has been shown to be involved in the performance of spatial tasks (Puumala et al., 1998; Packard, Kohlmaier, & Alexander, 1996; Packard & Teather, 1997).

5. Protection of the striatal dopaminergic system (Ramassamy et al., 1990; Ramassamy, Christen, Clostre, & Costentin, 1992).

6. Inhibition of monoamine oxidase activity (Pardon et al., 2000; White, Scates, & Cooper, 1996; Wu and Zhu et al., 1996).

Ginseng

Panax ginseng is one of the mostly widely used herbs in traditional Chinese medicine. There are numerous beneficial effects that have been attributed to ginseng, including its ability to modulate immune function and other functions such as memory, learning, and behavior (Petkov, 1978). In this regard, a number of different cognitive tests have shown the potential beneficial effects of ginseng on memory and learning performance in a variety of animal species (Jaenicke, Kim, Ahn, & Lee, 1991; Lasarova, Mosharrot, Petkov, Markovska, & Petkov, 1987; Petkov & Mosharrot, 1987; Petkov et al., 1993; Petkov et al., 1992). In addition several herbal mixtures that contain ginseng have been shown to improve cognitive performance. S-113m (Nishiyama et al., 1996; Nishiyama et al., 1995), which consists of *Biota orientalis, Panax schinseng,* and *Schizandra chinesis* (1:1:3 w/w/w); and d DX-9386 (Nishiyama, Zhou, & Saito, 1994a, 1994b; Nishiyama, Zhou, Takashina, & Saito, 1994; Smriga, Saito, & Nishiyama, 1995; Zhang, Saito, & Nishiyama, 1994; Zhang, Saito, Nishiyama, & Abe, 1994), which consists of *Panax schinseng, Polygala tenuifola, Acorus gramineus,* and *Paoria cocos* (1:1:25:50 w/w, dry).

Though the mechanism of action concerned with the beneficial properties of ginseng on cognitive function remains to be determined, it has been suggested that it may involve interactions with cholinergic and serotonergic neurons, which have been shown in numerous studies to be involved in memory functions (Balse et al., 1999; Lehmann et al., 2000). For example, ginseng supplementation reversed cholinergically mediated (Mingo et al., 1998) memory loss that was induced by electroconvulsive shock, presumably by enhancing choline acetyltransferase (Darnaudery, Koehl, Piazza, LeMoal, & Mayo, 2000; Herzog, Gandhi, Bhattacharya, & Walsh, 2000; Meck & Williams, 1999; Stancampiano, Cocco, Cugusi, Sarais, & Fadda, 1999). Other studies have shown that individual extracts from ginseng increase brain MAChR density, as well as ACh levels (Zhang, Qu, Liu, & Deng, 1990).

Ding Lang (*Policias fruticosum* L.)

Although ginseng is probably one of the best-known medicinal plants used as a traditional remedy, an abrupt reduction in its natural supply, as well as inherent difficulties in methods of cultivation, stimulated the study of other species of the Araliaceae family that could potentially elicit similar pharmacological responses. Subsequently, a medicinal remedy from an ornamental Vietnamese tree, Ding lang, was identified. In fact, the Ding lang root extract (DLRE) was found to be the most pharmacologically active. Among the actions promoted by DLRE was a beneficial effect on active and passive avoidance tests in aging rodents (Yen, 1990a). It was suggested that one possible mechanism behind this improvement may have been due to stimulation of neurotransmitter release, because in a previous study, DLRE was found to stimulate sexual performance of aged male rats (Yen, 1990b). This behavior is mediated by catecholamines and serotonin in the brain (Gessa & Tagliamonte, 1975).

As discussed earlier, age-related impairments in memory and learning tasks have been attributed to OS. A subsequent study by Yen (Yen, Kalasz, & Matkovics, 1990) showed that DLRE administration elevated the activity of the endogenous antioxidant enzyme superoxide dismutase in the striatum and cerebellum, while those of glutathione peroxidase and catalase were unaltered. Oxidative stress-induced declines in striatal functions have been shown to result in cognitive impairments, hence an increase in antioxidant status following DLRE may explain, in part, the beneficial effects observed in the initial study by Yen (1990a) on learning performance.

SUMMARY AND CONCLUSIONS

We have tried to show in this review that there is an overwhelming amount of data that suggests the involvement of several factors in brain aging that contribute to the well-known losses of neuronal function and behavior that have been reported for many years. These include the following:

1. Increased sensitivity to OS that may be the result of alterations in membrane constituencies, reductions in the synthesis of endogenous antioxidants such as reduced glutamine synthetase, increases in membrane lipid peroxidation (see above), and redox active iron (Gilissen, Jacobs, & Allman, 1999; Savory, Rao, Huang, Letada, & Herman, 1999);
2. Decrements in receptor-G protein uncoupling such that receptor sensitivity is reduced
3. Increases in inflammation (see above) possibly mitigating the effects of anti-inflammatory agents (Hauss-Wegrzyniak, Vraniak, & Weng, 1999)
4. Regional increases in membrane lipids such as CHL or SPH that would alter the biophysical properties of membranes (e.g., fluidity) and could have important implications for their adequate functioning and increase vulnerability to OS and inflammation

It is important to note that these changes are independent of putative A toxicity (which still has not been convincingly demonstrated in vivo) in both animals and humans). However, they parallel many of those that are observed in AD and possibly in other neurodegenerative diseases. In fact, there are no clear-cut findings that suggest Aβ alone is both sufficient and necessary for the induction of these deficits. Rather, it appears that the effects may be secondary to those involving inflammation or that at least one other genetic mutation (e.g., PS1) must be present to maximize the effects. Moreover, any deleterious effects on behavior that are expressed in Aβ-transgenics occur against a background of aging, suggesting once again that it is the aging nervous system that is of paramount importance here (see Joseph et al., 2001). Thus, it might be advantageous to focus upon research to reduce or forestall the age-related decrements, such as increased vulnerability to oxidative stress, that may provide a favorable environment for development of AD.

At the very least, effective methods should be explored to reduce the deleterious effects of aging that result in motor and cognitive deficits. We have tried to suggest in this review that these methods should involve dietary supplementations with fruits and vegetables and perhaps other compounds that are contained in the supplements described. The findings reviewed indicate that in addition to their known beneficial effects on cancer and heart disease, the phytochemicals present in antioxidant-rich foods may be beneficial in reversing the course of neuronal and behavioral aging. Hence, they may actually serve to mitigate the effects of other factors that may serve to predispose an individual to the development of diseases such as AD.

REFERENCES

Aisen, P. S. (1997). Inflammation and Alzheimer's disease: Mechanisms and therapeutic strategies. *Gerontology, 43,* 143–149.

al-Zuhair, H., Abd el-Fattah, A., & el-Sayed, M. I. (1998). The effect of meclofenoxate with *Ginkgo biloba* extract or zinc on lipid peroxide, some free-radical scavengers and the cardiovascular system of aged rats. *Pharmacology Research, 38,* 65–72.

Ariga, T., & Yu, R. K. (1999). Gm1 inhibits amyloid beta-protein-induced cytokine release. *Neurochemical Research, 24,* 219–226.

Armstrong, B. K., Mann, J. I., Adlestein, A. M., & Eskin, F. (1975). Commodity consumption and ischemic heart disease mortality, with special reference to dietary practices. *Journal of Chronic Disorders, 28,* 455–469.

Avdulov, N. A., Chochina, S. V., Igbavboa, U., Warden, C. S., Vassiliev, A.

V., & Wood, W. G. (1997). Lipid binding to amyloid beta-peptide aggregates: Preferential binding of cholesterol as compared with phosphatidylcholine and fatty acids. *Journal of Neurochemistry, 69,* 1746–1752.

Avrova, N. F., Chenykaeva, E. Y., & Obukhova, E. L. (1973). Ganglioside composition and content of rat-brain subcellular fractions. *Journal of Neurochemistry, 20,* 997–1004.

Baba, A. I., & Rotaru, O. (1983). Morphopathological findings in dog's acute toxoplasmosis. *Morphol Embryol (Bucur), 29,* 35–37.

Balse, E., Lazarus, C., Kelche, C., Jeltsch, H., Jackisch, R., & Cassel, J. C. (1999). Intrahippocampal grafts containing cholinergic and serotonergic fetal neurons ameliorate spatial reference but not working memory in rats with fimbria-fornix/cingular bundle lesions. *Brain Research Bulletin, 49,* 263–272.

Bartus, R. T. (1990). Drugs to treat age-related neurodegenerative problems: The final frontier of medical science? *Journal of the American Geriatric Society, 38,* 680–695.

Ben-Shachar, D., Zuk, R., & Glinka, Y. (1995). Dopamine neurotoxicity: Inhibition of mitochondrial respiration. *Journal of Neurochemistry, 64,* 718–723.

Bickford, P. (1993). Motor learning deficits in aged rats are correlated with loss of cerebellar noradrenergic function. *Brain Research, 620,* 133–138.

Bickford, P. C., Gould, T., Brederick, L., Chadman, K., Pollock, A., Young, D., Shukitt-Hale, B., & Joseph, J. (2000). Antioxidant-rich diets improve cerebellar physiology and motor learning in aged rats. *Brain Research, 866,* 211–217.

Bickford, P. C., Shukitt-Hale, B., & Joseph, J. (1999). Effects of aging on cerebellar noradrenergic function and motor learning: Nutritional interventions. *Mechanisms of Aging and Development, 111,* 141–154.

Blanchard, B. J., Hiniker, A. E., Lu, C. C., Margolin, Y., Yu, A. S., & Ingram V. M. (in press). Elimination of beta-amyloid neurotoxicity. *Journal of Alzheimer's Disease.*

Borgeat, P., Hamberg, M., & Samuelsson, B. (1976). Transformation of arachidonic acid and homo-gamma-linolenic acid by rabbit polymorphonuclear leukocytes. Monohydroxy acids from novel lipoxygenases. *Journal of Biological Chemistry, 251,* 7816–7820.

Brailowsky, S., & Montiel, T. (1997). Motor function in young and aged hemiplegic rats: Effects of a *Ginkgo biloba* extract. *Neurobiology of Aging, 18,* 219–227.

Bratton, D. L., Fadok, V. A., Richter, D. A., Kailey, J. M., Guthrie, L. A., & Henson, P. M. (1997). Appearance of phosphatidylserine on apoptotic cells requires calcium-mediated nonspecific flip-flop and is enhanced by loss of the aminophospholipid translocase. *Journal of Biological Chemistry, 272,* 26159–26165.

Cantuti-Castelvetri, I., & Joseph, J. A. (1999). Differential effect of dopamine catabolism and uptake inhibition on dopamine-induced calcium dysregulation and viability loss. *Free Radical Biology and Medicine, 27,* 1393–1404.

Cantuti-Castelvetri, I., Shukitt-Hale, B., & Joseph, J. A. (2000). Neurobehavioral aspects of antioxidants and aging. *International Journal of Developmental Neuroscience, 18,* 367–381.

Cao, G., Sofic, E., & Prior, R. L. (1996). Antioxidant capacity of tea and common vegetables. *Journal of Agriculture and Food Chemistry, 44,* 3426–3431.

Cao, G., Verdon, C. P., Wu, A. H. B., Wang, H., & Prior, R. L. (1995). Automated assay of oxygen radical absorbance capacity with the cobas fara II. *Clinical Chemistry, 41,* 1738–1744.

Carney, J. M., Smith, C. D., Carney, A. N., & Butterfield, D. A. (1994). Aging- and oxygen-induced modifications in brain biochemistry and behavior. *Annals of the New York Academy Sciences,* 44–53.

Chang, H. N., Wang, S. R., Chiang, S. C., Teng, W. J., Chen, M. L., Tsai, J. J., Huang, D. F., Lin, H. Y., & Tsai, Y. Y. (1996). The relationship of aging to endotoxin shock and to production of TNF-a. *Journal of Gerontology, 51,* M220–M222.

Choe, M., Jackson, C., & Yu, B. P. (1995). Lipid peroxidation contributes to age-related membrane rigidity. *Free Radical Biology and Medicine, 18,* 977–984.

Choi, J., & Yu, B. P. (1995). Brain synaptosomal aging: Free radicals and membrane fluidity. *Free Radical Biology and Medicine, 18,* 133–139.

Chopin, P., & Briley, M. (1992) Effects of four non-cholinergic cognitive enhancers in comparison with tacrine and galanthamine on scopolamine-induced amnesia in rats. *Psychopharmacology, 106,* 26–30.

Christen, Y. (2000). Oxidative stress and Alzheimer's disease. *American Journal of Clinical Nutrition, 71,* 621S–629S.

Cleary, J., Hittner, J. M., Semotuk, M., Mantyh, P., & O'Hare, E. (1995). Beta-amyloid(1-40) effects on behavior and memory. *Brain Research, 682,* 69–74.

Clostre, F. (1999). *Ginkgo biloba* extract (EGb 761). State of knowledge in the dawn of the year 2000. *Annales Pharmaceutiques Francaises, 57,* 1S8–88.

Cohen, S. A., & Muller, W. E. (1993). Effects of piracetam on n-methyl-d-aspartate receptor properties in the aged mouse brain. *Pharmacology, 47,* 217–222.

Cohen-Salmon, C., Venault, P., Martin, B., Raffalli-Sebille, M. J., Barkats, M., Clostre, F., Pardon, M. C., Christen, Y., & Chapouthier, G. (1997). Effects of *Ginkgo biloba* extract (EGb 761) on learning and possible actions on aging. *Journal of Physiology, 91,* 291–300.

Cutler, R., Joseph, J. A., Yamagami, K., Villalobos-Molina, R., & Roth, G. S. (1994). Area specific alterations in muscarinic stimulated low km GTPase activity in aging and Alzheimer's disease: Implications for altered signal transduction. *Brain Research, 664,* 54–60.

Darnaudery, M., Koehl, M., Piazza, P. V., Le Moal, M., & Mayo, W. (2000). Pregnenolone sulfate increases hippocampal acetylcholine release and spatial recognition. *Brain Research, 852,* 173–179.

Dean, R. L. D., Scozzafava, J., Goas, J. A., Regan, B., Beer, B., & Bartus, R. T. (1981). Age-related differences in behavior across the life span of the c57bl/6j mouse. *Experimental Aging Research, 7,* 427–451.

Deberdt, W. (1994). Interaction between psychological and pharmacological treatment in cognitive impairment. *Life Sciences, 55,* 2057–2066.

Delion, S., Chalon, S., Guilloteau, D., Besnard, J. C., & Durand, G. (1996). Alpha-linolenic acid dietary deficiency alters age-related changes of dopaminergic and serotoninergic neurotransmission in the rat frontal cortex. *Journal of Neurochemistry, 66,* 1582–1591.

Denisova, N., Cantuti-Castelvetri, I., Hassan, W., Paulson, K. E., & Joseph, J. A. (in press). Membrane sphingomyelin-cholesterol domains and their role in regulation of vulnerability to oxidative stress in PC12 cells. Implication for aging. *Free Radical Biology and Medicine.*

Denisova, N. A., Erat, S. A., Kelly, J. F., & Roth, G. S. (1998). Differential effect of aging on cholesterol modulation of carbachol-stimulated low-k(m) GTpase in striatal synaptosomes. *Experimental Gerontology, 33,* 249–265.

Denisova, N. A., Fisher, D., Provost, M., & Joseph, J. A. (1999). The role of glutathione, membrane sphingomyelin, and its metabolites in oxidative stress-induced calcium "dysregulation" in PC12 cells. *Free Radical Biology and Medicine, 27,* 1292–1301.

Denisova, N. A., Strain, J. G., & Joseph, J. A. (1997). Oxidant injury in PC12 cells—A possible model of calcium "dysregulation" in aging: I: Interactions with membrane lipids. *Journal of Neurochemistry, 69,* 1259–1266.

Devan, B. D., Goad, E. H. & Petri, H. L. (1996). Dissociation of hippocampal and striatal contributions to spatial navigation in the water maze. *Neurobiology of Learning and Memory, 66,* 305–323.

Diamond, B. J., Shiflett, S. C., Feiwel, N., Matheis, R. J., Noskin, O., Richards, J. A., & Schoenberger, N. E. (2000). *Ginkgo biloba* extract: Mechanisms and clinical indications. *Archives of Physical and Medical Rehabilitation, 81,* 668–678.

Diaz, C., & Schroit, A. J. (1996). Role of translocases in the generation of phosphatidylserine asymmetry. *Journal of Membrane Biology, 151,* 1–9.

Doll, R. (1990). An overview of the epidemiological evidence linking diet and cancer. *Proceedings Nutrition Society, 49,* 119–131.

Dornan, W. A., Kang, D. E., McCampbell, A., & Kang, E. E. (1993). Bilateral injections of beta a(25-35) + ibo into the hippocampus disrupts acquisition of spatial learning in the rat. *Neuroreport, 5,* 165–168.

Egashira, T., Takayama, F., & Yamanaka, Y. (1996). Effects of bifemelane on muscarinic receptors and choline acetyltransferase in the brains of aged rats following chronic cerebral hypoperfusion induced by permanent occlusion of bilateral carotid arteries. *Japanese Journal of Pharmacology, 72,* 57–65.

Elhusseiny, A., Cohen, Z., Olivier, A., Stanimirovic, D. B., & Hamel, E. (1999). Functional acetylcholine muscarinic receptor subtypes in human brain microcirculation: Identification and cellular localization. *Journal of Cerebral Blood Flow Metabolism, 19,* 794–802.

Floyd, R. A. (1999). Antioxidants, oxidative stress, and degenerative neurological disorders. *Proceedings of the Society of Experimental Biology Medicine, 222,* 236–245.

Fontana, A., Kristensen, F., Dubs, R., Gemsa, D., & Weber, E. (1982). Production of prostaglandin E and an interleukin–1 like factor by cultured astrocytes and C6 glioma cells. *Journal of Immunology, 129,* 2413–2419.

Fowler, C. J., Cowburn, R. F., & Joseph, J. A. (1997). Alzheimer's, aging and amyloid: An absurd allegory? *Gerontology, 43,* 132–142.

Gajewski, A., & Hensch, S. A. (1999). *Ginkgo biloba* and memory for a maze. *Psychological Reports, 84,* 481–484.

Garcia-Ruiz, C., Colell, A., Mari, M., Morales, A., & Fernandez-Checa, J. C. (1997). Direct effect of ceramide on the mitochondrial electron transport chain leads to generation of reactive oxygen species. Role of mitochondrial glutathione. *Journal of Biological Chemistry, 272,* 11369–11377.

Gessa, G. L., & Tagliamonte, A. (1975). The role of brain serotonin and dopamine in male sexual behavior. In M. Sandler and G. L. Gessa (Eds.), *Sexual behavior: Pharmacology and biochemistry* (pp. 117–128). New York: Raven Press.

Gilissen, E. P., Jacobs, R. E., & Allman, J. M. (1999). Magnetic resonance microscopy of iron in the basal forebrain cholinergic structures of the aged mouse lemur. *Journal of Neurological Sciences, 168,* 21–27.

Goodwin, J. S., Goodwin, J. M., & Garry, P. J. (1983). Association between nutritional status and cognitive functioning in a healthy elderly population. *Journal of the American Medical Association, 249,* 2917–2921.

Gould, T. J., & Bickford, P. C. (1997). Age-related deficits in the cerebellar beta adrenergic signal transduction cascade in Fischer 344 rats. *Journal of Pharmacology Experimental Therapeutics, 281,* 965–971.

Gudz, T. I., Tserng, K. Y., & Hoppel, C. L. (1997). Direct inhibition of mitochondrial respiratory chain complex III by cell-permeable ceramide. *Journal of Biological Chemistry, 272,* 24154–24158.

Halder, J., & Bhaduri, A. N. (1998). Protective role of black tea against oxidative damage of human red blood cells. *Biochemical and Biophysical Research Communications, 244,* 903–907.

Hastings, T. G., & Zigmond, M. J. (1994). Identification of catechol-protein conjugates in neostriatal slices incubated with [3H] dopamine: Impact of ascorbic acid and glutathione. *Journal of Neurochemistry, 63,* 1126–1132.

Hauss-Wegrzyniak, B., Vannucchi, M. G., & Wenk, G. L. (2000). Behavioral and utrastructural changes in by chronic neuroinflammation in young rats. *Brain Research, 859,* 157–166.

Hauss-Wegrzyniak, B., Vraniak, P., & Wenk, G. L. (1999). The effects of a novel NSAID on chronic neuroinflammation are age dependent. *Neurobiology of Aging, 20,* 305–313.

Hersch, S. M., Gutekunst, C. A., Rees, H. D., Heilman, C. J., & Levey, A. I. (1994). Distribution of M1-M4 muscarinic receptor proteins in the rat striatum: Light and electron microscopic immunocytochemistry using subtype-specific antibodies. *Journal of Neuroscience, 14,* 3351–3363.

Herzog, C. D., Gandhi, C., Bhattacharya, P., & Walsh, T. J. (2000). Effects of intraseptal zolpidem and chlordiazepoxide on spatial working memory and high-affinity choline uptake in the hippocampus. *Neurobiology of Learning and Memory, 73,* 168–179

Hofbauer, R., Frass, M., Gmeiner, B., Handler, S., Speiser, W., & Kapiotis, S. (1999). The green tea extract epigallocatechin gallate is able to reduce neutrophil transmigration through monolayers of endothelial cells. *Wiener Klinische Wochenschrift, 111,* 278–282.

Horie, T., Awazu, S., Itakura, Y., & Fuwa, T. (1992). Identified diallyl polysulfides from an aged garlic extract which protects the membranes from lipid peroxidation [Letter to the editor]. *Planta Medica, 58,* 468–469.

Horie, T., Murayama, T., Mishima, T., Itoh, F., Minamide, Y., Fuwa, T., & Awazu, S. (1989). Protection of liver microsomal membranes from lipid peroxidation by garlic extract. *Planta Medica, 55,* 506–508.

Hoyer, S., Lannert, H., Noldner, M., & Chatterjee, S. S. (1999). Damaged neuronal energy metabolism and behavior are improved by *Ginkgo biloba* extract (EGb761). *Journal of Neural Transmission (Budapest), 106,* 1171–1188.

Hughes, K. (1995). Diet and coronary heart disease—a review. *Annals, Academy of Medicine, Singapore, 24,* 224–229.

Igbavboa, U., Avdulov, N. A., Chochina, S. V., & Wood, W. G. (1997). Transbilayer distribution of cholesterol is modified in brain synaptic plasma membranes of knockout mice deficient in the low-density lipoprotein receptor, apolipoprotein E or both proteins. *Journal of Neurochemistry, 69,* 1661–1667.

Igbavboa, U., Avdulov, N. A., Schroeder, F., & Wood, W. G. (1996).

Increasing age alters transbilayer fluidity and cholesterol asymmetry in synaptic plasma membranes of mice. *Journal Neurochemistry, 66,* 1717–1725.

Ingram, D. K. (1990). Complex maze learning in rodents. In A. L. Goldstein (Ed.), *Biomedical advances in aging* (pp. 451–467). New York: Plenum.

Ingram, D. K., Jucker, M., & Spangler, E. 1994. Behavioral manifestations of aging. In U. Mohr, D. L. Cungworth, & C. C. Capen (Eds.), *Pathobiology of the aging rat* (pp. 149–170). Washington, DC: ILSI.

Ivaniv, O. P. (1998). [the results of using different forms of a *Ginkgo biloba* extract (EGb 761) in the combined treatment of patients with circulatory encephalopathy]. *Likarska Sprava,* 123–128.

Jaenicke, B., Kim, E. J., Ahn, J. W., & Lee, H. S. (1991). Effect of *Panax ginseng* extract on passive avoidance retention in old rats. *Archives of Pharmacology Research, 14,* 25–29.

Jakubic, J., & Wess, J. (1999). Use of a sandwich enzyme-linked immunosorbent assay strategy to study mechanisms of G protein-coupled receptor assembly. *Journal of Biological Chemistry, 274,* 1349–1358.

Jama, J. W., Launer, L. J., Witteman, J. C., den Breeijen, J. H., Breteler, M. M., Grobbee, D. E., & Hofman, A. (1996). Dietary antioxidants and cognitive function in a population-based sample of older persons. The Rotterdam Study. *American Journal of Epidemiology, 144,* 275–280.

Jope, R. S., Song, L., & Powers, R. E. (1997). Cholinergic activation of phosphoinositide signaling is impaired in Alzheimer's disease brain. *Neurobiology of Aging, 18,* 111–120.

Joseph, J. A., Bartus, R. T., Clody, D., Morgan, D., Finch, C., Beer, B., & Sesack, S. (1983). Psychomotor performance in the senescent rodent: Reduction of deficits via striatal dopamine receptor up-regulation. *Neurobiology of Aging, 4,* 313–319.

Joseph, J. A., Berger, R. E., Engel, B. T., & Roth, G. S. (1978). Age-related changes in the nigrostriatum: A behavioral and biochemical analysis. *Journal of Gerontology, 33,* 643–649.

Joseph, J. A., Erat, S., Denisova, N., & Villalobos-Molina, R. (1998). Receptor- and age-selective effects of dopamine oxidation on receptor-G protein interactions in the striatum. *Free Radical Biology and Medicine, 24,* 827–834.

Joseph, J. A., Hunt, W. A., Rabin, B. M., & Dalton, T. K. (1992). Possible "accelerated striatal aging" induced by ^{56}Fe-heavy-particle irradiation: Implications for manned space flights. *Radiation Research, 130,* 88–93.

Joseph, J. A., Kowatch, M. A., Maki, T., & Roth, G. S. (1990). Selective cross-activation/inhibition of second messenger systems and the reduction of age-related deficits in the muscarinic control of dopamine release from perfused rat striata. *Brain Research, 537*, 40–48.

Joseph, J. A., & Roth, G. S. (1993). Hormonal regulation of motor behavior in senescence. *Journal of Gerontology, 48*, 51–55.

Joseph, J. A., Shukitt-Hale, B., Denisova, N. A., Bielinski, D., Martin, A., McEwen, J. J., & Bickford, P. C. (1999). Reversals of age-related declines in neuronal signal transduction, cognitive, and motor behavioral deficits with blueberry, spinach, or strawberry dietary supplementation. *Journal of Neuroscience, 19*, 8114–8121.

Joseph, J.A., Shukitt Hale, B., Denisova, N.A, Martin, A., Perry, G., & Smith, M.A. (2001) Copernicus revisted: Amyloid beta in Alzheimer disease. *Neurobiology of Aging, 22*, 131–146.

Joseph, J. A., Shukitt-Hale, B., Denisova, N. A., Prior, R. L., Cao, G., Martin, A., Taglialatela, G., & Bickford, P. C. (1998). Long-term dietary strawberry, spinach, or vitamin E supplementation retards the onset of age-related neuronal signal-transduction and cognitive behavioral deficits. *Journal of Neuroscience, 18*, 8047–8055.

Joseph, J. A., Shukitt-Hale, B., McEwen, J., & Rabin, B. (1999). Magnesium activation of GTP hydrolysis or incubation in S-adenosyl-l-methionine reverses iron-56-particle-induced decrements in oxotremorine enhancement of K+-evoked striatal release of dopamine. *Radiation Research, 152*, 637–641.

Joseph, J. A., Strain, J. G., Jimenez, N. D., & Fisher, D. (1997). Oxidant injury in PC12 cells—a possible model of calcium deregulation in aging. I. Selectivity of protection against oxidative stress. *Journal Neurochemistry, 69*, 1252–1258.

Joseph, J. A., Villalobos-Molina, R., Denisova, N., Erat, S., Jimenez, N., & Strain, J. (1996). Increased sensitivity to oxidative stress and the loss of muscarinic receptor reponsiveness in senescence. *Annals of the New York Academy of Sciences, 786*, 112–119.

Kanowski, S., Herrmann, W. M., Stephan, K., Wierich, W., & Horr, R. (1996). Proof of efficacy of the *Ginkgo biloba* special extract EGb 761 in outpatients suffering from mild to moderate primary degenerative dementia of the Alzheimer type or multi-infarct dementia. *Pharmacopsychiatry, 29*, 47–56.

Kausler, D. (1982). *Experimental psychology and human aging.* New York: Wiley.

Kawaguchi, S., Kishikawa, M., Sakae, M., & Nakane, Y. (1995). Age-related changes in basal dendrite and dendritic spine of hippocampal pyramidal neurons (CA1) among samp1ta/ngs—quantitative analysis by the rapid Golgi method. *Mechanisms of Aging and Development, 83*, 11–20.

Kelly, J. F., Joseph, J. A., Denisova, N. A., Erat, S., Mason, R. P., & Roth,

G. S. (1995). Dissociation of striatal GTPase and dopamine release responses to muscarinic cholinergic agonists in F344 rats: Influence of age and dietary manipulation. *Journal of Neurochemistry, 64,* 2755–2764.

Kessler, A. R., & Yehuda, S. (1985). Learning-induced changes in brain membrane cholesterol and fluidity: Implications for brain aging. *International Journal of Neuroscience, 28,* 73–82.

Kleijnen, J. & Knipschild, P. (1992). *Ginkgo biloba* for cerebral insufficiency. *British Journal Clinical Pharmacology, 34,* 352–358.

Klein, J., Chatterjee, S. S., & Loffelholz, K. (1997). Phospholipid breakdown and choline release under hypoxic conditions: Inhibition by bilobalide, a constituent of *Ginkgo biloba. Brain Research, 755,* 347–350.

Kluger, A., Gianutsos, J. G., Golomb, J., Ferris, S. H., George, A. E., Frannssen, E., & Reisberg, B. (1997). Patterns of motor impairment in normal aging, mild cognitive decline, and early Alzheimer's disease. *Journal of Gerontology, 52,* 28–39.

Klunk, W. E., Xu, C. J., McClure, R. J., Panchalingam, K., Stanley, J. A., & Pettegrew, J. W. (1997). Aggregation of beta-amyloid peptide is promoted by membrane phospholipid metabolites elevated in Alzheimer's disease brain. *Journal of Neurochemistry, 69,* 266–272.

Kornhuber, J., Schoppmeyer, K., Bendig, C., & Riederer, P. (1996). Characterization of [3H] pentazocine binding sites in post-mortem human frontal cortex. *Journal of Neural Transmissions, 103,* 45–53.

Krischer, S. M., Eisenmann, M., Bock, A., & Mueller, M. J. (1997). Protein-facilitated export of arachidonic acid from pig neutrophils. *Journal of Biological Chemistry, 272,* 10601–10607.

La Rue, A., Koehler, K. M., Wayne, S. J., Chiulli, S. J., Haaland, K. Y., & Garry, P. J. (1997). Nutritional status and cognitive functioning in a normally aging sample: A 6-year reassessment. *American Journal of Clinical Nutrition, 65,* 20–29.

Landfield, P. W., & Eldridge, J. C. (1994). The glucocorticoid hypothesis of age-related hippocampal neurodegeneration: Role of dysregulated intraneuronal CA^{2+}. *Annals of the New York Academy of Sciences, 746,* 308–321.

Lasarova, M. B., Mosharrof, A. H., Petkov, V. D., Markovska, V. L., & Petkov, V. V. (1987). Effect of piracetam and of standardized ginseng extract on the electroconvulsive shock-induced memory disturbances in "step-down" passive avoidance. *Acta Physiologica et Pharmacologica Bulgarica, 13,* 11–17.

Lau, B. H., Yamasaki, T., & Gridley, D. S. (1991). Garlic compounds modulate macrophage and T-lymphocyte functions. *Molecular Biotherapy, 3,* 103–107.

Lehmann, O., Jeltsch, H., Lehnardt, O., Pain, L., Lazarus, C., & Cassel, J. C. (2000). Combined lesions of cholinergic and serotonergic neurons in the rat brain using 192 IgG-saporin and 5,7-dihydroxytryptamine; neurochemical and behavioural characterization. *European Journal of Neuroscience, 12*, 67–79.

Leibel, W. S., Firestone, L. L., Legler, D. C., Braswell, L. M., & Miller, K. W. (1987). Two pools of cholesterol in acetylcholine receptor-rich membranes from torpedo. *Biochimica et Biophysica Acta, 897*, 249–260.

Levey, A. I. (1996). Muscarinic acetylcholine receptor expression in memory circuits: Implications for treatment of Alzheimer's disease. *Proceedings for the National Academy of Sciences, USA, 93*, 13541–13546.

Levine, M. S., & Cepeda, C. (1998). Dopamine modulation of responses mediated by excitatory amino acids in the neostriatum. *Advances in Pharmacology, 42*, 724–729.

Lin, Y. L., & Lin, J. K. (1997). (-)-Epigallocatechin-3-gallate blocks the induction of nitric oxide synthase by down-regulating lipopolysaccharide-induced activity of transcription factor nuclear factor-kappa B. *Molecular Pharmacology, 52*, 465–472.

Lin, Y. L., Tsai, S. H., Lin-Shiau, S. Y., Ho, C. T., & Lin, J. K. (1999). Theaflavin-3,3'-digallate from black tea blocks the nitric oxide synthase by down-regulating the activation of NF-kappaB in macrophages. *European Journal of Pharmacology, 367*, 379–388.

Lopez, G. H., Ilincheta de Boschero, M. G., Castagnet, P. I., & Giusto, N. M. (1995). Age-associated changes in the content and fatty acid composition of brain glycerophospholipids. *Comparative Biochemistry and Physiology, 112*, 331–343.

Lynch, D. R., & Dawson, T. M. (1994). Secondary mechanisms in neuronal trauma [see comments]. *Current Opinions in Neurology, 7*, 510–516.

Marino, M. J., Rouse, S. T., Levey, A. I., Potter, L. T., & Conn, P. J. (1998). Activation of the genetically defined m1 muscarinic receptor potentiates n-methyl-d-aspartate (NMDA) receptor currents in hippocampal pyramidal cells. *Proceedings for the National Academy of Sciences, USA, 95*, 11465–11470.

Mason, R. P., Jacob, R. F., Walter, M. F., Mason, P. E., Avdulov, N. A., Chochina, S. V., Igbavboa, U., & Wood, W. G. (1999). Distribution and fluidizing action of soluble and aggregated amyloid beta-peptide in rat synaptic plasma membranes. *Journal of Biological Chemistry, 274*, 18801–18807.

Matsuoka, Y., Hasegawa, H., Okuda, S., Muraki, T., Uruno, T., & Kubota, K. (1995). Ameliorative effects of tea catechins on active oxygen-related nerve cell injuries. *Journal of Pharmacology and Experimental Therapeutics, 274*, 602–608.

Mattson, M. P., Goodman, Y., Luo, H., Fu, W., & Furukawa, K. (1997). Activation of nf-kappaB protects hippocampal neurons against oxidative stress-induced apoptosis: Evidence for induction of manganese superoxide dismutase and suppression of peroxynitrite production and protein tyrosine nitration. *Journal of Neuroscience Research, 49*, 681–697.

Mayne, S. T. (1996). Beta-carotene, carotenoids, and disease prevention in humans. *FASEB Journal, 10*, 690–701.

McDonald, R. J., & White, N. M. (1994). Parallel information processing in the water maze: Evidence for independent memory systems involving dorsal striatum and hippocampus. *Behavioral and Neural Biology, 61*, 260–270.

McGeer, P. L., & McGeer, E. G. (1995). The inflammatory response system of brain: Implications for therapy of Alzheimer's and other neurodegenerative diseases. *Brain Research Reviews, 21*, 195–218.

McLaurin, J., Franklin, T., Fraser, P. E., & Chakrabartty, A. (1998). Structural transitions associated with the interaction of Alzheimer's beta-amyloid peptides with gangliosides. *Journal of Biological Chemistry, 273*, 4506–4515.

Meck, W. H., & Williams, C. L. (1999). Choline supplementation during prenatal development reduces proactive interference in spatial memory. *Brain Research, 118*, 51–59.

Merrill, J. E., & Murphy, S. P. (1997). Inflammatory events at the blood brain barrier: Regulation of adhesion molecules, cytokines, and chemokines by reactive nitrogen and oxygen species. *Brain Behavior and Immmunity, 11*, 245–263.

Migheli, A., Cavalla, P., Piva, R., Giordana, M. T., & Schiffer, D. (1994). Bcl-2 protein expression in aged brain and neurodegenerative diseases. *Neuroreport, 5*, 1906–1908.

Mingo, N. S., Cottrell, G. A., Mendonca, A., Gombos, Z., Eubanks, J. H., & Burnham, W. M. (1998). Amygdala-kindled and electroconvulsive seizures alter hippocampal expression of the m1 and m3 muscarinic cholinergic receptor genes. *Brain Research, 810*, 9–15.

Mishra, O. P., & Delivoria-Papadopoulos, M. (1999). Cellular mechanisms of hypoxic injury in the developing brain. *Brain Research Bulletin, 48*, 233–238.

Moriguchi, T., Saito, H., & Nishiyama, N. (1997). Anti-aging effect of aged garlic extract in the inbred brain atrophy mouse model. *Clinical and Experimental Pharmacology and Physiology, 24*, 235–242.

Moriguchi, T., Takashina, K., Chu, P. J., Saito, H., & Nishiyama, N. (1994). Prolongation of life span and improved learning in the senescence accelerated mouse produced by aged garlic extract. *Biological and Pharmaceutical Bulletin, 17*, 1589–1594.

Morioka, N., Sze, L. L., Morton, D. L., & Irie, R. F. (1993). A protein fraction from aged garlic extract enhances cytotoxicity and proliferation of human lymphocytes mediated by interleukin-2 and concanavalin A. *Cancer Immunology, Immunotherapy, 37*, 316–322.

Muir, J. L. (1997). Acetylcholine, aging, and Alzheimer's disease. *Pharmacology, Biochemistry and Behavior, 56*, 687–696.

Murray, C. A., Clements, M. P., & Lynch, M. A. (1999). Interleukin-1 induces lipid peroxidation and membrane changes in rat hippocampus: An age-related study. *Gerontology, 45*, 136–142.

Nagahara, A. H., Gill, T. M., Nicolle, M., & Gallagher, M. (1996). Alterations in opiate receptor binding in the hippocampus of aged Long-Evans rats. *Brain Research, 707*, 22–30.

Neve, R. L., & Robakis, N. K. (1998). Alzheimer's disease: A re-examination of the amyloid hypothesis. *Trends in Neuroscience, 21*, 15–19.

Nishida, Y. & Nishino, S. (1999). Contribution of a metal-peroxide adduct to neurodegeneration is due to its oxidative protease activity. *Zeitschrift fur Naturforschung [C], 54*, 1107–1114.

Nishiyama, N., Moriguchi, T., & Saito, H. (1997). Beneficial effects of aged garlic extract on learning and memory impairment in the senescence-accelerated mouse. *Experimental Gerontology, 32*, 149–160.

Nishiyama, N., Zhou, Y., & Saito, H. (1994a). Ameliorative effects of chronic treatment using DX-9386, a traditional Chinese prescription, on learning performance and lipid peroxide content in senescence accelerated mouse. *Biological and Pharmaceutical Bulletin, 17*, 1481–1484.

Nishiyama, N., Zhou, Y., & Saito, H. (1994b). Beneficial effects of DX-9386, a traditional Chinese prescription, on memory disorder produced by lesioning the amygdala in mice. *Biological and Pharmaceutical Bulletin, 17*, 1679–1681.

Nishiyama, N., Zhou, Y., Takashina, K., & Saito, H. (1994). Effects of DX-9386, a traditional Chinese preparation, on passive and active avoidance performances in mice. *Biological and Pharmaceutical Bulletin, 17*, 1472–1476.

O'Hare, E., Weldon, D. T., Mantyh, P. W., Ghilardi, J. R., Finke, M. P., Kuskowski, M. A., Maggio, J. E., Shephard, R. A., & Cleary, J. (1999). Delayed behavioral effects following intrahippocampal injection of aggregated A-beta (1-42). *Brain Research, 815*, 1–10.

Olanow, C. W. (1992). An introduction to the free radical hypothesis in Parkinson's disease. *Annals of Neurology, 32*, S2–9.

Oliveira, M.G.M., Bueno, O.F.A., Pomarico, A.C., & Gugliano, E. B. (1997). Strategies used by hippocampal- and caudate-putamen-lesioned rats in a learning task. *Neurobiology of Learning and Memory, 68*, 32–41.

Oyama, Y., Chikahisa, L., Ueha, T., Kanemaru, K., & Noda, K. (1996). *Ginkgo biloba* extract protects brain neurons against oxidative stress induced by hydrogen peroxide. *Brain Research, 712*, 349–352.

Oyama, Y., Fuchs, P. A., Katayama, N., & Noda, K. (1994). Myricetin and quercetin, the flavonoid constituents of *Ginkgo biloba* extract, greatly reduce oxidative metabolism in both resting and CA(2+)-loaded brain neurons. *Brain Research, 635,* 125–129.

Oyama, Y., Hayashi, A., & Ueha, T. (1993). Ca(2+)-induced increase in oxidative metabolism of dissociated mammalian brain neurons: Effect of extract of *Ginkgo biloba* leaves. *Japanese Journal of Pharmacology, 61,* 367–370.

Packard, M. G., Kohlmaier, J. R., & Alexander, G. M. (1996). Posttraining intrahippocampal estradiol injections enhance spatial memory in male rats; interaction with cholinergic systems. *Behavioral Neuroscience, 110,* 626–632.

Packard, M. G., & Teather, L. A. (1997). Posttraining estradiol injections enhance memory in ovariectomized rats; cholinergic blockade and synergism. *Neurobiology, Learning and Memory, 68,* 172–188.

Pardon, M. C., Joubert, C., Perez-Diaz, F., Christen, Y., Launay, J. M., & Cohen-Salmon, C. (2000). In vivo regulation of cerebral monoamine oxidase activity in senescent controls and chronically stressed mice by long-term treatment with *Ginkgo biloba* extract (egb 761). *Mechanisms of Aging and Development, 113,* 157–168.

Perkins, A. J., Hendrie, H. C., Callahan, C. M., Gao, S., Unverzagt, F. W., Xu, Y., Hall, K. S., & Hui, S. L. (1999). Association of antioxidants with memory in a multiethnic elderly sample using the third national health and nutrition examination survey. *American Journal of Epidemiology, 150,* 37–44.

Perrig, W. J., Perrig, P., & Stahelin, H. B. (1997). The relation between antioxidants and memory performance in the old and very old. *Journal of the American Geriatric Society, 45,* 718–724.

Petkov, V. (1978). Effect of ginseng on the brain biogenic monoamines and 3',5'-AMP system. Experiments on rats. *Arzneimittel-Forschung, 28,* 388–393.

Petkov, V. D., Cao, Y., Todorov, I., Lazarova, M., Getova, D., Stancheva, S., & Alova, L. (1992). Behavioral effects of stem-leaves extract from *panax ginseng* C.A. Meyer. *Acta Physiologica et Pharmacologica Bulgarica, 18,* 41–48.

Petkov, V. D., Kehayov, R., Belcheva, S., Konstantinova, E., Petkov, V. V., Getova, D., & Markovska, V. (1993). Memory effects of standardized extracts of panax ginseng (g115), *Ginkgo biloba* (GK 501) and their combination gincosan (phl-00701). *Planta Medica, 59,* 106–114.

Petkov, V. D., & Mosharrof, A. H. (1987). Effects of standardized ginseng extract on learning, memory and physical capabilities. *American Journal of Chinese Medicine, 15,* 19–29.

Pinto, J. T., Qiao, C., Xing, J., Rivlin, R. S., Protomastro, M. L., Weissler, M. L., Tao, Y., Thaler, H., & Heston, W. D. (1997). Effects of garlic thioallyl derivatives on growth, glutathione concentration, and polyamine formation of human prostate carcinoma cells in culture [see comments]. *American Journal Clinical Nutrition, 66,* 398–405.

Planas, A. M., Soriano, M. A., Justicia, C., & Rodriguez-Farre, E. (1999). Induction of cyclooxygenase-2 in the rat brain after a mild episode of focal ischemia without tissue inflammation or neural cell damage. *Neuroscience Letters, 275,* 141–144.

Poirier, J. (1999). Apolipoprotein E: A pharmacogenetic target for the treatment of Alzheimer's disease. *Molecualr Diagnostics, 4,* 335–341.

Poon, L. W. (1985). Differences in human memory with aging: Nature, causes and clinical implications. In J. E. Birren & K. W. Schaie (Eds.), *Handbook of the psychology of aging* (pp. 427–462). New York: Van Nostrand Reinhold.

Porsolt, R. D., Martin, P., Lenegre, A., Fromage, S., & Drieu, K. (1990). Effects of an extract of *Ginkgo biloba* (egb 761) on "learned helplessness" and other models of stress in rodents. *Pharmacology, Biochemistry and Behavior, 36,* 963–971.

Prior, R. L., Cao, G., Martin, A., Sofic, E., McEwen, J., O'Brien, C., Lischner, N., Ehlenfeldt, M., Kalt, W., Krewer, G., & Mainland, M. (1998). Antioxidant capacity as influenced by total phenolic and anthocyanin content, maturity and variety of vaccinium species. *Journal of Agriculture and Food Chemistry, 46,* 2586–2593.

Pu, L., Igbavboa, U., Wood, W. G., Roths, J. B., Kier, A. B., Spener, F., & Schroeder, F. (1999). Expression of fatty acid binding proteins is altered in aged mouse brain. *Molecular and Cellular Biochemistry, 198,* 69–78.

Puumala, T., Greijus, S., Narinen, K., Haapalinna, A., Riekkinen, P., Sr., & Sirvio, J. (1998) Stimulation of alpha-1 adrenergic receptors facilitates spatial learning in rats. *European Journal of Neuropsychopharmacology, 8,* 17–26.

Rabin, O., Drieu, K., Grange, E., Chang, M. C., Rapoport, S. I., & Purdon, A. D. (1998). Effects of EGb 761 on fatty acid reincorporation during reperfusion following ischemia in the brain of the awake gerbil. *Molecular and Chemical Neuropathology, 34,* 79–101.

Rai, G. S., Shovlin, C., & Wesnes, K. A. (1991). A double-blind, placebo controlled study of *Ginkgo biloba* extract ('tanakan') in elderly outpatients with mild to moderate memory impairment. *Current Medical Research and Opinion, 12,* 350–355.

Ramassamy, C., Christen, Y., Clostre, F., & Costentin, J. (1992). The *Ginkgo biloba* extract, EGb761, increases synaptosomal uptake of 5-hydroxytryptamine; in vitro and ex vivo studies. *Journal of Pharmacy and Pharmacology, 44,* 943–945.

Rapin, J. R., Lamproglou, I., Drieu, K., & DeFeudis, F. V. (1994). Demonstration of the "anti-stress" activity of an extract of *Ginkgo biloba* (EGB761) using a discrimination learning task. *General Pharmacology, 25,* 1009–1016.

Reiter, C. D., Teng, R. J., & Beckman, J. S. (2000). Superoxide reacts with nitric oxide to nitrate tyrosine at physiological pH via peroxynitrite. *Journal of Biological Chemistry, 275,* 32460–32466.

Rodriguez de Turco, E. B., Droy-Lefaix, M. T., & Bazan, N. G. (1993). Decreased electroconvulsive shock-induced diacylglycerols and free fatty acid accumulation in the rat brain by *Ginkgo biloba* extract (EGb 761); selective effect in hippocampus as compared with cerebral cortex. *Journal of Neurochemistry, 61,* 1438–1444.

Rosenman, S., Shrikant, P., Dubb, L., Benveniste, E., & Ransohoff, R. (1995). Cytokine-induced expression of vascular cell adhesion molecule-1 (VCAM-1) by astrocytes and astrocytoma cell lines. *Journal of Immunology, 154,* 1888–1899.

Rossner, S., Ueberham, U., Schliebs, R., Perez-Polo, J. R., & Bigl, V. (1998). The regulation of amyloid precursor protein metabolism by cholinergic mechanisms and neurotrophin receptor signaling. *Progress in Neurobiology, 56,* 541–569.

Roth, G. S., Joseph, J. A., & Mason, R. P. (1996). Membrane alterations as causes of impaired signal transduction in Alzheimer's disease and aging. *Trends in Neuroscience, 18,* 203–205.

Rozovsky, I., Finch, C. E., & Morgan, T. E. (1998). Age-related activation of microglia and astrocytes: In vitro studies show persistent phenotypes of aging, increased proliferation, and resistance to downregulation. *Neurobiology of Aging, 19,* 97–103.

Sano, M., Ernesto, C., Thomas, R. G., Klauber, M. R., Schafer, K., Grundman, M., Woodbury, P., Growdon, J., Cotman, C. W., Pfeiffer, E., Schneider, L. S., & Thal, L. J. (1997). A controlled trial of selegiline, alpha-tocopherol, or both as treatment for Alzheimer's disease. The Alzheimer's disease cooperative study [see comments]. *New England Journal of Medicine, 336,* 1216–1222.

Savory, J., Rao, J. K., Huang, Y., Letada, P. R., & Herman, M. M. (1999). Age-related hippocampal changes in Bcl-2:Bax ratio, oxidative stress, redox-active iron and apoptosis associated with aluminum-induced neurodegeneration: Increased susceptibility with aging. *Neurotoxicology, 20,* 805–817.

Sayre, L. M., Zagorski, M. G., Surewicz, W. K., Krafft, G. A., & Perry, G. (1997). Mechanisms of neurotoxicity associated with amyloid beta deposition and the role of free radicals in the pathogenesis of Alzheimer's disease: A critical appraisal. *Chemical Research in Toxicology, 10,* 518–526.

Schafer, M. K., Schwaeble, W. J., Post, C., Salvati, P., Calabresi, M., Sim, R. B., Petry, F., Loos, M., & Weihe, E. (2000). Complement c1q is dramatically up-regulated in brain microglia in response to transient global cerebral ischemia. *Journal of Immunology, 164,* 5446–5542.

Scheuer, K., Rostock, A., Bartsch, R., & Muller, W. E. (1999). Piracetam improves cognitive performance by restoring neurochemical deficits of the aged rat brain. *Pharmacopsychiatry, 32,* 10–16.

Schipper, H. (1996). Astrocytes, brain aging, and neurodegeneration. *Neurobiology of Aging, 17,* 467–480.

Schmidt, R., Hayn, M., Reinhart, B., Roob, G., Schmidt, H., Schumacher, M., Watzinger, N., & Launer, L. J. (1998). Plasma antioxidants and cognitive performance in middle-aged and older adults: Results of the austrian stroke prevention study. *Journal of the American Geriatric Society, 46,* 1407–1410.

Schor, N. F., Tyurina, Y. Y., Fabisiak, J. P., Tyurin, V. A., Lazo, J. S., & Kagan, V. E. (1999). Selective oxidation and externalization of membrane phosphatidylserine: Bcl-2-induced potentiation of the final common pathway for apoptosis. *Brain Research, 831,* 125–130.

Schroeder, F., Frolov, A. A., Murphy, E. J., Atshaves, B. P., Jefferson, J. R., Pu, L., Wood, W. G., Foxworth, W. B., & Kier, A. B. (1996). Recent advances in membrane cholesterol domain dynamics and intracellular cholesterol trafficking. *Proceedings of the Society of Experimental Biology and Medicine, 213,* 150–177.

Seif-El-Nasr, M., & El-Fattah, A. A. (1995). Lipid peroxide, phospholipids, glutathione levels and superoxide dismutase activity in rat brain after ischaemia: Effect of *Ginkgo biloba* extract. *Pharmacological Research, 32,* 273–278.

Sharoni, Y., Giron, E., Rise, M., & Levy, J. (1997). Effects of lycopene-enriched tomato oleoresin on 7,12-dimethyl- benz[a]anthracene-induced rat mammary tumors. *Cancer Detection and Prevention, 21,* 118–123.

Shimada, A., Hosokawa, M., Ohta, A., Akiguchi, I., & Takeda, T. (1994). Localization of atrophy-prone areas in the aging mouse brain: Comparison between the brain atrophy model SAM-P/10 and the normal control SAM-R/1. *Neuroscience, 59,* 859–869.

Shimada, A., Ohta, A., Akiguchi, I., & Takeda, T. (1992). Inbred SAM-P/10 as a mouse model of spontaneous, inherited brain atrophy. *Journal of Neuropathology and Experimental Neurology, 51,* 440–450.

Shukitt-Hale, B. (1999). The effects of aging and oxidative stress on psychomotor and cognitive behavior. *Age, 22,* 9–17.

Shukitt-Hale, B., Mouzakis, G., & Joseph, J. A. (1998). Psychomotor and spatial memory performance in aging male fischer 344 rats. *Experimental Gerontology, 33,* 615–624.

Sigurdsson, E. M., Lee, J. M., Dong, X. W., Hejna, M. J., & Lorens, S. A. (1997). Bilateral injections of amyloid-beta 25-35 into the amygdala of young Fischer rats: Behavioral, neurochemical, and time dependent histopathological effects. *Neurobiology of Aging, 18,* 591–608.

Sirinathsinghji, D. J. (1998). Transgenic mouse models of Alzheimer's disease. *Biochemical Society Transactions, 26,* 504–508.
Slotte, J. P., & Bierman, E. L. (1988). Depletion of plasma-membrane sphingomyelin rapidly alters the distribution of cholesterol between plasma membranes and intracellular cholesterol pools in cultured fibroblasts. *Biochemical Journal, 250,* 653–658.
Smith, M. A., Richey Harris, P. L., Sayre, L. M., Beckman, J. S., & Perry, G. (1997). Widespread peroxynitrite-mediated damage in Alzheimer's disease. *Journal of Neuroscience, 17,* 2653–2657.
Smith, M. A., Wehr, K., Harris, P. L. R., Siedlak, S. L., Connor, J. R., & Perry, G. (1998). Abnormal localization of iron regulatory protein in Alzheimer's disease. *Brain Research, 788,* 323–326.
Smriga, M., Saito, H., & Nishiyama, N. (1995). Hoelen (Poria cocos Wolf) and ginseng (*Panax ginseng* C. A. Meyer), the ingredients of a Chinese prescription DX-9386, individually promote hippocampal long-term potentiation in vivo. *Biological and Pharmaceutical Bulletin, 18,* 518–522.
Snowdon, D. A., Gross, M. D., & Butler, S. M. (1996). Antioxidants and reduced functional capacity in the elderly: Findings from the nun study. *Journals of Gerontology. Series A, Biological Sciences and Medical Sciences, 51,* M10–16.
Soderberg, M., Edlund, C., Alafuzoff, I., Kristensson, K., & Dallner, G. (1992). Lipid composition in different regions of the brain in Alzheimer's disease/senile dementia of Alzheimer's type. *Journal of Neurochemistry, 59,* 1646–1653.
Sparks, D. L. (1997). Coronary artery disease, hypertension, ApoE, and cholesterol: A link to Alzheimer's disease? *Annals of the New York Academy of Sciences, 826,* 128–146.
Stancampiano, R., Cocco, S., Cugusi, C., Sarais, L., & Fadda, F. (1999). Serotonin and acetylcholine release response in the rat hippocampus during a spatial memory task. *Neuroscience, 89,* 1135–1143.
Stanimirovic, D., & Satoh, K. (2000). Inflammatory mediators of cerebral endothelium: A role in ischemic brain inflammation. *Brain Pathology, 10,* 113–126.
Steele, C. D. (2000). The genetics of Alzheimer disease. *Nursing Clinics of North America, 35,* 687–694.
Steffen, B., Breier, G., Butcher, E., Schulz, M., & Engelhardt, B. (1996). ICAM-1, VCAM-1, and MADCAM-1 are expressed on choroid plexus epithelium but not endothelium and mediate binding of lymphocytes in vitro. *American Journal of Pathology, 148,* 1819–1838.
Stella, N., Estelles, A., Siciliano, J., Tence, M., Desagher, S., Piomelli, D., Glowinski, J., & Premont, J. (1997). Interleukin-1 enhances the ATP-evoked release of arachidonic acid from mouse astrocytes. *Journal of Neurosciences, 17,* 2939–2946.

Stephenson, D., Yin, T., Smalstig, E. B., Hsu, M. A., Panetta, J., Little, S., & Clemens, J. (2000). Transcription factor nuclear factor-kappa B is activated in neurons after focal cerebral ischemia. *Journal of Cerebral Blood Flow and Metabolism, 20,* 592–603.

Stoll, S., Scheuer, K., Pohl, O., & Muller, W. E. (1996). *Ginkgo biloba* extract (EGb 761) independently improves changes in passive avoidance learning and brain membrane fluidity in the aging mouse. *Pharmacopsychiatry, 29,* 144–149.

Suganuma, H., Hirano, T., & Inakuma, T. (1999). Amelioratory effect of dietary ingestion with red bell pepper on learning impairment in senescence-accelerated mice (samp8). *Journal of Nutritional Science and Vitaminology, 45,* 143–149.

Suganuma, M., Okabe, S., Oniyama, M., Tada, Y., Ito, H., & Fujiki, H. (1998). Wide distribution of [3H](-)-epigallocatechin gallate, a cancer preventive tea polyphenol, in mouse tissue. *Carcinogenesis, 19,* 1771–1776.

Suganuma, M., Okabe, S., Sueoka, N., Sueoka, E., Matsuyama, S., Imai, K., Nakachi, K., & Fujiki, H. (1999). Green tea and cancer chemoprevention. *Mutation Research, 428,* 339–344.

Sunshine, C., & McNamee, M. G. (1994). Lipid modulation of nicotinic acetylcholine receptor function: The role of membrane lipid composition and fluidity. *Biochimica et Biophysica Acta, 1191,* 59–64.

Suzuki, H., Park, S. J., Tamura, M., & Ando, S. (1998). Effect of the long-term feeding of dietary lipids on the learning ability, fatty acid composition of brain stem phospholipids and synaptic membrane fluidity in adult mice: A comparison of sardine oil diet with palm oil diet. *Mechanims of Aging and Development, 16,* 119–128.

Svennerholm, L., & Gottfries, C. G. (1994). Membrane lipids, selectively diminished in Alzheimer brains, suggest synapse loss as a primary event in early-onset form (type I) and demyelination in late-onset form (type II). *Journal of Neurochemistry, 62,* 1039–1047.

Tacconi, M. T., Lligona, L., Salmona, M., Pitsikas, N., & Algeri, S. (1991). Aging and food restriction: Effect on lipids of cerebral cortex. *Neurobiology of Aging, 12,* 55–59.

Verlangieri, A. J., Kapeghian, J. C., el-Dean, S., & Bush, M. (1985). Fruit and vegetable consumption and cardiovascular mortality. *Medical Hypotheses, 16,* 7–15.

Wallace, J. E., Krauter, E. E., & Campbell, B. A. (1980). Motor and reflexive behavior in the aging rat. *Journal of Gerontology, 35,* 364–370.

Wang, H., Cao, G., & Prior, R. L. (1996). Total antioxidant capacity of fruits. *Journal of Agriculture and Food Chemistry, 44,* 701–705.

Wattenberg, L. W., & Coccia, J.B. (1991). Inhibition of 4-(methylnitrosamino)-1-(3-pyridyl)-1-butanone carcinogenesis in mice by d-limonene and citrus fruit oils. *Carcinogenesis, 12,* 115–117.

Welford, A. T. 1977. Motor performance. In J. E. Birren and K. W. Schaie (Eds.), *Handbook of the psychology of aging* (pp. 450–497). New York: Van Nostrand Reinhold.

Wells, K., Farooqui, A. A., Liss, L., & Horrocks, L. A. (1995). Neural membrane phospholipids in Alzheimer disease. *Neurochemical Research, 20,* 1329–1333.

West, R. L. (1996). An application of pre-frontal cortex function theory to cognitive aging. *Psychology Bulletin, 120,* 272–292.

White, H. L., Scates, P. W., & Cooper, B. R. (1996) Extracts of *Ginkgo biloba* leaves inhibit monoamine oxidase. *Life Sciences, 58,* 1315–1321

Willett, W. C. (1994). Diet and health: What should we eat? *Science, 264,* 532–537.

Winkler, J., Connor, D. J., Frautschy, S. A., Behl, C., Waite, J. J., Cole, G. M., & Thal, L. J. (1994). Lack of long-term effects after beta-amyloid protein injections in rat brain. *Neurobiology of Aging, 15,* 601–607.

Wood, G. W., Schroeder, F., Avdulov, N. A., Chochina, S. V., & Igbavboa, U. (1999). Recent advances in brain cholesterol dynamics: Transport, domains and Alzheimer's disease. *Lipids, 34,* 225–234.

Wood, G. W., Schroeder, F., Rao, A. M., Igbavboa, U., & Avdulov, N. A. (1996). Membranes and ethanol: Lipid domains and lipid-protein interactions. In R. A. Deitrich & V. G. Erwin (Eds.), *Pharmacological effects of ethanol on the nervous system* (pp. 13–27). Boca Raton, FL: CRC Press.

Wood, W. G., Strong, R., Williamson, L. S., & Wise, R. W. (1984). Changes in lipid composition of cortical synaptosomes from different age groups of mice. *Life Sciences, 35,* 1947–1952.

Woodroofe, M. N. (1995). Cytokine production in the central nervous system. *Neurology, 45*(6 Suppl.6), S6–S10.

Wu, W. R., & Zhu, X. Z. (1999). Involvement of monoamine oxidase inhibition in neuroprotective and neurorestorative effects of *Ginkgo biloba* extract against MPTP-induced nigrostriatal dopaminergic toxicity in C57 mice. *Life Sciences, 65,* 157–164.

Yagi, H., Irino, M., Matsushita, T., Katoh, S., Umezawa, M., Tsuboyama, T., Hosokawa, M., Akiguchi, I., Tokunaga, R., & Takeda, T. (1989). Spontaneous spongy degeneration of the brain stem in sam-p/8 mice, a newly developed memory-deficient strain. *Journal of Neuropathology and Experimental Neurology, 48,* 577–590.

Yamada, K., Komori, Y., Tanaka, T., Senzaki, K., Nikai, T., Sugihara, H., Kameyama, T., & Nabeshima, T. (1999). Brain dysfunction associated with an induction of nitric oxide synthase following an intracerebral injection of lipopolysaccharide in rats. *Neuroscience, 88,* 281–294.

Yamagami, K., Joseph, J. A., & Roth, G. S. (1992). Decrement of muscarinic receptor-stimulated low km GTPase in striatum and hippocampus from the aged rat. *Brain Research, 576,* 327–331.

Yanagisawa, K., Odaka, A., Suzuki, N., & Ihara, Y. (1995). Gm1 ganglioside-bound amyloid beta-protein (A-Beta): A possible form of preamyloid in Alzheimer's disease [see comments]. *Nature Medicine, 1,* 1062–1066.

Yen, T. T. (1990a) Improvement of learning ability in mice and rats with the root extract of ding lang (Policias fruticosum L.). *Acta Physiologica Hungarica, 75,* 69–76.

Yen, T. T. (1990b) Stimulation of sexual performance in male rats with the root extract of ding lang (*Policias fruticosum* L.). *Acta Physiologica Hungarica, 75,* 61–67.

Yen, T. T., Kalasz, H., & Matkovics, B. (1990). The effects of Ding lang root extract on the activities of peroxide metabolism enzymes in the rat. In B. Matkovics, L. Karmazsin, and H. Kalasz (Eds.), *Radicals, ions and tissue damage* (pp. 293–298). Budapest, Hungary: Akademiai Kiado.

Youdim, K. A., & Joseph, J. A. (2001). A possible emerging role of phytochemicals in improving age-related neurological dysfunctions: A multiplicity of effects. *Free Radical Biology and Medicine, 30,* 583–594.

Youdim, K. A., Martin, A., & Joseph, J. A. (2000). Essential fatty acids and the brain: Possible health implications. *International Journal of Developmental Neuroscience, 18,* 383–399.

Youdim, K. A., Shukitt-Hale, B., Martin, A., Wang, H., Denisova, N., Bickford, P. C., & Joesph, J. A. (2000). Short-tern dietary supplementation of blueberry polyphenolics: Beneficial effects on aging brain performance and peripheral tissue function. *Nutritional Neuroscience, 3,* 383–391.

Youdim, M. B. H., & Riederer, P. (1997). Understanding Parkinson's disease. *Scientific American, 276,* 52–59.

Yu, B. P. (1994). Cellular defenses against damage from reactive oxygen species. *Physiological Reviews, 74,* 139–162.

Yufu, F., Egashira, T., & Yamanaka, Y. (1994). Age-related changes of cholinergic markers in the rat brain. *Japanese Journal of Pharmacology, 66,* 247–255.

Zaidi, A., & Michaelis, M. L. (1999). Effects of reactive oxygen species on brain synaptic plasma membrane CA(2+)-ATPase. *Free Radical Biology and Medicine, 27,* 810–821.

Zhang, J. T., Qu, Z. W., Liu, Y., & Deng, H. L. (1990). Preliminary study on antiamnestic mechanism of ginsenoside Rg1 and Rb1. *Chinese Medical Journal, 103,* 932–938.

Zhang, Y., Appelkvist, E. L., Kristensson, K., & Dallner, G. (1996). The lipid compositions of different regions of rat brain during development and aging. *Neurobiology of Aging, 17,* 869–875.

Zhang, Y., Moriguchi, T., Saito, H., & Nishiyama, N. (1998). Functional relationship between age-related immunodeficiency and learning deterioration. *European Journal of Neuroscience, 10,* 3869–3875.

Zhang, Y., Saito, H., & Nishiyama, N. (1994). Improving effects of DX-9386, a traditional Chinese medicinal prescription, on thymectomy-induced impairment of learning behaviors in mice. *Biological and Pharmaceutical Bulletin, 17,* 1199–1205.

Zhang, Y., Saito, H., Nishiyama, N., & Abe, K. (1994). Effects of DX-9386, a traditional Chinese medicinal prescription, on long-term potentiation in the dentate gyrus in rats. *Biological and Pharmaceutical Bulletin, 17,* 1337–1340.

Zornetzer, S. F. & Rogers, J. (1983). Animal models for assessment of geriatric mnemonic and motor deficits. In T. Crook, S. Ferris, & R. Bartus (Eds.), *Behavioral assessment in geriatric pharmacology.* New Canaan, CT: Powley Associates.

CHAPTER 10

The Genetics of Behavioral Aging

GERALD E. MCCLEARN
CENTER FOR DEVELOPMENTAL AND HEALTH GENETICS
PENNSYLVANIA STATE UNIVERSITY

The topic of genetics of behavioral aging obviously engages the disciplines of genetics, behavioral sciences, and gerontology. The two-way interfaces among these disciplines—behavioral aging, gerontological genetics, and behavioral genetics—are thriving interdisciplinary areas:

1. Behavioral aging is a key domain of concern in gerontology; age-related changes in personality, incidence of depression, impairments in functional competence (ADL), and decline in cognitive functioning and development of dementia are familiar themes in gerontological science, with enormous implications for quality of life.
2. Various genetic perspectives have been directed toward the phenomena of aging. Population genetic principles are intrinsic to species comparisons calculated to provide insights into the evolution of aging; molecular genetics considerations of mutation, DNA repair, antioxidant defense, and so on are key to the current approaches to the study of the physiological and biochemical mechanisms of aging; modern extensions of basic Mendelian genetics inquire into the genetic origins of categorical age-related disorders such as dementias; quantitative genetic principles underly the various approaches analyzing kin resemblance in noncategorical, continuously distributed phenotypes of age and aging.
3. Although philosophical and political objections (frequently characterized in terms of a "nature vs. nurture" debate) have been raised against the suggestion that behavioral attributes might be affected by genetic factors, the weight of empirical evidence, both from humans and from animal models is conclusive: Genetic factors have been shown to be influential in a sweeping panorama of behavioral phenotypes, ranging from taxes and kineses to complex cognitive processing (Plomin, DeFries, McClearn, & McGuffin, 2000).

The combination of these domains constitutes a three-way interdiscipline—the genetics of behavioral aging—that is extraordinarily rich in diverse theories, methods, empirical data bases, and scientific conventions.

GERONTOLOGICAL GENETICS OF BEHAVIOR

The empirical data pertaining to genetic influences on aging of behavioral phenotypes have been extensively reviewed previously (Goodrick, 1978; Kallman & Jarvik, 1959; McClearn & Foch, 1985; Omenn, 1977; Pedersen, 1996; Plomin & McClearn, 1990). Given the breadth of coverage of these various reviews, the present chapter will not attempt a comprehensive survey, but will concentrate instead on a frame of reference for interpretation of the data, on selected illustrative data, and on a few conjectures about some likely directions of future research.

A particularly lamentable aspect of the "nature vs. nurture" view was the conclusion drawn by some that these two identified domains are antagonistic and require an either-or decision: that is, something is due to heredity or it is not (and similarly, one must be either a hereditarian or an environmentalist). Evidence of any environmental influence was sometimes interpreted to deny the possibility of any genetic involvement and vice versa. Although it lingers still in some quarters, the basic bankruptcy of this perspective became clear early in the 20th century, when the quantitative genetic model was introduced and subsequently was elegantly elaborated.

In its simplest form, the basic assumption is that an aggregate of multiple genetic factors and another of multiple environmental factors influence the location of an individual's measured attribute, or phenotype, along a continuous dimension. Each gene (or locus, a term derived from the location on the chromosome that a particular gene occupies) may exist in alternative forms or alleles. Different alleles have different molecular structures, and may have vastly different functional properties. The genotype of an individual for any single locus in the polygenic system is specified by the two alleles it possesses, one derived from each parent. Environment is defined by exclusion (any influence not arising from the DNA), so that together, G (the genetic aggregate) and E (the environmental aggregate) provide a comprehensive accounting of all pertinent influences on P, the phenotype (ignoring for the moment covariance and interaction terms that will be explored later). It is particularly important to note the breadth of the definition of environmental factors, which embrace the spectrum from biochemical milieux to sociocultural forces. Because of the explicit inclusion of both genetic and environmental factors in the model, the usual appellation of "quantitative genetics" is somewhat misleading. A description as a "quantitative genetic and environmental" model would clearly be more accurate, but also rather awkward. Because the targeted phenomena are the differentiae among individuals, a more felicitious characterization would be that of a "differential" model.

Individuals differ in the particular genetic elements they possess and in the environmental factors to which they have been exposed. Thus, the phenotype of an individual will be located along a continuum, depending upon his or her unique mix of the two influences. It is important to emphasize that the location of each individual on this dimension is due *both* to genes and to environments. The phenotype cannot be due either to one or the other—without both, there would be no organism. A conceptualization appropriate for analysis of this continuous distribution is that of variance decomposition. The question is how much of the variability of a group of individuals can be attributed to genetic differences among them, and how much to environmental differences. Given the basic and simple model

$$P = G + E$$

where P represents the measured phenotype, G refers to the genetic influences and E to the environmental ones (and, to repeat, ignoring interaction and covariance terms until later) the variance displayed by a group of individuals can be represented by

$$V_P = V_G + V_E$$

Each of these terms is divisible further. V_G, for example, may be decomposed into a term V_A, representing additive genetic variance and V_D, representing the influence of dominance, or V_{NA}, which includes not only the nonadditive feature of dominance but also that of intergene interactions called epistasis. V_E can be subdivided into components representing long- or short-term environmental influences or environmental factors shared or not shared by particular individuals (V_{ES} and V_{ENS}), among other distinctions.

A basic statistic of quantitative inheritance is *heritability*, the proportion or percentage of the total phenotypic variance that is attributable to genetic sources. This may be further distinguished as "narrow sense" heritability (V_A/V_P) or "broad sense" heritability (V_G/V_P), which terms are differentially useful for diverse descriptive or predictive purposes (see, for example, Falconer & Mackay, 1996). It is important to note that heritability is a descriptive statistic, and the estimate depends upon the number and relative frequencies of different alleles in the population and on the range of environmental circumstances to which members of the population are exposed. Another gene pool or different environments could give different results.

An unfortunate consequence of failure to appreciate the conditionality of an estimate of heritability has been an assumption by some that high heritability of a phenotype implies an impossibility of manipulation by environmental means. Clearly, a high heritability implies a relative absence of environmental factors contributing to individuality in the environmental range to which that particular population has been exposed. It does not preclude the possibility that an effective environmental factor (say, educational or nutritional preventive intervention or remediation) might be devised.

A variety of research designs permits the estimation of these components of individuality, and many of them have been deployed in gerontological genetics research.

ANIMAL MODEL RESEARCH

In the case of animal models, it is possible to manipulate genotypes systematically for particular purposes. Molecular genetic procedures can result in overexpression or in "knockout" of specific genes, and these techniques are destined to provide increasing proportions of the knowledge base on the genetics of aging processes. But most of the pertinent literature to date has been produced by methods that derive from quantitative genetics, methods that have long histories of productive deployment in a variety of biological disciplines and in agricultural application.

Inbred Strains

The procedure of mating relatives results in homogenizing of the genotype. More technically, inbreeding leads to increasing homozygosity (that is, an increasing number of genetic loci will be occupied by alleles that are alike). Strictly speaking, this is an ideal situation that is only asymptotically approached (see Falconer & Mackay, 1996), but after about 20 consecutive generations in the case of sibling mating, this state is approximated, the genotypes are relatively fixed and therefore relatively stable. (Mutational events can, of course, result in changes, and such changes can result in the appearance of sub-strains.) The relative genotypic stability of inbred strains across time and across laboratories has provided a foundation—"reagent grade" animals—for biomedical animal-model research in general, and in the arena of the genetics of aging specifically. Because of the stochastic features of the inbreeding process, the particular genotype fixed within any particular inbred strain is largely a matter of chance. Because of this feature and the fact that most of the extant strains were derived from different foundation populations with different allelic frequencies, each strain can be regarded as genetically unique. Thus, if two inbred strains are reared, maintained, and tested in the same circumstances, any phenotypic difference found between them is ipso facto evidence of genetic influence on that phenotype. This is a basic piece of information, but it reveals little of the details of the genetic system involved. Additional information can be obtained by further genotype manipulation via controlled matings. The mating of individuals from two different strains results in F_1 (first filial) hybrid offspring that are heterozygous for all loci for which the parent strains differ. That is to say, the F_1 will have an intermediate gene dosage at all these loci. Nevertheless, the F_1 is a genetically homogeneous group: all F_1s are heterozygous at the same loci. Thus, the variance observed within any of these groups—parent strains and F_1—is attributable to environmental sources.

If F_1 animals are mated inter se, however, their gametes will each be a different sampling of the genes of the progenitor strains, and the resulting progeny will be genetically heterogeneous. In this F_2 (second filial) generation, both genetic and environmental sources of variance are present. Thus, subtracting an estimate of the environmental variance from the F_2 variance yields (with some assumptions) an estimate of the genetic variance. Divided by the total F_2 phenotypic variance, this gives an estimate of the proportion of the total variance that is due to genetic factors. This is a very simple example of the variance decomposition approach of quantitative genetics.

Inbred strains were identified early as powerful tools for the study of the genetics of behavioral aging, and several investigators at about the same time cast a wide behavioral net in reviewing the possibilities and prospects. Sprott (1972), for example, called attention to differing behavioral attributes of likely relevance to the study of aging of two strains that have been widely employed in biological and biomedical research since the early part of the century—the C57BL/6 and DBA/2 and their F_1. Phenotypic categories discussed included feeding behavior (alcohol preference, sucrose preference, phenylthiocarbamide taste sensitivity); aggression (male-male); mating behavior; "emotionality" (measured by defecation in test apparatus); learning (maze performance, passive and active avoidance situations); and activity. Sprott noted that whereas the strain differences identified in these domains clearly indicated genetic influences, they had mostly been observed in young adult animals, and relatively little was known about their late-life manifestations.

Goodrick (1975) addressed aging phenomena in a cross-sectional study of C57BL/6 and another widely used strain, A, at 5 months of age and at 23 months (A) or 26 months (C57BL/6) of age. Phenotypes included operant learning, activity, sensory discrimination, and alcohol preference. Overall, relative to the young animals, the older ones were less proficient in nest building, drank more water, exhibited less exploratory behavior, were less active, ingested less quinine solution in a discrimination test, and drank less alcohol solution in a preference test. No evidence of age differences was found for a measure of emotionality or for operant performance. Strain differences were also evident in many of these phenotypes. Of particular interest are the situations that yielded interactions between strain and age, suggestive of a genetically influenced difference in rate of aging. Examples of this outcome are provided in Figures 10.1 and 10.2 for measures of exploratory and open field activity. Such interactions were also found for a measure of open field activity, wheel activity, light contingent bar pressing, quinine discrimination, sucrose discrimination, and alcohol preference.

These omnibus studies illustrate convincingly that there exists a large number of behavioral variables displaying geneticallly influenced age differences or changes. Many other studies have reported on particular phenotypes. Wood (1976), for example, examined further age-related differences in voluntary alcohol ingestion using the C57BL/6 and BALB/c strains tested at 7–9 months, 14–16 months, and 22–24 months of age. The BALB/c strain was chosen because of previous work (Kakihana & McClearn, 1963) that had shown early-life developmental decline in alcohol preference in this strain. Figure 10.3 shows the pattern of strain by age interaction for ethanol preference averaged over the several different concentrations that

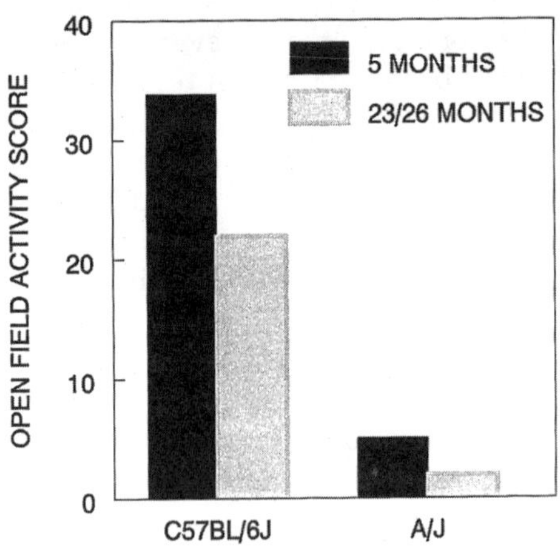

FIGURE 10.1 Mean scores of C57BL/6 and DBA/2 mice at 5 months of age and 23–26 months of age, assessed cross-sectionally for exploration, measured by time-sampling every 10 seconds for 15 minutes of the position of the mouse in brightly lit or dark parts of an open field. Twelve males and twelve females were tested in each group. Drawn from data presented in Goodrick (1975).

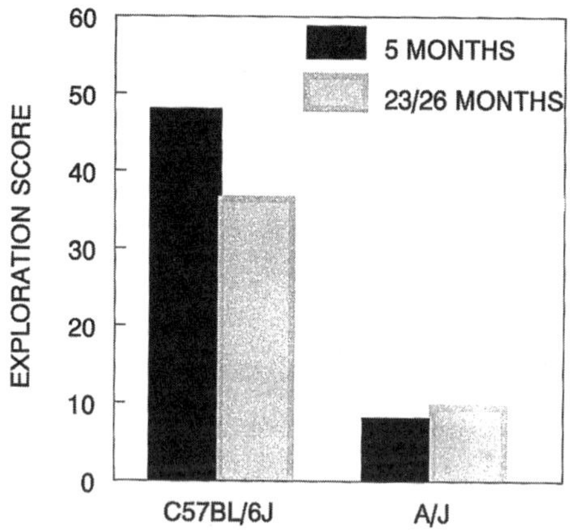

FIGURE 10.2 Mean scores of C57BL/6 and DBA/2 mice at 5 months of age and 23–26 months of age assessed cross-sectionally for locomotor activity for 15 minutes in an open field. Twelve males and twelve females were tested in each group. Drawn from data presented in Goodrick (1975).

had been used. There is a clear and regular decline from a high preference level in young C57BL/6 mice, but a continuing low level of alcohol avidity on the part of the BALB/c animals.

Activity and Exploration

Various behavioral measures are often considered together as representing a domain of activity and exploration. Among other concepts, curiosity, exploratory drive, anxiety, and activity drive have been invoked variously to account for the behaviors. There is no agreed-upon taxonomy in the area, but it is clear that several dimensions are represented by the measures that are typical in research in the area. McClearn and Meredith (1964) identified five factors from factor and cluster analyses of 21 measures that were obtained from five test situations administered to mice of a systematically derived genetically heterogeneous stock (of advantage for correlational studies; see McClearn & Hofer, 1999). It is certain that genetic influences on this type of measure can be very pronounced. Some of the most dramatic differences among inbred strains have been described for measures in this domain. Age-relatedness of various of these measures is easily established, and differences in rate of age change were intimated. Simmel, Haber, and Hirshfield (1976) investigated two strains (C57BL/10 and LG) and their F_1 in an arena apparatus. Distinguishing exploratory

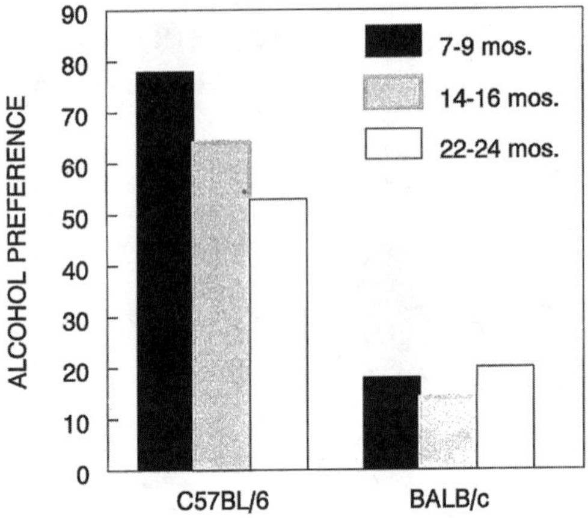

FIGURE 10.3 Mean alcohol preference scores of male C57BL/6 and BALB/c mice at 7–9, 14–16, and 22–24 months of age. The values shown express preference as the ratio of alcohol solution consumed to total liquid consumed, and are average results derived from observations on eight concentrations of alcohol solution ranging from 4% to 18%. Six animals were tested in each age/strain group. Drawn from data presented in Wood (1976).

behavior and activity indices, they concluded that age influences locomotor activity more than it does stimulus exploration. Strain differences were large, but no interactions of strain with age were discerned.

Ingram (1990) provided an expanded discussion of the relative implications of situations in which strains differ in phenotypic level but display parallel changes with age, and those in which the age trajectories diverge or converge. Different outcomes were obtained for various psychomotor phenotypes in A and C57BL/6 mice from 3 months to 24 months. The time it took to fall from a balance beam, for example, declined more or less in parallel for both strains; clinging time to a tightrope was the same in the strains when young, but the A animals retained the initial level of performance, whereas the C57BL/6 declined.

Learning and Memory

Because of the salience of cognitive processes in human gerontological research it was inevitable that there has been a concentration on learning and memory in animal models of aging. A wide variety of learning situations has been utilized in this pursuit. There are numerous taxonomies that can characterize the various tests and procedures. Here a distinction will be made between the two general classes of appetitive and aversive situations.

Aversive learning, where the learned response removes or avoids some noxious stimulus, has been widely employed in studies of behavioral aging. Sprott (1972) tested male C57BL/6 and DBA/2 mice and their F_1 in a passive-avoidance conditioning situation. Cross-sectional observations were made at 5 weeks of age and at 4 to 5 months of age and with varying levels of motivation. The animal was placed on a platform above a grid floor. On the first occasion, a shock of 0.1, 1.0, 2.0, or 4.0 mA was applied for one second. Daily trials were given until the animals achieved a criterion of refraining for 60 seconds from stepping down onto the floor. Under the motivational condition of 0.1 mA shock, young C57BL/6 mice were superior to the DBA/2. However, for the older mice, at 4.0 mA, the DBA/2 were greatly superior to the C57BL/6, reflecting an improvement of the former with age, and a decrement on the part of the latter. The F_1 animals were very similar to their C57BL/6 parent throughout. Sprott emphasized that strain differences observed under particular conditions often do not generalize to other conditions.

In a parallel study, Stavnes and Sprott (1975) measured active avoidance performance of male C57BL/6 and DBA/2 mice at the approximate ages of 21, 45, 145, and 560 days. In this situation, the animals were placed upon the shock-grid floor and after 5 seconds, were subjected to a 60 sec 0.1 mA foot shock unless they jumped to a platform. Most DBA/2 mice were escapers, rather than avoiders, jumping to the platform after the onset of shock. The percentage of escape responses remained stable over the age range; the peak avoiding behavior in this strain occurred at 45 days of age, declining greatly at the later ages. C57BL/6 mice, on the other hand, displayed relatively greater avoidance behavior, peaking also at 45 days, but also declining to a low level at 560 days. In this strain, the percentage of escapers rose systematically from low levels in the young to high levels in the most aged group.

In an effort to identify useful model systems for the study of aging of appetitive learning performance, Warren (1986) evaluated several situations longitudinally in male C57BL/6 and DBA/2 mice at 100, 200, 400, 600, and 700 days of age. The specific phenotypes included brightness discrimination, performance in the relatively simple Lashley I maze and in the more complicated Lashley III maze, food-seeking behavior, activity in an arena, latent learning (while learning a particular task, incidentally learning something useful for a future different task), and multiple T-maze performance. A principal feature of the results was the task-specificity of age effects. In brief, old C57BL/6 but not old DBA/2 mice were impaired on a visual discrimination problem. In latent learning, old C57BL/6 animals were superior to young ones, but the reverse was true in DBA/2 animals. In a food-seeking task, C57BL/6 animals failed at all ages; older DBA/2 mice were inferior to younger ones.

This theme of the specificity and particularity of test situations is persuasively illustrated for appetitive learning in a subsequent report by Warren (1988), who trained 60-day-old male and female C57BL/6, DBA/2, and F_1 mice on the Lashley III maze with hunger or thirst as motivation and water, oatmeal, mash, or cheese as the incentive; 120-day-old animals were tested under the oatmeal and water conditions. At 60 days, hybrid vigor (heterosis) was evident in that the performance of the F_1 animals was superior to that of either parent for all conditions except that of hunger motivation and cheese reward, where the F_1 performance was intermediate to the parents' performance. This specificity of outcome depending on incentive is noteworthy. At 120 days, the F_1 performance was intermediate in both test circumstances, contrary to the 60-day results. The author suggested that a different set of genes was influencing maze learning at the two ages. The age span of this study is not very large, but the implications for longer age spans are obvious.

Another related issue that arises in interpreting studies on the aging of learning ability is the well-known fact that the performance of an animal in the test situation is a function not only of fundamental "cognitive" ability but also of numerous other factors and the equally recognized fact that it is not easy to distinguish among them. The potentially confounding factors have been variously identified. (Sprott & Stavnes, 1975, pp. 149–150) identified "motivation . . . speed of performance, physiological factors such as weight, size and perceptual difficulties." Sarter (1987, p. 765) analyzed a variety of learning situations employed in aging research and suggested that "most of the findings indicating an age-related decline are better attributed to the altered motivational status and/or emotional reactiveness than to impaired cognitive processes of senescent animals." Similarly, Crady and Quinton (1989) attempted to distinguish between learning/memory and performance parameters in a visual discrimination situation with foot-shock motivation. They concluded that old mice can learn this task as well as younger adults but the rate of learning is slower, whereas their physical performance on the task is persistently inferior to adult mice. Ingram (1985) also reviewed noncognitive performance factors in rodent models of learning and memory and noted especially the additional complications of genetic factors, unremarked by Sarter or by Crady and Quinton. Ingram concluded that rather than inhibiting understanding of functional age changes, genetic complexities offered powerful opportunities.

Selective Breeding

Another particularly powerful form of genotype manipulation is that of phenotypic selective breeding. Although the rationalizing model was provided in 1918 by Fisher, selective breeding has been employed for millennia in the domestication of animals and plants and has played a central role in the generation of today's food crops and food animals. (In an engaging historical reference, Gimpel [1976] identifies the increasing size of parchment in the Middle Ages as evidence of the efficacy of pragmatic selection for increased body size of sheep.)

If the locations of individuals on a phenotypic continuum are influenced by genetic factors, then the mating of animals with phenotypes that deviate substantially in the same direction from the mean of their generation will result in offspring with genotypes that are enriched in respect to alleles at the loci causing, say, high levels of the phenotype. Their phenotypic mean, therefore, will be elevated with respect to the mean of their parents' generation, although, except in the case of a heritability of 1.0, lower than that of their parents themselves. If this procedure is continued through successive generations, the result will be a line of animals with phenotypic distributions that are increasingly divergent from the original foundation population.

Thus, by selective breeding, animal models can be generated to phenotypic specification. In research applications, it is typical to select bidirectionally, yielding animal groups with very different mean phenotypes (and of the underlying alleles) that are powerful tools for the study of the physiological and anatomical mechanisms that mediate the genetic influence.

Different biological and biomedical research domains have benefited to different degrees from these tailor-made models. In behavioral science, one of the most significant selective breeding studies was that of Tryon (1940), who selectively bred rats for errors committed in negotiating a 14-unit multiple T-maze, under conditions of hunger motivation and food reward. The resulting "maze-bright" and "maze-dull" strains have subsequently found employment in a variety of studies exploring the behavioral and neurobiological bases of the strain differences. One of these studies addressed age differences. McGaugh and Cole (1965) hypothesized that the well-described effect of massed versus distributed practice would vary both by strain and by age. Animals of the maze bright and maze dull strains (now renamed S1 and S3, respectively) of two age groups (29 to 33 days and 142 to 164 days) were tested in a Lashley III maze under conditions of 30 seconds or 30 minutes between trials. The results were as follows: No strain differences in error scores appeared between young members of these strains in this particular maze when tested under massed practice conditions; distribution of practice facilitated the maze performance of older animals in both strains; with distributed practice, young S1 animals were superior to young S3 animals.

As a general summary, this sampling of animal model results has demonstrated the existence, indeed the near ubiquity, of genetic influence on behavioral aging processes. A recurring theme has been the particularity of the results, with outcomes depending upon details of the testing situation and upon the genotypes of the subject animals. Some implications of this sensitivity will be discussed later.

HUMAN RESEARCH

In human research, the observations that permit variance decomposition are measures of the degree of phenotypic resemblance of individuals of differing degrees of biological relatedness, from the zero of randomly paired individuals, through the intermediate relationships of siblings and of parents to offspring, to the genetic identity of monozygotic twins.

Because of the difficulty in obtaining longevity or late-life information on successive human generations, parent-offspring analyses in human gerontological genetics have been limited, and the twin method has been particularly useful. The basic logic is simple. Identical (monozygotic or MZ) twins are derived from a single fertilized egg and are consequently identical genetically. Fraternal (dizygotic or DZ) twins are genetically the same as ordinary siblings, sharing on average half of their genetic material. A greater phenotypic similarity of MZs can then be interpreted as indicative of genetic influence if one can assume, among other things, that the impact of environmental influences is not such as to generate greater MZ similarity. It is easy to identify or to speculate on ways in which MZ twins are treated more similarly (dressing, for an obvious example), but the crucial issue is whether these matters affect the phenotype in question. The "equal environmental influence assumption" is sometimes hard to evaluate, but where it has been possible, it appears not to be a vitiating problem (see Plomin et al., 2000). Nonetheless, it is always necessary to retain a degree of caution in interpreting twin data, and converging evidence from other designs such as adoption studies is always desirable.

In application to gerontology, the pioneering twin research was that of Kallman, Jarvik and their associates (see Blum, Fossage, & Jarvik, 1972; Jarvik, Blum, & Varma, 1972; Jarvik, Kallman, Falek, & Klaber, 1957, for example). They administered a broad psychometric battery to MZ and DZ twins who were 60 years of age or more. Analysis was largely focused on the magnitude of intrapair differences—in general, MZ pairs differed less than did DZ pairs. In a 20-year follow-up, the differences had converged, largely because the surviving MZ pairs had become less similar. A decline in performance on speeded tests was seen as normal, but decline in nonspeeded tests was indicative of impending death, introducing the notions of terminal decline and terminal drop.

Striking advances in model-fitting analyses in multivariate data in general (see, e.g., Duncan, 1975; Loehlin, 1992; Maruyama, 1998) and in quantitative genetics in particular (see Neale & Cardon, 1992) have provided twin researchers with greatly refined procedures for estimating variance components. These analyses characterize the current wave of twin research in gerontology.

A few twin studies have had the opportunity to combine the logic of twin studies with that of adoption studies. One such is the Swedish Adoption Study of Aging (SATSA; Pedersen, Friberg, Floderus-Myrhed, McClearn, & Plomin, 1984), which involves MZ and DZ twins (most over 50 years of age, with an average at the time of first testing of 65.6 years) who were reared apart (for greater or lesser parts of their childhood; average age of separation was 2.8 years, with 48% separated during the first year of life) along with twins reared conventionally. This capability has provided enhanced power to distinguish between the environmental components of variance. For example, shared environmental effects are indicated if MZ twins who were reared apart are less similar than MZs reared together; DZ twins provide similar information. Thus, the comparisons of the structural equation analyses basically involve both zygosity and rearing circumstances. The components extracted from such analyses can variously include additive and nonadditive genetic influence, and shared and non-shared environmental influence, depending on the model employed. SATSA assays a broad variety of behavioral and biomedical phenotypes and of putative environmental influences. Within the behavioral domain, there is an emphasis on personality and on cognitive variables.

Personality

In the realm of personality, an example of the outcome of variance decomposition via structural equation modeling is the analysis by Plomin, Pedersen, McClearn, Nesselroade, & Bergeman (1988) of the phenotypes assessed by the widely studied EAS temperaments (Emotionality-distress; Emotionality-fear; Emotionality-anger; Activity and Sociability). Figure 10.4 shows estimates of the percentage of variance attributable to additive genetic (Ga), dominance (Gd), shared environmental (Es), and non-shared environmental (Ens) sources (which also includes measurement error). The narrow-sense heritabilities differ greatly, with only Emotionality-distress, Emotionality-anger and Sociability having measurable additive genetic variance. Broad-sense heritabilities, assessing both additive genetic and dominance variance, range from about .20 to about .40.

Various other personality measures were similarly assessed by Pedersen, Lichenstein, and colleagues (1989) who used a modified version of the Framingham Scale. This instrument provided an overall type-A behavior

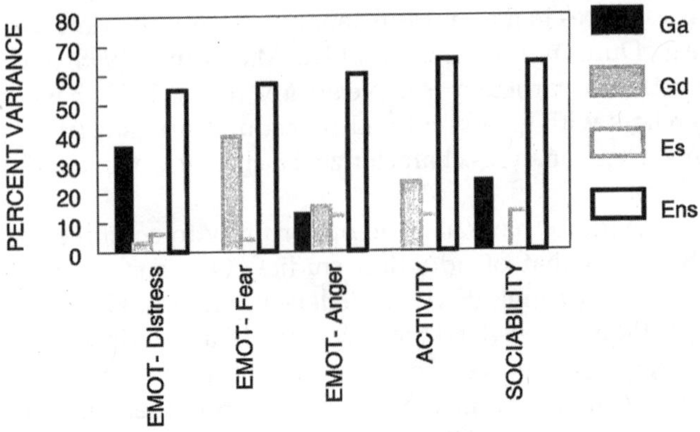

FIGURE 10.4 Variance components for several personality phenotypes assessed in the Swedish Adoption/Twin Study of Aging. (Ga = Additive Genetic; Gd = Dominance Genetic; Es = Shared Environment; Ens = Non-shared environment). Analyses were based on responses of 99 pairs of MZ twins reared apart, 229 Dz pairs reared apart, 160 MZ pairs reared together, and 212 DZ pairs reared together. The measures were derived from the EAS Temperament Survey; 3 Emotionality scales are Distress, Fear, and Anger; other scales assess Activity and Sociability. Data from Plomin et al. (1988).

index, with three subscales derived by principal components analysis: Pressure (life stress); Hard-driving (self-imposed demands in interpersonal interactions); and Ambitious (self-imposed demands in interactions not involving other people). In addition, a measure of Hostility and another measure of lack of assertiveness (inhibition of aggression) were administered. In a separate study, Pedersen, Gatz, Plomin, Nesselroade, and McClearn (1989), investigated three dimensions of perceptions of Locus of Control. Results of both of these studies are given in Table 10.1.

Considering these personality measures, genetic influence is detectable for all, with the exception of the Luck scale of the Locus of Control instrument, which has no detectable genetic influence whatsoever. The heritability estimates vary, ranging from 12% to 43%. There is an evident concentration, however, in the range from 27% to 43%. This level of influence is substantial; nevertheless, most of the variance is clearly due to environmental factors. A striking and counterintuitive result is the relative absence of influence of shared rearing environment. That environmental factors unique to individuals are the primary origin of variability in most of these phenotypes gives a general direction for attempts to identify effective environmental factors. Furthermore, the exceptional cases in which shared environments have a detectable effect invite scrutiny of shared family environments (10% to 30% of the variance in a complex system is no small influence, after all).

TABLE 10.1 Percentages of Variance from Different Sources and Broad-Sense Heritability

Personality measure	Ga	Gd	Ens	Es	Broad-sense heritability
Framingham	27	0	62	11	27
Pressure	28	0	60	12	28
Hard-driving	0	43	57	0	43
Ambitious	0	37	63	0	37
Hostility	20	0	59	20	20
Aggression inhibition		12	69	19	12
Luck	0	0	69	31	0
Responsibility	34	0	66	0	34
Life direction	31	0	69	0	31

Note: From "Individual Differences in Locus Control" by N. L. Pedersen, M. Gatz, et al., 1989, *Journals of Gerontology: Psychological Sciences, 44,* p. 100. Adapted with permission. "Genetic and Environmental Influences" by N. L. Pedersen, P. Lichtenstein, et al., 1989, *Psychosomatic Medicine, 50,* p. 428. Copyright © The Gerontological Society of America. Reproduced by permission of the publisher.

Cognition

One of the most actively pursued areas of behavioral genetics research is that of human cognitive processes. A review by Bouchard and McGue in 1981 and a revision of the published evidence from more than 100 studies by McGue, Bouchard, Iacono, and Lykken (1993) gives persuasive evidence of genetic influence on measures of general intelligence. Most of the evidence, obtained from resemblance of twins, siblings, half-siblings, cousins, and parents/offspring was obtained from individuals less than 20 years of age. In general, the heritability of IQ is estimated at about 51% from ages 4 to 20. The effective environmental component appears to be non-shared, however. In their review, McGue, Bouchard, et al. (1993) examine the direct evidence obtained from relationships between adopted siblings. The average IQ correlation in childhood from seven studies was 0.25, indicating a substantial role at that age of shared environmental factors. From three studies of adult adoptees, however, the average correlation was –.01. The influence of a shared rearing environment in generating similarities among biologically unrelated individuals had disappeared in adulthood.

From the point of view of gerontological genetics, it is essential, of course, to extend twin observations into late adulthood. Several longitudinal programs are now in progress. The SATSA program, for example, includes an extensive battery of cognitive tests, from which a general intelligence index was computed by principal component analysis (Pedersen, Plomin, Nesselroade, & McClearn, 1992). Eighty one percent of the phenotypic variance was explained by genetic sources, with the remaining 19% accounted for by non-shared environmental sources. This extraordinary value is one of the largest ever described in the behavioral genetics literature and is exceeded by few anatomical or physiological phenotypes (the estimated heritability for the prototype trait of body weight is 70% [Plomin et al., 2000]). Similar results from the Minnesota Twin Study of Adult Development and Aging (MTSADA) were reported by McGue, Hirsch, and Lykken (1993). This report covered an age range from 11 to 88 years, with a preponderance of subjects in the 11–12 years and 60–88 years categories. Analysis of these age groups concluded that IQ heritability increases from about 50% in preadolescents to about 80% in older adults.

Finkel, Pedersen, McGue, and McClearn (1995) compared MTSADA and SATSA data in parallel analyses with three defined age groups (27 to 50 years; 50 to 65 years; 65 to 88 years). Heritabilities of the youngest groups were the same for the two populations. For the older group of Swedish twins, however, there was a significant reduction to a heritability of 54%. A subsequent extension into older ages has been made in the OCTO-Twin study, which addresses genetic and environmental influences on an array of age-related variables in Swedish octogenarian and nonagenarian twins (median age 82.3 years at the time of first measurement). McClearn et al. (1997) evaluated general intelligence through a principal components analysis of measures of specific cognitive abilities and from a short version of the Wechsler Adult Intelligence Scale. Heritability estimates for the former and latter indices were 62% and 53% respectively. Shared environmental influences were estimated to be 11% and 15% respectively. This result appears to confirm a reduction in heritability of general intelligence in the old-old. It should be noted, however, that this level of genetic influence is still remarkably high. The reappearance of evidence of shared environmental influence is also noteworthy.

The congruence of the results of these two studies is important because, as noted earlier, heritability estimates are logically specific to the population investigated. The gene pools and the environmental circumstances of the two populations are certainly not as different as could be selected, but they are far from identical. As a consequence, the joint findings of high heritability of IQ well into older age ranges appear to indicate at least some range of generality to their estimates.

Temporal Considerations

Many of these twin results (and those of the preceding animal studies) indicate differences in genetic influence at different ages. Several analyses have focused on issues of variability, change, and stability in advanced age. Plomin, Pedersen, Lichtenstein, and McClearn (1994) applied longitudinal model-fitting analyses to the SATSA cognitive data from the first two measurement occasions, 3 years apart. The high heritability of general intelligence that was found on the first occasion was also found for the second. The stability across occasions was very high: the test–retest correlation was .92, and genetic factors accounted for 90% of this stability.

Not surprisingly, not all phenotypes yield such simple results. McGue and Christensen (1997), for example, investigated depression in Danish twins aged 75 years and older with an instrument that yielded an Affect subscale, a Somatic subscale, and an overall index. Heritabilities were estimated to be 27%, 31%, and 34%, respectively for these three measures. All heritable effects on the Affect and Somatic subscales could be attributed to a single genetic factor (as defined from the multivariate analysis—not a single gene!). Heritability did not vary over the age range.

Carmelli and Reed (2000) also examined symptoms of depression in a longitudinal study of male American twins from the National Heart, Lung, and Blood Institute Twin Study. Heritability was estimated to be 25% at 63 years of age (range from 59 to 70) and 10 years later 55%. The stability of symptoms was found to be due primarily to continuity of genetic influences. The heritability estimate on the first occasion was very similar to that of the overall measure in the McGue and Christensen study (1997), but the second occasion was rather higher. From the same study population Carmelli and Reed (2000), conducted a study of hand-grip-strength. Additive genetic, shared environmental, and non-shared environmental components were respectively 35%, 39%, and 26% at baseline and 22%, 45%, and 33% at the second occasion. Grip strength declined significantly in the 10-year interval, but the test-retest correlation was 0.62. It was estimated that genetic and shared environmental influences accounted for 35% and 48% of this stability, respectively.

Harris, Pedersen, Stacey, McClearn, and Nesselroade (1992) utilized similar analytical procedures to evaluate in the SATSA data the role of genetic and environmental influences on the widely observed correlation between the self-reported variables of Life Satisfaction and Health. The phenotypic correlations were 0.38 for the younger members of the SATSA sample (<65 years), and 0.47 for the older age group (65 years and older). In the younger group, all of the correlation could be attributed to environmental sources; in the older group about half (47%) of the correlation could be attributed to genetic factors, and 53% to non-shared environmental influences.

The varying results from this sample of studies are reminiscent of the particularity observed in the animal studies. Together, these databases make it clear that the question of whether heritability increases or decreases with advancing age, of whether genetic factors or environmental ones contribute to stability or change, or whether phenotypic correlations are due to genes or environments cannot receive a simple answer. It depends upon the phenotype, upon the gene pool of the population being studied, and upon the array of environmental circumstances to which they are exposed.

There is a rich body of empirical fact and of theory to provide a context for interpreting these whole-organism, quantitative trait results—the burgeoning field of molecular developmental genetics. This intricate field of investigation is concerned with the regulation of gene expression, with a natural emphasis on the changing engagement of genes in early developmental processes, and has revealed amazing intricacies of processes and their timing. There have long been intimations of age-related differences in gene expression in later life with late-onset diseases such as Huntington's disease and the various dementias. It is the case, of course, that a responsible gene could have been producing gene product from early life, with some cumulative consequence that ultimately reaches a critical threshold. Alternatively, it might be that relevant loci are either turning on or off, or are being down-regulated or up-regulated. For any given phenotype, particularly a complex one with polygenic influence, all of the preceding might pertain. Even though the specific mechanisms may not yet be known, the successes of the molecular developmental geneticists have provided gerontologists with enormously powerful heuristic models.

Specific Abilities

Throughout much of the indicated research, a finer grain of cognitive functioning has also been considered in addition to global intelligence. Specific cognitive abilities are variously conceptualized and measured in an active research area that is beyond the scope of the present review. One useful taxonomy identifies verbal and spatial abililties, perceptual speed, and memory. In SATSA, heritabilities of these specific abilities were reported as 58%, 46%, 58%, and 38%, respectively (Pedersen et al., 1992). In OCTO-Twin, the comparable values were 55%, 32%, 62%, and 52%, respectively. Shared environmental components of 20% and 13% were found for verbal and spatial abilities, respectively, but none for speed of processing or memory. An expanded array of tasks in the OCTO-Twin battery permitted a detailed analysis of six facets of memory function (Johansson et al., 1999). Figure 10.5 shows the results. Heritability estimates range from .04 to .49. Shared environmental influences are detectable for Digits

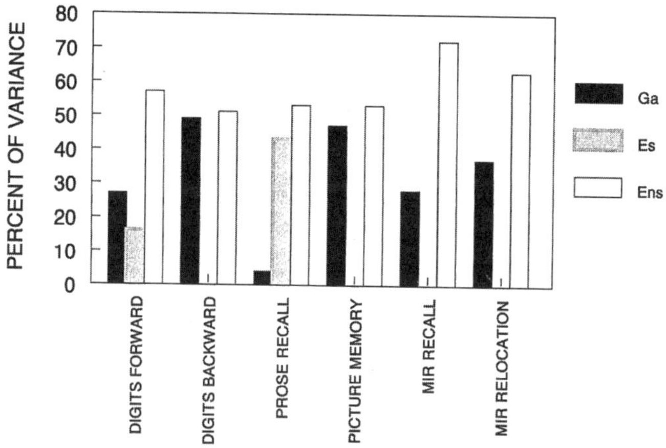

FIGURE 10.5 Variance components for several measures of memory assessed in the Swedish Adoption/Twin Study of Aging. (Ga = Additive Genetic; Es = Shared Environment; Ens = Non-shared Environment). Measures included Digit Span Forward, Digit Span Backward, Prose Recall (memory for 100-word story), Thurstone's Picture Memory Test, and Memory-in-Reality (involving location of items in a model home). Complete data were available for approximately half of the subjects enumerated in Figure 10.4. Data from Johansson et al. (1999).

Forward (ability to remember spoken digits for varying periods of time), and are very substantial for Prose Recall (immediate free recall of a brief story), which displays little if any genetic influence.

The finer structure of cognition was explored in another manner by Petrill et al. (2001), addressed the question of whether the same genetic and environmental structure underlies cognitive functioning through the entire continuum. Equivocal results had been obtained in earlier studies on this issue in young subjects. In older adults (the SATSA sample), Saudino, Plomin, Pedersen, and McClearn (1994) estimated group heritabilities (the extent to which the difference between the mean of a selected extreme group and the unselected population mean is due to genetic factors). They concluded that the etiology of extreme high and extreme low ability was the same as that for the normal range. Petrill et al. (2001) examined the Wechsler Adult Intelligence Scale data from the older OCTO-Twin sample (average age 82.3 years), and found a contrasting result, as shown in Figure 10.6.

The heritability of general intelligence previously reported in this group (53%) clearly cloaks considerable structural heterogeneity. With cutoffs successively at the 90th, 80th, 70th, and 60th percentiles, heritability is as high as that reported in the younger SATSA sample. With a 40th

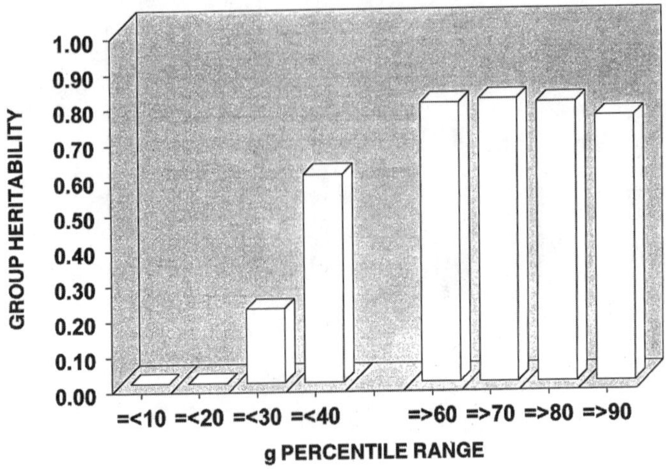

FIGURE 10.6 Group heritability estimates of different levels of cognitive functioning. Each bar represents group heritability estimate for subjects performing at or above the 60th, 70th, 80th, or 90th percentile, or at or below the 40th, 30th, 20th, or 10th percentile. Subjects were 110 pairs of MZ twins and 130 pairs of same-sex DZ twins (all nondemented) participating in the OCTO-Twin study of Swedish octogenarians and nonagenarians. The cognitive performance measure was a short form of the Wechsler Adult Intelligence Scale–Information and Block Design subtests. Data from Petrill et al. (2001).

and a 30th percentile cutoff, the heritability estimates drop, and below the 20th percentile, there is no evidence of genetic influence whatsoever. With possible implications for the terminal drop phenomenon, the contrast of these results with that of younger populations suggests a change in the etiology of low cognitive performance in the old-old. It remains to be seen how many apparently uniform phenotypic continua will similarly show increasing genetic heterogeneity in advanced age.

Single Locus Genetics

The foregoing has been concerned with polygenic systems underlying continuously distributed phenotypes. Phenotypes that are di- or trichotomous—typical of Mendelian genetics—can be regarded as limiting cases of the quantitative genetic model, where the number of genes in the genetic aggregate equals one. In the case of so-called major genes (those loci at which allelic differences of the single gene lead to categorical differences at the phenotypic level) genetical analysis can proceed by traditional Mendelian methods. The distribution of the categorical phenotypes within families yields interpretations in terms of the well-known phenomena of dominance and recessivity and, in some cases, permits localization of the loci on chromosomes through linkage analysis. There are many examples of single locus influence on age-related phenotypes (see, for example, several chapters in Harrison [1990] for reviews and examples).

With respect to behavior, there is keen interest at present in loci that influence the risk of developing dementia. The age-associated dementias are a heterogeneous complex with diverse etiologies (Hardy & Duff, 1993). Alzheimer's disease (AD) is a preponderant form, accounting for perhaps half of cases. Twin studies (Bergeman, 1997; Breitner et al., 1995; Gatz et al., 1997; Raiha, Kaprio, Koskenvuo, Rajala, & Sourander, 1996) have provided evidence for genetic influence on the likelihood of developing AD in Finnish, Swedish, Norwegian, and American populations. In addition, several specific loci have been identified. Three loci, for example, are implicated in early-onset AD: *PS1* for presenilin-1 on chromosome 14 (St. George-Hyslop et al., 1992); *PS2* for presenilin-2 on chromosome 1 (Hardy & Hutton, 1995); and a locus for beta-amyloid on chromosome 21 (St. George-Hyslop et al., 1987; see also Campion et al., 1999; Crook et al., 1997, 1998; Lenden, Ashall, & Goate, 1997). These early-onset cases constitute a small fraction of the Alzheimer's cases. Accordingly, research activity has been particularly intense in relation to observation of a relationship between the *ApoE* locus on chromosome 19 and late-onset AD (Corder et al., 1993). The meta-analysis of Farrer et al. (1997), involving 5,930 AD patients and 8,607 controls, summarizes the general findings. In Caucasians, the risks for the different genotypes derived from the ε2, ε3, and ε4 alleles at this locus are as shown in Table 10.2.

The risk of developing AD if heterozygous for the ε4 allele is apparent, and the risk if homozygous for that allele is much higher. This association is stronger in Japanese, but weaker among African Americans and Hispanics. The ε4 effect is present between the ages of 40 and 90, but becomes less pronounced after 70 years of age. Nonetheless, as Myers et al. (2000) have pointed out, the ε4 allele is neither necessary nor sufficient to determine Alzheimer's disease. About half of AD patients do not possess even one ε4 allele.

Of the AD cases not relatable to *ApoE* status, some may be due to the cumulative small effects of polygenes. That other major loci may be involved, however, is indicated by the recent simultaneous publications by Myers et al. (2000), Bertram et al. (2000), and Ertekin-Taner et al. (2000) describing a new susceptibility locus for AD on chromosome 10. It is estimated that the relative risks associated with this locus are about equal to those associated with *ApoE*.

In addition to the risk of developing the disease, there is some evidence that the ε4 allele is associated with rate of progression. Craft et al. (1998)

TABLE 10.2 Odds Ratios for Developing Alzheimer's Disease for Different *ApoE* Genotypes

ApoE genotype	Odds/Ratio
ε2ε2	0.6
ε2ε3	0.6
ε2ε4	2.6
ε3ε4	3.2
ε4ε4	14.9

Note: From "Effects of Age, Sex, and Ethnicity" by L. A. Farrer et al., 1997, *Journal of the American Medical Association, 278*, p. 1349. Adapted with permission.

examined newly diagnosed probable AD patients at baseline and then annually for 1 to 6 years on a Dementia Rating Scale. Homozygous ε4ε4 individuals displayed a higher rate of cognitive decline than did the other genotypes. Also pertinent is the observation (Del Bo et al., 1997) of the association of the ε4 allele with a faster rate of decline in cognitive functioning of Down syndrome patients. However, evidence concerning rate of progression is not unequivocal. Holmes, Levy, McLoughlin, Powell, and Lovestone (1996) in an English sample of 164 AD patients found that possession of an ε4 allele was associated with an earlier age of onset but *not* with severity or with more rapid progression.

A related topic that has promoted strenuous research efforts is the possible effect of the ε4 allele in nondemented individuals. A substantial body of data is accumulating (of which only a sampling can be cited here), suggesting that, possession of an ε4 allele may indeed have deleterious consequences within the normal range of cognitive functioning. Bondi et al. (1995), administered a verbal learning test to nondemented older adults. Those with at least one ε4 allele performed less well than those with none. Some of the former, but none of the latter, developed AD or possible AD during a follow-up period. Consistent results were obtained by Yaffe, Cauley, Sands, and Browner (1997) who compared nondemented community-dwelling women with and without an ε4 allele on several cognitive tests at baseline and 6 years later. Those with one or more ε4 alleles had significantly poorer performance on all tests. Chey, Kim and Cho (2000) demonstrated a similar outcome in a population of nondemented older Korean adults. Differential effects on cognitive functioning are suggested in a report by Bondi, Salmon, Galasko, Thomas, and Thal (1999) who described inferior performance of ε4-possessing older adults on a delayed recall memory task, but not on a variety of other tasks. Flory, Manuck,

Ferrell, Ryan, and Muldoon (2000) extended the age range in a study of healthy middle-aged (24 to 60 years old) adults. Those with at least one ε4 performed more poorly on several learning and memory tasks, but attention span did not differ according to genotype. The authors conclude that ε4 is either a marker for age-related cognitive decline or a marker for lifelong poorer performance.

These striking results are not without exception. Small et al. (2000) examined randomly selected, community-based older adults and found no evidence of ε4 effect on measures of episodic memory, psychomotor speed, and attention. These authors conclude that ε4 is *not* a risk factor for cognitive impairment in normal aging.

COACTIVITY OF GENES AND ENVIRONMENT

The simple formulation $V_P = V_G + V_E$, serves for many analytical purposes, but there are some potential complications that must be kept in mind. A more complete statement adds three more broad terms:

$$V_P = V_G + V_E + V_I + V_{GE} + 2Cov_{GE}$$

Where V_I refers to interactions among genes, V_{GE} refers to interactions of genes with environments, and $2Cov_{GE}$ refers to a covarying of genes with environment. This is still a simplified representation, in that, for example, V_G can be divided further into V_A and V_D, and V_E can be subdivided into V_{ES} and V_{ENS} as already noted. The interaction terms can likewise be decomposed. Reference should be made to Falconer and Mackay (1996) for detailed presentation.

Gene–Gene Interaction

The interaction of genes with other genes is termed epistasis. Basically, this term refers to situations in which the effect of a difference in genotype at a particular locus depends upon the genotype at some other locus. There are may examples of such interactions throughout the various specialties of genetics. In recent years, the proliferation of examples at the molecular genetics level are illuminating the basic mechanisms through which the interactions are occurring.

At the level of complex phenotypes, a classic example is that of Coleman and Hummel (1975) who demonstrated the interaction of a specific identified locus that "causes" diabetes in mice with an unknown number of loci represented in the genotype of different inbred strains. When the *db/db* genotype (homozygous for the recessive alleles) is located in the C57BL/6 strain, there was a rise to about 185 mg% of blood glucose levels at 4 to 5 months of age, with a subsequent drop to 129 mg% at 6 months, and hypertrophy of the pancreatic islet cells. The same *db/db* genotype on the background of the C57BL/Ks strain attained a blood glucose level of 400 mg% by 6 months of age and showed atrophy of the islet cells. This dramatic difference in effect of a single locus genotype when on different but related genetic backgrounds serves a cautionary note about identifying a particular gene as "the gene for" some phenotype.

In a current example of direct relevance to the present topic, Kamboh, Sanghera, Ferrell, & DeKosky, (1995) report a gene-gene interaction involving *ApoE*. The risk of AD associated with the ε4 allele is significantly affected by the genotype of another locus *(ACT)* that codes for α1-antichymotrypsin. The risk associated with ε4 allele dosage was unchanged for individuals heterozygous for the *A* and *T* alleles of the *ACT* locus. Homozygous *TT* individuals showed no greater risk if they possessed two rather than only one ε4 allele at the *ApoE* locus; this genotype was described as protective against the added effect of the second ε4 allele. For *AA* individuals, the risk associated with ε4 was increased twofold, and individuals homozygous ε4/ε4 and *AA* were extremely susceptible. Clearly, even such a robust effect as that of the ε4 allele must be interpreted in the genetic context in which it occurs. Such epistatic dependencies may account for the different effect size of the ε4 allele in different populations (Farrer et al., 1997; Osuntokun et al., 1995; Sahota et al., 1997; Tang et al., 1998). Alternatively, there may be a subtle gene–environment interaction of the sort discussed in the following section.

Gene–Environment Interaction

Gene–environment interaction occurs when the effect of genotype depends on environmental circumstances, or, conversely, when the effect of an environmental factor depends upon the genotype on which it impinges. The many examples of strain differences cited previously can be regarded as examples at the quantitative genetic level of such interactions. Animals of different genotypes respond differently to the particular environmental circumstances—intertrial interval, shock level, difficulty of maze—of the test situation. Another example involved the chronic administration of the specific nutritional environment of food with elevated levels of aluminum content (Fosmire, Focht, & McClearn, 1993). The study was motivated by conflicting evidence on aluminum as a risk factor in Alzheimer's disease and sought to demonstrate genetic influence on the impact of an environmental variable. The point was clearly made by virtue of the fact that only two of five inbred strains presented with this diet showed substantial elevation of brain aluminum levels. Thus, susceptibility to the effects of adverse environments (or, equally, to the beneficial effects of therapeutic or preventive environments) may depend greatly upon genotype.

Two pertinent examples relate to *ApoE* status. Yaffe, Haan, Byers, Tangen, and Kuller (2000) showed that estrogen use among women 65 years of age and older reduced risk of cognitive impairment among ε4-negative women, but it did not reduce the risk among ε4-positive women. An example of interaction of *ApoE* status with a self-selected environment is provided by Dufoil et al. (2000). Cognitive performance of French subjects aged 59–71 was assessed at time of entry into the study and 4 years later. Alcohol consumption was significantly associated with decreased risk of cognitive deterioration in non-ε4 individuals, but with enhanced risk in those with an ε4 allele. Among smokers, those with ε4 were at decreased risk and non-ε4 carriers were at increased risk.

A dramatic demonstration of the scope for gene-environment interactions is provided by Vieira and colleagues (2000) who evaluated quantitative trait loci (QTLs) affecting longevity in *Drosophila melanogaster* reared in five different environments distinguished by temperature or food availability. (The term quantitative trait locus refers to a locus identified by association with the phenotype but localized only to a region of the chromosome, not to a definite location.) The variety of interactions was astounding. Some of the loci influenced only one sex; some were influential in only a subset of the environments and not in others; some influenced only one sex in one of the environments. As a brief summary, the authors noted that *all* genetic variance in this situation was associated with genotype X sex or genotype X environment interactions.

The analytic models for quantitatively distributed phenotypes are relatively inefficient at identification of the genotype-environment interactions, and relatively few have been described. An explicit attempt to identify interaction of genotype with rearing environment in personality development was undertaken by Bergeman, Plomin, McClearn, Pedersen, and Friedberg (1988). Eleven significant interactions were identified, which example will illustrate: Individuals with a genotype associated with high extraversion (assessed by measurement of twin partner) are not affected by a "controlling" or "restrictive" rearing environment; those with a genotype associated with low extraversion are affected by these environmental features. Though the total amount of variance accounted for by these interactions amounted only to 7%, the outcome is heuristically valuable.

Gene–Environment Covariance

A covariance of genes and environments arises when individuals with genotypes that influence a phenotype in a certain direction encounter environments with similar influences. Behavioral geneticists distinguish three types: passive, evocative, and active (Plomin et al., 2000). Parents with genotypes making for higher cognitive function, for an example of the passive type, could provide children with genes and a supportive environment (books, schools, encouragement) that would operate in the same direction. Evocative covariance occurs when some (genetically influenced) attribute of the individual evokes a differential response from the environment. Active covariance occurs when on the basis of genetically influenced propensities, the individual seeks out or constructs particular aspects of the environment. Some examples from invertebrate research illustrate the active type convincingly. Rodriguez, Sokolowski, and Shore (1992), for example, established strains of *Drosophila* by collecting pupae from two microhabitats (on or off fruit). Strain by environment interactions influenced habitat choice behavior, with a positive correlation between habitat suitability and larval habitat choice behavior.

Cavener (1979) studied preference for ethanol in *Drosophila melanogaster.* Two groups of flies, homozygous for different alleles at the alcohol dehydrogenase locus, were involved. These two genotypes (Adh^F/Adh^F and Adh^S/Adh^S; abbreviated *FF* and *SS*, respectively) were on genetically varied backgrounds. *FF* larvae and adults have much higher ADH activity level than do *SS* larvae and adults. No significant differences were found in oviposition site choices by females, but in preference tests (preference for medium with or without alcohol), the *FF* larvae show a 2 to 1 preference for the medium containing alcohol. *SS* larvae were indifferent, showing a 50-50 preference.

In human situations, the selection or manipulation of environments can lead to the superficially paradoxical result of a genetic influence on environment. As an example, (Plomin, Lichtenstein, Pedersen, McClearn, & Nesselroade, 1990) found that 40% of the variance of the total score measuring the occurrence of significant life events is due to genetic differences among individuals from the SATSA sample. Kendler, Neale, Kessler, Heath, and Eaves (1993) also examined life events in subjects in the Virginia Twin Registry, finding that genetic and shared environmental sources each accounted for about 20% of the total variance.

Family environmental circumstances of the SATSA twins were investigated by Plomin, McClearn, Pedersen, Nesselroade, and Bergeman (1989) who showed an average heritability of 24% for the Moos Family Environment Scales. Such genetic influence on self-reported environment features could, of course, be mediated through the evocative dynamic mentioned earlier, or it could represent genetically influenced bias in social perception and memory.

Yet another way in which genetic and environmental forces are intertwined is illustrated by the research (Smith, Banerjee, Gold, & Glowa, 1992), which shows not only that behavioral stressors can result in increased gene expression in certain regions of the brain, but that classical conditioning can have a similar effect.

SUMMARY

Each of the various research designs and analytical methods that have generated the data presented here has its limitations, but collectively they paint a broad picture of strong hereditary influence on behavioral aging. The examples that have been given reveal the complexities at the phenotypic level and hint at the nature of the complexities of the mechanisms underlying those phenotypic manifestations. The future research directions will undoubtedly engage integrative notions of complex biological systems. The building blocks for this integrative effort will be information about the individual elements of the polygenic systems that influence the complex phenotypes. That information is already growing at a phenomenal rate, yet additional power is promised by the ability to identify quantitative trait loci, to manipulate single genes by transgenic procedures, to assemble genotypes to specification, and, with microchip arrays, to examine the ebb and flow of gene expression across developmental stages. This will give us unprecedented and, until very recently, unimaginable capabilities to identify the dynamics of interactions and co-actions of the various compartments of genetics and environment factors. A decade hence, a review of this topic—the genetics of behavioral aging—will have much more to say.

ACKNOWLEDGMENT

Supported by the National Institute on Aging (grants AG08861, AG14731, AG06543, and AG10175) of the National Institutes of Health.

REFERENCES

Bergeman, C. S. (1997). *Aging: Genetic and environmental influences.* Newbury Park, CA: Sage.

Bergeman, C. S., Plomin, R., McClearn, G. E., Pedersen, N. L., & Friberg, L. T. (1988). Genotype-environment interaction in personality development: Identical twins reared apart. *Psychology and Aging, 3,* 399–406.

Bertram, L., Blacker, D., Mullin, K., Keeney, D., Jones, J., Basu, S., Yhu, S., McInnis, M. G., Go, R. C. P., Vekrellis, K., Selkoe, D. J., Saunders, A.

J., & Tanzi, R. E. (2000). Evidence for genetic linkage of Alzheimer's disease to chromosome 10q. *Science, 290,* 2302–2303.

Blum, A. D., Fosshage, J. L., & Jarvik, L. F. (1972). Intellectual changes and sex differences in octogenarians: A twenty-year longitudinal study of aging. *Developmental Psychology, 7,* 178–187.

Bondi, M. W., Salmon, D. P., Galasko, D., Thomas, R. G., & Thal, L. J. (1999). Neuropsychological function and apolipoprotein E genotype in the preclinical detection of Alzheimer's disease. *Psychology and Aging, 14,* 295–303.

Bondi, M. W., Salmon, D. P., Monsch, A. U., Galasko, D., Butters, N., Klauber, M. R., Thal, L. J., & Saitoh, T. (1995). Episodic memory changes are associated with the APOE-epsilon 4 allele in nondemented older adults. *Neurology, 45,* 2203–2206.

Bouchard, T. J., Jr. & McGue, M. (1981). Familial studies of intelligence: A review. *Science, 250,* 223–238.

Breitner, J. C., Welsh, K. A., Gau, B. A., McDonald, W. M., Steffens, D. C., Saunders, A. M., Magruder, K. M., Helms, M. J., Plassman, B. L., Folstein, M. F., et al. (1995). Alzheimer's disease in the National Academy of Sciences-National Research Council Registry of aging twin Bererans III. Detection of cases, longitudinal results, and observations on twin concordance. *Archives of Neurology, 52,* 763–771.

Campion, D., Dumanchin, C., Hannequin, D., Dubois, B., Belliard, S., Puel, M., Thomas-Anterion, C., Michon, A., Martin, C., Charbonnier, F., Raux, G., Camuzat, A., Penet, C., Mesnage, V., Martinez, M., Clerget-Darpoux, F., Brice, A., & Frebourg, T. (1999). Early-onset autosomal dominant Alzheimer's disease: Prevalence, genetic heterogeneity, and mutation spectrum. *American Journal of Human Genetics, 65,* 664–670.

Carmelli, D., & Reed, T. (2000). Stability and change in genetic and environmental influences on hand-grip strength in older male twins. *Journal of Applied Physioilogy, 89,* 1879–1883.

Cavener, D. (1979). Preference for ethanol in *Drosophila melanogaster* associated with the alcohol dehydrogenase polymorphism. *Behavior Genetics, 9,* 359–365.

Chey, J., Kim, J. W., & Cho, H. Y. (2000). Effects of apolipoprotein E phenotypes on the neuropsychological functions of community-dwelling elderly individuals without dementia. *Neuroscience Letter, 289,* 230–234.

Coleman, D. L., & Hummel, K. P. (1975). Influence of genetic background on the expression of mutations at the diabetes locus in the mouse II. Studies on background modifiers. *Israeli Journal of Medical Science, 11,* 708–713.

Corder, E. H., Saunders, A. M., Strittmatter, W. J., Shmechel, D. E., Gaskell, P. C., Small, G. W., Roses, A. D., Haines, J. L., & Pericak-Vance, M. A.

(1993). Gene dose of apolipoprotein E type 4 allele and the risk of Alzheimer's disease in late onset families. *Science, 261*, 921–923.
Crady, D. D., & Quinton, E. E. (1989). Dissociation of learning and performance deficits in aged mice. *Experimental Aging Research, 15*, 143–150.
Craft, S., Teri, L., Edland, S. D., Kuwull, W. A., Schellenberg, G., McCormick, W. C., Bowen, J. D., & Larson, E. B. (1998). Accelerated decline in apolipoprotein E-epsilon4 homozygotes with Alzheimer's disease. *Neurology, 51*, 149–153.
Crook, R., Ellis, R., Shanks, M., Thal, L. J., Perez-Tur, J., Baker, M., Hutton, M., Haltia, T., Hardy, J., & Galasko, D. (1997). Early-onset Alzheimer's disease with a presenilin-1 mutation at the site corresponding to the Volga German presenilin-2 mutation. *Annals of Neurology, 42*, 124–128.
Crook, R., Verkkoniemi, A., Perez-Tur, J., Mehta, N., Baker, M., Houlden, H., Farrer, M., Hutton, M., Lincoln, S., Hardy, J., Gwinn, K., Somer, M., Paetau, A., Kalmio, H., Ylikoski, R., Poyhonen, M., Kucera, S., & Haltia, M. (1998). A variant of Alzheimer's disease with spastic paraparesis and unusual plaques due to deletion of exon 9 of presenilin 1. *Nature Medicine, 4*, 452–455.
Del Bo, R., Comi, P., Bresolin, N., Castelli, E., Conti, E., Degiuli, A., Ausends, C. D., & Scarlato, G. (1997). The apolipoprotein E epsilon4 allele causes a faster decline of cognitive performances in Down's syndrome subjects. *Journal of Neurological Science, 145*, 87–91.
Dufouil, C., Tzourio, C., Brayne, C., Berr, C., Amouyel, P., & Alpérovitch, A. (2000). Influence of apolipoprotein E genotype on the risk of cognitive deterioration in moderate drinkers and smokers. *Epidemiology, 11*, 280–284.
Duncan, O. D. (1975). *Introduction to structural equation models.* New York: Academic Press.
Ertekin-Taner, N., Graff-Radford, N., Younkin, L. H., Eckman, C., Baker, M., Adamson, J., Ronald, J., Blangero, J., Hutton, M., & Younkin, S. G. (2000). Linkage of plasma Ab42 to a quantitative locus on chromosome 10 in late-onset Alzheimer's disease pedigrees. *Science, 290*, 2303–2304.
Falconer, D. C., & Mackay, T. F. C. (1996). *Introduction to quantitative genetics* (4th ed.). Harlow, UK: Longman.
Farrer, L. A., Cupples, L. A., Haines, J. L., Hyman, B., Kukull, W. A., Mayeux, R., Myers, R. H., Pericak-Vance, M. A., Risch, N., & van Duijn, C. M. (1997). Effects of age, sex, and ethnicity on the association between apolipoprotein E genotype and Alzheimer's disease. A meta-analysis. APOE and Alzheimer's disease Meta Analysis Consortium. *Journal of the American Medical Association, 278*, 1349–1356.
Finkel, D., Pedersen, N. L., McGue, M., & McClearn, G. E. (1995). Heritability of cognitive abilities in adult twins: Comparison of Minnesota and Swedish data. *Behavior Genetics, 25*, 421–431.

Fisher, R. A. (1918). The correlation between relatives on the supposition of Mendelian inheritance. *Transactions of the Royal Society of Edinburgh, 52,* 399–433.

Flory, J. D., Manuck, S. B., Ferrell, R. E., Ryan, C. M., & Muldoon, M. F. (2000). Memory performance and the apolipoprotein E polymorphism in a community sample of middle-aged adults. *American Journal of Medical Genetics, 96,* 707–711.

Fosmire, G. J., Focht, S. J., & McClearn, G. E. (1993). Genetic influences on tissue deposition of aluminum in mice. *Biological Trace Element Research, 37,* 115–121.

Gatz, M., Pedersen, N. L, Berg, S., Johansson, B., Johansson, K., Mortimer, J. A., Posner, S. F., Viiatanen, M., Winblad, B., & Ahlbom, A. (1997). Heritability for Alzheimer's disease: The study of dementia in Swedish twins. *Journals of Gerontology Series A: Biological Science and Medical Science, 52,* M117–M125.

Gimpel, J. (1976). *The medieval machine.* New York: Holt, Rinehart & Winston.

Goodrick, C. L. (1975). Behavioral differences in young and aged mice: Strain differences for activity measures, operant learning, sensory discrimination, and alcohol preference. *Experimental Aging Research, 1,* 191–207.

Goodrick, C. L. (1978). Behavior genetics and aging. In E. L. Schneider (Ed.), *The genetics of aging* (pp. 403–415). New York: Plenum Press.

Hardy, J., & Duff, K. (1993). Heterogeneity in Alzheimer's disease. *Annals of Medicine, 25,* 437–440.

Hardy, J. A., & Hutton, M. (1995). Two new genes for Alzheimer's disease. *Trends in Neuroscience, 18,* 436.

Harris, J. R., Pedersen, N. L., Stacey, C., McClearn, G. E, & Nesselroade, J. R. (1992). Age differences in the etiology of the relationship between life satisfaction and self-rated health. *Journal of Aging and Health, 4,* 349–367.

Harrison, D. E. (Ed.) (1990). *Genetic effects on aging II.* Caldwell, NJ: The Telford Press.

Holmes, C., Levy, R., McLoughlin, D. M., Powell, J. F., & Lovestone, S. (1996). Apolipoprotein E: Non-cognitive symptoms and cognitive decline in late onset Alzheimer's disease. *Journal of Neurology, Neurosurgery, and Psychiatry, 61,* 580–583.

Ingram, D. K. (1985). Analysis of age-related impairments in learning and memory in rodent models. *Annals of the New York Academy of Sciences, 444,* 312–331.

Ingram, D. K. (1990). Perspectives on genetic variability in behavioral aging of mice. In D. E. Harrison (Ed.), *Genetic effects on aging II* (pp. 205–231). Caldwell, NJ: The Telford Press.

Jarvik, L. F., Blum, J. E., & Varma, A. D. (1972). Genetic components and intellectual functioning during senescence: A 20-year study of aging twins. *Behavior Genetics, 2,* 159–171.

Jarvik, L. F., Kallman, F. J., Falek, A., & Klaber, M. M. (1957). Changing intellectual functions in senescent twins. *Acta Genetica et Statistica Medica, 7,* 421–430.

Johansson, B., Whitfield, K., Pedersen, N. L., Hofer, S. M., Ahern, F., & McClearn, G. E. (1999). Origins of individual differences in episodic memory in the oldest-old: A population-based study of identical and same-sex fraternal twins aged 80 and older. *Journal of Gerontology: Psychological Sciences, 54B,* P173–P179.

Kakihana, R., & McClearn, G. E. (1963). Development of alcohol preference in BALB/c mice. *Nature, 199,* 511–512.

Kallman, F. J., & Jarvik, L. F. (1959). Individual differences in constitution and genetic background. In J. E. Birren (Ed.), *Aging and the individual.* University of Chicago Press.

Kamboh, M. I., Sanghera, D. K., Ferrell, R. E., & DeKosky, S. T. (1995). *APOE*4*-associated Alzheimer's disease risk is modified by a1-antichymotrypsin polymorphism. *Nature Genetics, 10,* 486–488.

Kendler, K. S., Neale, M., Kessler, R., Heath, A., & Eaves, L. (1993). A twin study of recent life events and difficulties. *Archives of General Psychiatry, 50,* 789–796.

Lenden, C. L., Ashall, F., & Goate, A. (1997). Exploring the etiology of Alzheimer's disease using molecular genetics. *Journal of the American Medical Association, 277,* 825–831.

Loehlin, J. C. (1992). *Latent variable models* (2nd ed.). Hillsdale, NJ: Lawrence Erlbaum.

Maruyama, G. M. (1998). *Basics of structural equation modeling.* Thousand Oaks: Sage.

McClearn, G. E., & Foch, T. T. (1985). Behavioral genetics. In J. E. Birren & K. W. Schaie (Eds.), *Handbook of the psychology of aging* (2nd ed., pp. 113–143). New York: Van Nostrand Reinhold.

McClearn, G. E. & Hofer, S. M. (1999). Genes as gerontological variables: Genetically heterogeneous stocks and complex systems. *Neurobiology of Aging, 20,* 147–156.

McClearn, G. E., Johansson, B., Berg, S., Pedersen, N. L., Ahern, F., Petrill, S. A., & Plomin, R. (1997). Substantial genetic influence on cognitive abilities in twins 80 or more years old. *Science, 276,* 1560–1563.

McClearn, G. E., & Meredith, W. (1964). Dimensional analysis of activity and elimination in a genetically heterogeneous group of mice *(Mus musculus). Animal Behaviour, 12,* 1–10.

McGaugh, J. L., & Cole, J. M. (1965). Age and strain differences in the effect of distribution of practice on maze learning. *Psychonomic Science, 2,* 253–254.

McGue, M., Bouchard, T. J., Jr., Iacono, W. G., & Lykken, D. T. (1993). Behavioral genetics of cognitive ability: A life-span perspective. In R. Plomin & G. E. McClearn (Eds.), *Nature, nurture, and psychology* (pp. 59–76). Washington, DC: American Psychological Association.

McGue, M., & Christensen, K. (1997). Genetic and environmental contributions to depression symtomatology: Evidence from Danish twins 75 years of age and older. *Journal of Abnormal Psychology, 106,* 439–448.

McGue, M., Hirsch, B., & Lykken, D. T. (1993). Age and self-perception of ability: A twin study analysis. *Psychology and Aging, 8,* 72–80.

Myers, A., Holmans, P., Marshall, H., Kwon, J., Meyer, D., Ramic, D., Shears, S., Booth, J., DeVrieze, F. W., Crook, R., Hamshere, M., Abraham, R., Tunstall, N., Rice, F., Carty, S., Lillystone, S., Kehoe, P., Rudrasingham, V., Jones, L., Lovestone, S., Perez-Tur, J., Williams, J., Owen, M. J., Hardy, J., & Goate, A. M. (2000). Susceptibility locus for Alzheimer's disease on chromosome 10. *Science, 290,* 2304–2305.

Neale, M. C., & Cardon, L. R. (1992). *Methodology for genetic studies of twins and families.* Dordrecht, The Netherlands: Kluwer Academic Publishers.

Omenn, G. S. (1977). Behavior genetics. In J. E. Birren & K. W. Schaie (Eds.), *Handbook of the psychology of aging* (pp. 190–218). New York: Van Nostrand Reinhold.

Osuntokun, B. O., Sahota, A., Ogunniyi, A. O., Gureje, O., Baiyewu, O., Adeyinka, A., Oluwole, S. O., Komolafe, O., Hull, K. S., Unverzugt, F. W., Hui, S. L., Yang, M., & Hendrie, H. C. (1995). Lack of an association between apolipoprotein E ε4 and Alzheimer's disease in elderly Nigerians. *Annals of Nuerology, 38,* 463–465.

Pedersen, N. (1996). Gerontological behavior genetics. In J. E. Birren & K. W. Schaie (Eds.), *Handbook of the psychology of aging* (4th ed., pp. 59–77). San Diego: Academic Press.

Pedersen, N. L., Friberg, L., Floderus-Myrhed, B., McClearn, G. E., & Plomin, R. (1984). Swedish early separated twins: Identification and characterization. *Acta Medicae Geneticae et Gemellologaie, 33,* 243–250.

Pedersen, N. L., Gatz, M., Plomin, R., Nesselroade, J. R., & McClearn, G. E. (1989). Individual differences in locus of control during the second half of the life span for identical and fraternal twins reared apart and reared together. *Journal of Gerontology: Psychological Sciences, 44,* P100–105.

Pedersen, N. L., Lichtenstein, P., Plomin, R., DeFaire, U., McClearn, G. E., & Matthews, K. A. (1989). Genetic and environmental influences for type A-like measures and related traits: A study of twins reared apart and twins reared together. *Psychosomatic Medicine, 51,* 428–440.

Pedersen, N. L., Plomin, R., Nesselroade, J. R., & McClearn, G. E. (1992).

A quantitative genetic analysis of cognitive abilities during the second half of the life span. *Psychological Science, 3,* 346–353.

Petrill, S. A., Johansson, B., Pedersen, N. L., Berg, S., Plomin, R., Ahern, F., & McClearn, G. E. (2001). Low cognitive functioning in non-demented 80+ year old twins is not genetic. *Intelligence, 29,* 75–83.

Plomin, R., DeFries, J. C., McClearn, G. E., & McGuffin, P. (2000). *Behavioral genetics* (4th ed.). New York: Worth.

Plomin, R., Lichtenstein, P., Pedersen, N. L., McClearn, G. E., & Nesselroade, J. R. (1990). Genetic influence on life events during the last half of the life span. *Psychology and Aging, 5,* 25–30.

Plomin, R., & McClearn, G. E. (1990). Human behavioral genetics of aging. In J. E. Birren & K. W. Schaie (Eds.), *Handbook of the psychology of aging* (3rd ed., pp. 66–77). New York: Academic Press.

Plomin, R., McClearn, G. E., Pedersen, N. L., Nesselroade, J. R., & Bergeman, C. S. (1989). Genetic influence on adults' ratings of their current environment. *Journal of Marriage and the Family, 51,* 791–803.

Plomin, R., Pedersen, N. L., Lichtenstein, P., & McClearn, G. E. (1994). Variability and stability in cognitive abilities are largely genetic later in life. *Behavior Genetics, 24,* 207–215.

Plomin, R., Pedersen, N. L., McClearn, G. E., Nesselroade, J. R., & Bergeman, C. S. (1988). EAS temperaments during the last half of the life span: Twins reared apart and twins reared together. *Psychology and Aging, 3,* 43–50.

Raiha, I., Kaprio, J., Koskenvuo, M., Rajala, T., & Sourander, L. (1996). Alzheimer's disease in Finnish twins. *Lancet, 347,* 573–578.

Rodriguez, L., Sokolowski, M. B., & Shore, J. S. (1992). Habitat selection by *Drosophila melanogaster* larvae. *Journal of Evolutionary Biology, 5,* 61–70.

St. George-Hyslop, P., Haines, J., Rogaev, E., Mortilla, M., Vaula, G., Pericak-Vance, M., Foncin, J-F., Montesi, M., Bruni, A., Sorbi, S., Rainero, I., Pinessi, L., Pollen, D., Polinsky, R., Nee, L., Kennedy, J., Macciardi, F., Rogaeva, E., Liang, Y., Alexandrova, N., Lukiw, W., Schlumpf, K., Tanzi, R., Tsuda, T., Farrer, L., Cantu, J-M., Duara, R., Amaducci, L., Bergamini, L., Gusella, J., Roses, A., & Crapper McLachlan, D. (1992). Genetic evidence for a novel familial Alzheimer's disease locus on chromosome 14. *Nature Genetics, 2,* 330–334.

St. George-Hyslop, P. H., Tanzi, R. E., Polinsky, R. J., Haines, J. L., Nee, L., Watkins, P. C., Myers, R. H., Conneally, P. M., & Gusella, J. F. (1987). The genetic defect causing familial Alzheimer's disease maps on chromosome 21. *Science, 235,* 885–889.

Sahota, A., Yang, M., Gao, S., Hui, S. L., Baiyewu, O., Gureje, O., Oluwole, S., Ogunniyi, A., Hall, K. S., & Hendrie, H. C. (1997). Apolipoprotein E-associated risk for Alzheimer's disease in the African-American population is genotype dependent. *Annals of Neurology, 42,* 659–661.

Sarter, M. (1987). Measurement of cognitive abilities in senescent animals. *International Journal of Neuroscience, 32,* 765–774.

Saudino, K. J., Plomin, R., Pedersen, N. L., & McClearn, G. E. (1994). The etiology of high and low cognitive ability during the second half of the life span. *Intelligence, 19,* 359–371.

Simmel, E. C., Haber, S. B., & Harshfield, G. (1976). Age, sex, and genotype effects on stimulus exploration and locomotor activity in young mice. *Experimental Aging Research, 2,* 253–259.

Small, B. J., Graves, A. B., McEvoy, C. L., Crawford, F. C., Mullan, M., & Mortimer, J. A. (2000). Is APOE-epsilon4 a risk factor for cognitive impairment in normal aging? *Neurology, 54,* 2082–2088.

Smith, M. A., Banerjee, S., Gold, P. W., & Glowa, J. (1992). Induction of *c-fos* mRNA in rat brain by conditioned and unconditioned stressors. *Brain Research, 578,* 135–141.

Sprott, R. L. (1972). Passive-avoidance conditioning in inbred mice: Effects of shock intensity, age, and genotype. *Journal of Comparative and Physiological Psychology, 80,* 327–334.

Sprott, R. L., & Stavnes, K. (1975). Avoidance learning, behavior genetics, and aging: A critical review and comment on methodology. *Experimental Aging Research, 1,* 145–168.

Stavnes, K., & Sprott, R. L. (1975). Effects of age and genotype on acquisition of an active avoidance response in mice. *Developmental Psychobiology, 8,* 437–445.

Tang, M-X., Stern, Y., Marder, K., Bell, K., Gurland, B., Lantigua, R., Andrews, H., Feng, L., Tycko, B., & Mayeux, R. (1998). The APOE-ε4 allele and the risk of Alzheimer's disease among African Americans, Whites, and Hispanics. *Journal of the American Medical Association, 279,* 751–755.

Tryon, R. C. (1940). Genetic differences in maze-learning ability in rats. *39th yearbook of the National Society for the Study of Education* (Part I, pp. 111–119). Bloomington, IL: Public School.

Vieira, C., Pasyukova, E. G., Zeng, Z-B., Hackett, J. B., Lyman, R. F., & Mackay, T. F. C. (2000). Genotype-environment interaction for quantitative trait loci affecting life span in *Drosophila melanogaster. Genetics, 154,* 213–227.

Warren, J. M. (1986). Appetitive learning by old mice. *Experimental Aging Research, 12,* 99–105.

Warren, J. M. (1988). Age, incentives, and maze learning by hybrid mice. *Behavior Genetics, 18,* 167–173.

Wood, W. G. (1976). Ethanol preference in C57BL/6 and BALBc mice at three ages and eight ethanol concentrations. *Experimental Aging Research, 2,* 425–434.

Yaffe, K., Cauley, J., Sands, L., & Browner, W. (1997). Apolipoprotein E phenotype and cognitive decline in a prospective study of elderly community women. *Archives of Neurology, 54,* 1110–1114.

Yaffe, K., Haan, M., Byers, A., Tangen, C., & Kuller, L. (2000). Estrogen use, APOE, and cognitive decline: Evidence of gene-environment interaction. *Neurology, 54,* 1949–1954.

CHAPTER 11

Biological Implications of the Demography of Aging

S. Jay Olshansky
School of Public Health
University of Illinois at Chicago and Center on Aging
University of Chicago

Bruce A. Carnes
NORC/Center on Aging
University of Chicago

THE DEMOGRAPHY OF AGING

The aging of individuals and the populations to which they belong is the subject of intense interest and study among demographers, geriatricians, physicians, and scientists from a broad range of disciplines that inform the biological and social sciences. Although there have always been people who have lived very long lives, even as far back as Egyptian times, the phenomenon of population aging as we know it today is new, experienced by only a few species, and then only under an unusual set of living conditions where individuals are insulated from the hostile environment. Important issues of public policy are directly related to the aging of individuals and populations, including the future solvency of age-entitlement programs such as Social Security and Medicare, the future of marriage and retirement, and the modern practice of medicine in a world where nearly everyone who is born in the developed world has an opportunity to live beyond the age of 65 (Carnes, Olshansky, Gavrilov, Gavrilova, & Grahn, 1999; Martin & Preston, 1994).

Population aging refers to demographic changes in the age structure of a population, which are characterized primarily by increases in the size and proportional distribution of older individuals relative to younger individuals (Olshansky, Carnes, & Cassel, 1993). Prior to the 20th century, the age structure of humans (and most other species) could be depicted by a pyramid, with a large number of young people and relatively few individuals who survived to the outer limits of the human life span. The shift in the age structure from a pyramid to a more rectilinear configuration is a product of the ongoing change in the age distribution of death from the young to the old (Omran, 1971). As the influence of infectious and parasitic diseases on death rates at younger ages diminished in the last century, the saved population had the opportunity to live decades longer. The modern world has therefore experienced something unique—an opportunity to enjoy the personal and societal benefits that can accompany a population's living to older ages. However, this phenomenon has also made it possible for the first time to witness the full effects of an aging process expressed in a large, genetically diverse population (Carnes & Olshansky, 2001).

Individual aging defines the observed life span of individuals as characterized by the duration of time that elapses between birth and death, irrespective of demographic changes that may be occurring at the level of populations. The mortality transition that contributed to the modern rise in the number and proportional distribution of elderly people has been well documented in the scientific literature (Olshansky & Ault, 1986; Omran, 1971, 2000; Rogers & Hackenberg, 1989). The important point here is that the simultaneous demographic phenomenon of an aging world and a longer-lived population has had, and will continue to have, a profound influence on a variety of issues related to the biology of aging (Carnes et al., 1999; Carnes & Olshansky, 2001). Both phenomena have contributed to the rise in geriatric medicine as the diseases common in old age have become prevalent (Cassel et al., 2001); they have already given rise to ethical dilemmas about the rationing of scarce health care resources (Ubel, 1999); and they have led to a renewed interest in finding ways to forestall the aging process (Olshansky & Carnes, 2001). Although aging may be predestined, there are important attributes of the aging process that are modifiable. Understanding the biological laws that govern age patterns of disease and death in humans and other species will help to illuminate the important links that exist between the demography and the biology of aging (Carnes & Olshansky, 1997; Finch & Kirkwood, 2000).

THE LAW OF MORTALITY

In 1825 an English actuary by the name of Benjamin Gompertz made an important discovery. Gompertz's job was to calculate the risk of death for people of different ages in order to determine how much to charge for life insurance annuities, a practice that continues to this day. Based on observed vital statistics from various parts of England where he lived, Gompertz discovered that the risk of death increased with age at a predictable rate. His calculations led him to conclude that the death rate doubled about every 10 years between the ages of 20 and 60, which was the primary age range of people who were purchasing insurance annuities at that time. The mathematical formula Gompertz used to describe the exponential rise in mortality in the middle years of the human life span has become known colloquially as the Gompertz equation, $\lambda(t) = \alpha\exp(\beta t)$ (This is the modern formulation of the Gompertz hazard function, $\lambda(t)$ where α and β are the Gompertz parameters.) It has remained an integral part of mortality computations conducted by actuaries and demographers since then (Gompertz, 1825).

What made Gompertz's discovery so interesting was not that he devised a formula that accurately portrayed the dying-out process of humans, although this has been widely viewed as one of his most important accomplishments. Gompertz, and many scientists who came after him, believed that his equation, or some variation of it, could be used to characterize age patterns of death rates for all living things. In fact, for more than 100 years following his discovery, numerous investigators from a wide range of scientific disciplines used the Gompertz equation as the basis for a debate about whether there is a universal law of mortality (for example, Brownlee, 1919; Deevey, 1947; Greenwood, 1928; Loeb & Northrop, 1916; Makeham, 1867; Pearl, 1922). The scientist who expended the greatest effort in search of the universal law of mortality was Raymond Pearl, a biologist at Johns Hopkins University in the early 20th century. Based on studies of mortality distributions among humans and in *Drosophila* (Pearl & Parker, 1921; Pearl, 1922), Pearl was convinced early in his career that the common age pattern of death observed among these species, when compared on a uniform time scale, would provide evidence for such a law. Despite 20 years of effort and numerous attempts to scale mortality distributions among animals with varying life spans, Pearl was never able to get the mortality distributions of different species to match up perfectly. Frustrated by this, Pearl and Minor (1935) eventually declared that no evidence for a law of mortality could be found.

Later in the same century, instead of searching for a universal law of mortality, scientists began developing alternative mathematical models to the Gompertz equation (for example, Beard, 1959; Heligman & Pollard, 1980; Perks, 1932; Pollard & Valkovics, 1992; Sacher & Trucco, 1962; Simms, 1948; Weibull, 1951). Summaries of these efforts may be found in Economos (1982), Gavrilov and Gavrilova (1991), Mildvan and Strehler (1960), Pollard and Streatfield (1979), and Strehler and Mildvan (1960). It has since been discovered that historical efforts to reveal similar age patterns of mortality across species was hampered by several problems, the most difficult of which was the lack of reliable mortality data and pathology assessments to determine why death occurred (Deevey, 1947). The reason cause of death is important is because extrinsic (that is, non-biological) forces of mortality have been shown to contaminate the mortality schedule by removing members of the population prematurely, before the consequences of aging can be expressed (Carnes & Olshansky, 1997, 1993; Carnes, Olshansky, & Grahn, 1996; Deevey, 1947). A second problem was that early in the last century, the theoretical and quantitative tools required to make use of cause-of-death statistics had not yet been developed. It wasn't until the late 20th century that the search for Gompertz and Pearl's universal law of mortality was tested once again (Carnes et al., 1996). In this latest study, it was discovered that once extrinsic causes of death are eliminated from the death rates of humans, dogs, and mice, the mortality schedules of these species became indistinguishable when evaluated on a comparable time scale—just as predicted by Raymond Pearl in 1922. In other words, there is scientific evidence to suggest that both Gompertz and Pearl were right—that there is a common age pattern to the dying-out process of a variety of species when only biological (that is, aging-related) causes of death are examined. Whether this so-called law of mortality is universal—applying to most forms of life—will continue to be the subject of future scientific research.

IS THERE BIOLOGY IN THE LIFE TABLE?

As Benjamin Gompertz inquired in 1825 and as was echoed in the research of Brownlee (1919) and Greenwood (1928), the question of whether there is biology in the life table is central to an understanding of the biological implications of the demography of aging. In demography, the question of why the age pattern of death looks the way it does has direct implications for important issues, including how much lower death rates can decline and how high life expectancy can rise. An answer to the question of whether there is biology in the life table may be found within two lines of scientific inquiry that ran parallel but completely independent of each other for more than a century—evolution biology and the actuarial/demographic sciences.

It has been known from the actuarial/demographic sciences since the time of Gompertz that the risk of death is extremely high at birth, declines to its lowest point at sexual maturity (about age 13 in humans), and then rises exponentially thereafter until very old ages as shown in Figure 11.1. This is what Gompertz observed in 1825; it is what numerous other actuaries observed for other human populations for more than a century following Gompertz (for example, see Makeham, 1867; Olshansky & Carnes, 1997); and it has been observed repeatedly for a variety of other species

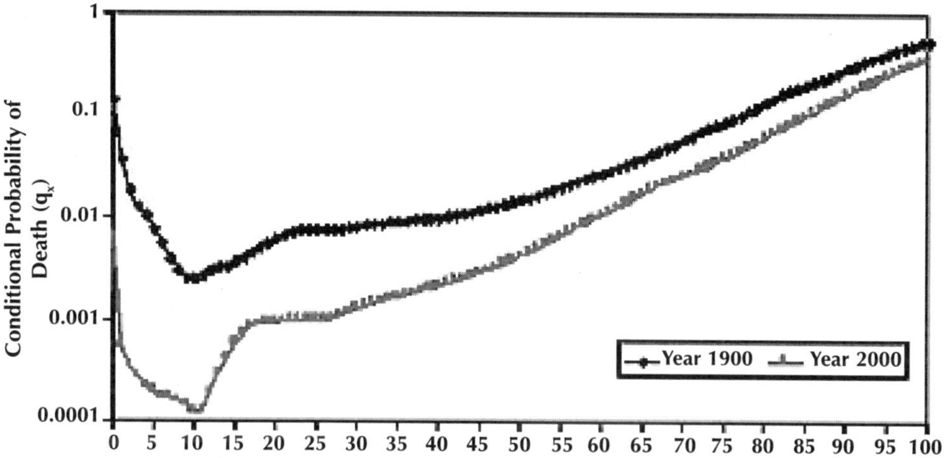

FIGURE 11.1 Age as a factor in probability of death.

during the 20th century (Carnes et al., 1996; Deevey, 1947; Finch, Pike, & Witten, 1990). Although it has been observed that life expectancy among humans rose rapidly in the last century, the mortality curve did not change appreciably—it merely shifted downward, with a substantial portion of the deaths that used to occur early in life now redistributed from younger to older ages. Thus, from both the actuarial/demographic and biological sciences it is now known that throughout most of the life span there is a uniformity to the dying-out process of many forms of life for which reliable data may be obtained (Carey & Liedo, 1995; Deevey, 1947; Finch et al., 1990; Fukui, Xiu, & Curtsinger, 1993; Olshansky et al., 1996).

Although Gompertz had speculated on a biological force (such as the loss of some vital substance throughout life) that might have contributed to the age patterns of death he observed in humans, neither he nor any of the actuaries or demographers who addressed this issue could ever explain why age patterns of death were so uniform across species and time. The biological explanation for this observation may be found within the central organizing principle that governs all life—the theory of evolution set forth by Charles Darwin (1859) and Alfred Russell Wallace (1855) and expanded upon by evolutionary theorists in the 20th century (Hamilton, 1966; Kirkwood, 1977; Medawar, 1952; Williams, 1957). It is interesting to note that scientists from evolution biology and from the actuarial/demographic sciences have, until recently, worked independently of one another, with neither group referencing papers from the other disciplines or recognizing the complementary nature of their work. As it turns out, the evolutionary theory of senescence offers highly specific and testable research hypotheses that have been used to answer Gompertz's question about why the age pattern of death looks so uniform and whether there is biology in the life table.

In the early 1990s, scientists from the biological and demographic sciences were working together to address the question of how high the life expectancy of humans can rise. The product of that effort was an empirical article based entirely on the actuarial/demographic sciences where it was demonstrated that the rise in life expectancy at birth will likely decelerate in the coming decades (Olshansky, Carnes, & Cassel, 1990)—a phenomenon that had been discussed and demonstrated previously in the demographic literature (Keyfitz, 1985). This mathematical approach to predicting the future course of life expectancy led its authors to rediscover the same question that had intrigued Gompertz more than 165 years earlier. Is there an underlying biology of life and death that explains not just why age patterns of death look the way the do, but also why the measure of life expectancy grows less sensitive as it rises, making it increasingly more difficult to raise it further once it has already reached high levels? The answer is yes.

The biology that drives the shape of the mortality curve of humans and other living things may be understood only within the context of the one force that drives all life—evolution. Although Darwin did not pay much attention to the question of why we age, Alfred Russell Wallace made specific reference in his early work to the evolutionary forces that lead to aging (personal communication in Weismann, 1891). Wallace suggested that old age was nature's way of removing the old to make room for the young, who would be competing for limited resources for survival. The same point was expanded upon by the scientist most responsible for launching the evolutionary theory of senescence, German biologist August Weismann (1891). (See Kirkwood and Cremer [1993] for a detailed examination of the evolutionary theory of aging as set forth by August Weismann.) According to Weismann, it is not possible for animals to avoid exposure to a hostile environment, which in turn is expected to produce a constant barrage of small injuries to the body. Because the perfect repair of damage to the body is not practically achievable, whether caused by external or internal forces, Weismann concluded that older members of a species should be replaced by younger ones. This line of reasoning served as the rationale supporting the need for both reproduction and death. Weismann went on to argue that individuals are disposable once their reproductive roles are completed and that the underlying biological cause of senescence was the inability of individual cells to continually replicate. Both these concepts served as forerunners of the modern theory of senescence and the contemporary view, known as the Hayflick limit (Hayflick & Moorehead, 1961), that somatic cells can replicate only a limited number of times.

The next step in the development of the evolutionary theory of senescence was made by the British Nobel laureate Sir Peter Medawar. Like Weismann before him, Medawar (1952) emphasized the importance of extrinsic causes of death as the central force that influenced the rise of senescence, but then supplemented the theory with an emphasis on the role of genetics. Medawar used the temporal link between reproduction and the force of natural selection as the basis for suggesting that senescence and aging-related diseases are products of larger proportions of the population surviving into the postreproductive period, where the force of selection is at or near zero. Medawar suggested that with a reduction in early-age mortality from infectious and parasitic diseases, the population saved from early death would then live with greater frequency into the postreproductive phase of the life span. The result, he suggested, would be a proliferation of aging-related diseases and disorders. Medawar had used a combination of evolutionary theory and his knowledge of genetics to provide the first biological explanation for why senescence should proliferate in a population that is surviving with regularity into later stages of the life span wherein the force of selection is weak.

Williams (1957) provided the next piece of the evolutionary puzzle that explains why senescence occurs. Like Medawar, Williams focused on the question of how it is possible for genes with adverse health effects to be present and increase in a population. His answer was based on a rather innovative twist to an established genetic phenomenon. Geneticists now know that single genes perform more than one function at any given time, a phenomenon known as pleiotropy. Unlike Medawar who suggested that harmful genes expressed in the postreproductive period could accumulate in a species' genome without penalty, Williams proposed that genes acting normally early in life could act abnormally later in life, that is, genes were thought to function pleiotropically in time—a phenomenon that has come to be known as antagonistic pleiotropy. The genes that give rise to senescence are therefore expected to accumulate in the gene pool because natural selection cannot remove them, and there is no penalty for their presence among species that rarely live beyond their reproductive years. These genetic-based evolutionary theories of senescence serve as the biological basis for understanding the temporal nature of death in sexually reproducing organisms and represent the bridge between the demography and the biology of aging.

THE LINK BETWEEN THE BIOLOGY AND THE DEMOGRAPHY OF AGING

The biological implications of the demography of aging have now been brought into focus by the recently developed discipline of biodemography (Carnes & Olshansky, 1993; Carnes et al., 1996; Olshansky & Carnes, 1994, 1997, 2001; Wachter & Finch, 1997). The age-old questions of why humans die when they do and whether there is biology in the life table have now been answered by theoretical and empirical research addressed specifically to this topic.

Humans and other sexually reproducing species experience a common age pattern of death because the aging of individuals, and by implication the aging of populations, is fundamentally linked to the timing of reproduction. The theoretical basis for this view is derived from evolutionary biology but is expanded upon within the new field of biodemography. It is now known that the age trajectory of death is a species-specific phenomenon that is calibrated to the onset and length of a species' reproductive window (Carnes et al., 1996). For example, in humans the reproductive window is about 35 years as it extends beyond puberty and menopause (see Figure 11.2), but this window is different for each species. The reproductive window, in turn, is a genetically determined and tightly controlled attribute that is established as part of a life-history strategy that has been molded by the environment within which each species arose. For species that experience puberty shortly after birth and have relatively short reproductive windows (such as mice and rats), the slope of the mortality curve following puberty is steep, leading to short life expectancies. For species that experience puberty at a later age and have longer reproductive windows, the slope of their mortality curve following puberty is less steep, and they tend to live longer.

It is known from biodemography that for each species there is a fundamental link between the timing of sexual maturation, the length of the reproductive window, and the onset and rate of increase in the death rate from biological causes of death. We now know the answer to Gompertz's question: There is biology in the life table (Brownlee, 1919), and it is a biology that is driven by evolutionary forces that operate through genetic mechanisms. Although there is evidence to suggest that common age patterns of mortality exist for several mammals, whether that pattern holds constant for other species in the form of a universal law of mortality has yet to be determined. In any case, from the evidence provided here, the biological implications of the demography of aging are as interesting and important as the demographic implications of the biology of aging. Continued advances in the biology of aging will provide not only a more complete understanding of the mechanisms of senescence, but will also

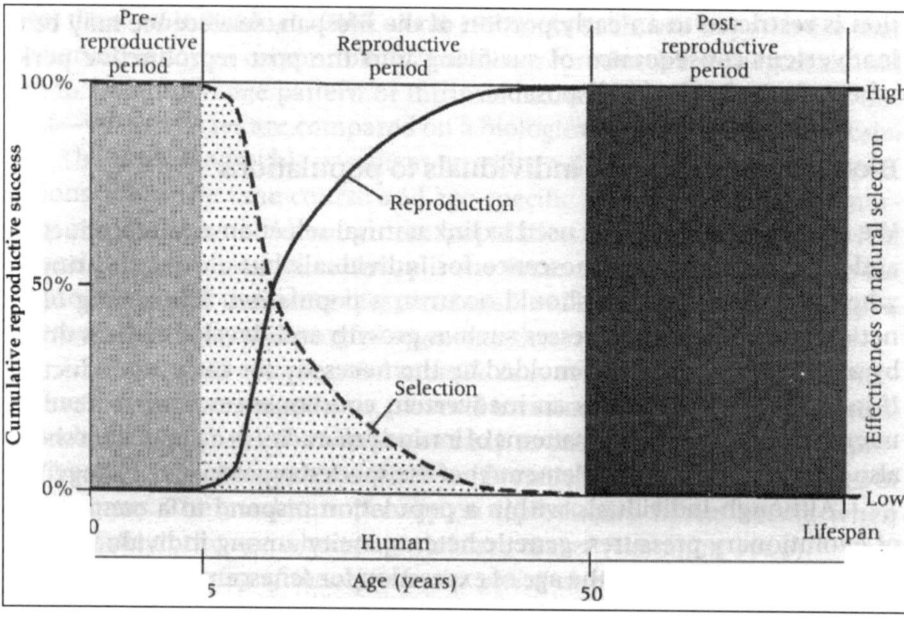

FIGURE 11.2 Depiction of the human reproductive window.
Reprinted with the permission of the Population Council, from Bruce A. Carnes, S. Jay Olshansky, & Douglas Grahn (1996), "Continuing the Search for a Law of Mortality," *Population and Development Review, 22*(2), p. 235.

shed light on how demographic shifts in the age structure of populations in the coming decades will alter the expression of aging in a rapidly growing and more diverse older population.

ACKNOWLEDGMENTS

Funding for this work was provided by the National Institutes of Health/ National Institutes on Aging Grants AG 13698-01 and AG 00894-01.

REFERENCES

Beard, R. E. (1959). Actuarial aspects of human lifespans. In G. E. W. Wolstenholme & M. O'Connor (Eds.), *CIBA Foundation Colloquia on Ageing, Vol. 5.* Boston: Little, Brown.

Brownlee, J. (1919). Note on the biology of a life-table. *Journal of theRoyal Statistical Society, 82,* 34–77.

Carey, J. R., & Liedo, P. (1995). Sex-specific life table aging rates in large Medfly cohorts. *Experimental Gerontology, 30,* 315–325.

Carnes, B. A., & Olshansky, S. J. (1993). Evolutionary perspectives on human senescence. *Population and Development Review, 19,* 793–806.

Carnes, B. A., & Olshansky, S. Jay. (1997). Biodemographic perspective: A biologically motivated partitioning of mortality. *Experimental Gerontology, 32,* 615–631.

Carnes, B. A., & Olshansky, S. Jay. (2001). Heterogeneity and its biodemographic implications for longevity and mortality. *Experimental Gerontology, 36,* 419–430.

Carnes, B. A., Olshansky, S. J., Gavrilov, L., Gavrilova, N., & Grahn, D. (1999). Human longevity: Nature vs. nurture—fact or fiction. *Perspectives in Biology and Medicine, 42,* 422–441.

Carnes, B. A., Olshansky, S. J., & Grahn, D. (1996). Continuing the search for a law of mortality. *Population and Development Review, 22,* 231–264.

Cassel, C. K., Cohen, H. J., Larson, E. B., Meier, D. E., Resnick, N. M., Rubenstein, L. Z., & Sorensen, L. B. (Eds.). (2001). *Geriatric medicine.* New York: Springer.

Darwin, C. (1998). *The origin of species* (G. Suriano, Ed.). New York: Grammercy. (Original work published 1859)

Deevey, E. S., Jr. (1947). Life tables for natural populations of animals. *Quarterly Review of Biology, 22,* 283–314.

Economos, A. (1982). Rate of aging, rate of dying and the mechanism of mortality. *Archives of Gerontological Geriatrics, 1,* 3–27.

Finch, C., & Kirkwood, T. B. L. (2000). *Chance, development, and aging.* New York: Oxford University Press.

Finch, C. E., Pike, M. C., Witten, M. (1990). Slow mortality rate accelerations during aging in some animals approximate that of humans. *Science, 24,* 902–905.

Fukui, H. H., Xiu, L., & Curtsinger, J. W. (1993). Slowing of age-specific mortality rates in *Drosophila melanogaster. Experimental Gerontology 28,* 585–599.

Gavrilov, L. A., & Gavrilova, N. S. (1991). T*he biology of life span: A quantitative approach.* Switzerland: Harwood Academic.

Gompertz, B. (1825). On the nature of the function expressive of the law of human mortality and on a new mode of determining life contingencies. *Philosophical Transactions of the Royal Society of London, 115,* 513–585.

Greenwood, M. (1928). Laws of mortality from the biological point of view. *Journal of Hygiene, 28,* 267–294.

Hamilton, W.D. (1966). The moulding of senescence by natural selection. *Journal of Theoretical Biology, 12,* 12–45.

Hayflick, L., & Moorehead, P. S. (1961). The serial cultivation of human diploid cell strains. *Experimental Cell Research, 25,* 585–621.

Heligman, L., & Pollard, J. H. (1980). The age pattern of mortality. *Journal of the Institute of Actuaries, 107*, 49–80.

Keyfitz, N. (1985). *Applied mathematical demography* (2nd ed.). New York: Springer.

Kirkwood, T .B L. (1977). Evolution of aging. *Nature, 270*, 301–304.

Loeb, J., & Northrop, J. H. (1916). Is there a temperature coefficient for the duration of life? *Proceedings of the National Academy of Sciences, USA, 2*, 456–457.

Makeham, W. M. (1867). On the law of mortality. *Journal of the Institute of Actuaries, 13*, 325–358.

Martin, L. G., & Preston, S.H. (1994). *Demography of aging*. Washington, DC: National Academy Press.

Medawar, P. B. (1952). *An unsolved problem in biology*. London: Lewis.

Mildvan, A., & Strehler, B. L. (1960). A critique of theories of mortality. In B. L. Strehler, J. D. Ebert, A. B. Gloss, & N. W. Shock (Eds.), *The biology of aging* (Pub. No. 6). Washington, DC: American Institute of Biological Sciences.

Olshansky, S. J., & Ault, A. B. (1986). The fourth stage of the epidemiologic transition: The age of delayed degenerative diseases. *Milbank Memorial Fund Quarterly, 64*, 355–391.

Olshansky, S. J., & Carnes, B. A. (1994). Demographic perspectives on human senescence. *Population and Development Review, 20*, 57–80.

Olshansky, S. J., & Carnes, B. A. (1997). Ever since Gompertz. *Demography, 34*, 1–14.

Olshansky, S. J., & Carnes, B. A. (2001). *The quest for immortality: Science at the frontiers of aging*. New York: W. W. Norton.

Olshansky, S. J., Carnes, B. A., & Cassel, C. (1990). In search of Methuselah: Estimating the upper limits to human longevity. *Science, 250*, 634–640.

Olshansky, S. J., Carnes, B. A., & Cassel, C. A. (1993, April). The aging of the human species. *Scientific American*, 46–52.

Omran, A. R. (1971). The epidemiologic transition: A theory of the epidemiology of population change. *Milbank Memorial Fund Quarterly, 49*, 509–538.

Omran, A. R. (2000). The epidemiologic transition revisited thirty years later. *World Health Statistics Quarterly, 53*(2–4), 99–119.

Pearl, R. (1922). A comparison of the laws of mortality in Drosophila and in man. *American Naturalist, 56*, 398–405.

Pearl, R., & Minor, J. R. (1935). Experimental studies on the duration of life. XIV. The comparative mortality of certain lower organisms. *Quarterly Review of Biology, 10*, 60–79.

Pearl, R., & Parker, S. L. (1921). Experimental studies on the duration of life. *American Naturalist, 55*, 481–509.

Perks, W. (1932). On some experiments in the graduation of mortality statistics. *Journal of the Institute of Actuaries, 63,* 12–57.

Pollard, J. H., & Valkovics, E. (1992). The Gompertz distribution and its applications. *Genus, 48,* 15–27.

Pollard, J. H., & Streatfield, K. (1979). Factors affecting mortality and the length of life. Paper presented at the joint convention of the Institute of Actuaries of Australia (Christchurch, New Zealand).

Rogers, R., & Hackenberg, R. (1989). Extending epidemiologic transition theory: A new stage. *Social Biology, 34,* 234–243.

Sacher, G. A., & Trucco, E. (1962). The stochastic theory of mortality. *Annals of the New York Academy of Sciences, USA, 96,* 985–1007.

Simms, H. S. (1948). Logarithmic increase in mortality as a manifestation of aging. *Journal of Gerontology, 1,* 13–26.

Strehler, B. L., & Mildvan, A. S. (1960). General theory of mortality and aging (a stochastic model relates observations on aging, physiologic decline, mortality, and radiation). *Science, 132,* 14–19.

Ubel, P. (1999). *Pricing life: Why it's time for health care rationing.* Boston: MIT Press.

Wachter, K., & Finch, C. (Eds.). (1997). *Between Zeus and the salmon: The biodemography of longevity.* Washington, DC: National Academy Press.

Wallace, A. R. (1855). *On the law which has regulated the introduction of new species.*

Weibull, W. (1951). A statistical distribution function of wide applicability. *Journal of Applied Mechanics, 18,* 293–297.

Weismann, (1891). *Essays upon heredity and kindred biological problems.* Oxford, England: Clarendon Press.

Williams, G. C. (1957). Pleiotropy, natural selection and the evolution of senescence. *Evolution, 11,* 398–411.

Index